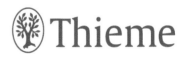

Thieme Review for the USMLE® Step 2:
CS for IMGs

Mohamed M. Elawdy, MD, MSc, ECFMG certified
Specialist (A) in Urology
Sohar Hospital
Ministry of Health
Sohar, Oman;
Urology and Nephrology Center
Mansoura, Egypt;
International Fellow
Thomas Jefferson University Hospital
Philadelphia, Pennsylvania, USA

Dara B. Oken, MEd
Pronunciation Modification Trainer
Articulation LLC;
Adult ELL Teacher
Minneapolis Adult Education
Minneapolis Center for Adult Learning
Minneapolis, Minnesota, USA

144 illustrations

Thieme
New York • Stuttgart • Delhi • Rio de Janeiro

Library of Congress Cataloging-in-Publication Data is available with the publisher.

Thieme Medical Publishers New York
333 Seventh Avenue
New York, New York 10001 USA
+1 800 782 3488, customerservice@thieme.com

Georg Thieme Verlag KG
Rüdigerstrasse 14, 70469 Stuttgart, Germany
+49 [0]711 8931 421, customerservice@thieme.de

Thieme Publishers Delhi
A-12, Second Floor, Sector-2, Noida-201301
Uttar Pradesh, India
+91 120 45 566 00, customerservice@thieme.in

Thieme Publishers Rio de Janeiro,
Thieme Publicações Ltda.
Edifício Rodolpho de Paoli, 25º andar
Av. Nilo Peçanha, 50 – Sala 2508,
Rio de Janeiro 20020-906 Brasil
+55 21 3172-2297

Cover design: Thieme Publishing Group
Typesetting by DiTech Process Solutions, India

Printed in USA by King Printing Company, Inc.   5 4 3 2 1

ISBN 978-1-68420-196-9

Also available as an e-book:
eISBN 978-1-68420-197-6

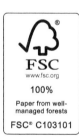

FSC
www.fsc.org
100%
Paper from well-managed forests
FSC® C103101

To all of my colleagues who reviewed this book and the Thieme team.

Mohamed M. Elawdy

In memory of my father, Dr. Martin Oken, and his gifts to medicine.

Dara B. Oken

Contents

Videos

Audios

Audio 2.1   The audio contains the core of the CIS and can be used as a quick review before the exam.

Audio 9.1   The audio contains the core of psychiatry and can be used as a quick review before the exam.

Audio 10.1   The audio contains the core of neurology and can be used as a quick review before the exam.

Preface

The United States Medical License Examination (USMLE) Step 2 Clinical Skills (CS) is one of three exams (Step 1, Step 2 CK, and Step 2 CS) that one must pass to qualify for ECFMG certification. This certification is a requirement for both international medical graduates (IMGs) and US medical graduates to apply for residency training.

The USMLE website includes exam candidate requirements, exam description, scoring, and other important general information regarding the CS exam. Please be sure to read the most up-to-date CS Bulletin of Information carefully.

The CS exam is scored on the basis of three sub-components. Each of the following three sub-components must be passed in order to achieve an overall "passing" result:

- Integrated Clinical Encounter (ICE)
- Communication and Interpersonal Skills (CIS)
- Spoken English Proficiency (SEP)

Although one may be able to pass the CS exam with good training and practice, it is a challenging exam. It is a day long exam with 12 patient encounters, each followed by Patient Note (PN) documentation. The exam utilizes Standardized Patients (SPs), actors who lack any actual physical signs. Each encounter is limited to 15 minutes, and the PN is limited to 10 minutes. For IMGs, there are additional challenges like SEP component, the high cost of traveling, accommodation, visa application fees that is in addition to the exam fees, and the difficulty of procuring an exam date at one of the only five exam centers in the United States.

As an IMG myself, and as someone whose exam preparations were limited due to the lack of resources such as adequate guidance, I had two unsuccessful attempts in the CS exam before I ultimately passed in my third attempt. Through this learning process, I became acutely aware of what I needed to do to be successful, and what lack of information there is in the existing commercial resources. This was the prime motivator for me to start writing this book, so that I may help others pass the exam and they may not have to learn through their mistakes.

The exam is unique and unconventional; it requires an unparalleled preparation resource that not only *provides* medical information but also shows how to *use* this information. This book will assist the exam candidate to overcome specific challenges encountered during the exam by using a unique format tailored specifically to the requirements of the CS exam.

The available commercial resources for the CS exam are few, and they have many limitations. They present CS cases individually without organizing them into body-system chapters. They contain no specific questions for analyzing possible differential diagnoses, physical exam steps for each case, checklist, or a self-assessment scoring system. Although practice is the key to passing the CS exam, these resources do not provide authentic role-plays for this purpose. In addition, they do not provide any guidance for the SEP component, and most of them have been edited by medical professionals rather than those who have experience as examinees.

We worked extensively to compensate for the limitations in the presently available commercial resources, and to fill in the gaps. We have put great effort into making CS for IMGs a comprehensive and user-friendly resource that will help candidates pass the CS exam in the first attempt.

How is *CS for IMGs* organized?

The central strength of this book is its organization which provides a solid foundation that can be utilized in all CS cases. The book starts with "The Basics" and then offers different types of cases that are divided into individual chapters:

The Basics:

A. Integrated Clinical Encounter (ICE): In this chapter, the fundamentals of medical history and physical exam that are relevant to the CS exam are covered. This provides a simple and reproducible approach that can be utilized in all CS cases. There are also reproducible mnemonics, as well as tips on how to write complete and effective PNs.

B. Communication Interpersonal Skills (CIS): The CIS for the CS exam is written concisely in order to be easily understood by the reader. It also provides tips for "model answers" to the questions commonly asked by SPs.

C. Spoken English Proficiency (SEP): It is a comprehensive overview of key sounds and patterns in English. There are tips to guide you through some language-specific challenges, and examples include pertinent sentences and questions you will likely use with the SPs.

Systematically arranged chapters:

Practice cases have been organized according to appropriate body systems and disciplines. These have been arranged into individual chapters. The proper approach to history, physical exam, and workup are explained. Each chapter contains a number of practice cases that are commonly tested in the actual CS exam.

Miscellaneous chapter: In this chapter, unclassified cases, medical check-up, medication refill, and infrequent cases are covered.

The book concludes with an Appendix that details screening protocols, medications that are commonly seen in the CS along with the associated side effects, different mnemonics, and more.

In an effort to help you emulate role-plays to closely resemble the actual CS exam, we have included instructions for the SP role and the "Doorway Information." Each practice case begins with an introduction that gives you some basic information about the case. An answer key is provided that includes the recommended line of questioning for history-taking, the possible differential diagnoses, the physical exam technique, a sample closure, and a suggested PN. This is a unique system that will give you a solid strategy to approach various types of cases. This is a more user-friendly method than what has been traditionally proposed in other commercial CS books.

To further understand how this book is structured, here is an analogy: Imagine this book was built just as a building is constructed. The *basics* represent the solid "foundation" that will be used for all cases and serve all levels. This includes general medical history, general physical exam, closure, counseling, and communication skills. *Individual chapters* represent the "levels/floors," and contain specific history-taking questions, focused clinical exam maneuvers, and suggested workup that are common to a particular group of cases. Finally, *each individual case* represents the individual "apartment units." Just as each apartment unit in a building has unique furniture and decorations, each case has various differential diagnoses, specific questions to ask, analysis of complaints, special clinical tests, and recommended special workups. This unique arrangement facilitates rapid retrieval of the content.

Step-by-step studying strategy for success in CS exam
Several months to a year before the exam:
Immerse yourself in the English component. Do not hesitate to take live or online courses to improve your English. It is an investment in your ability to communicate. Make a commitment to gradually improve your English, not only for the exam but for the upcoming residency interviews and your medical career in the United States. Efficient typing skills also require significant time to be mastered. Please read the SEP chapter and our recommendation for the PN and watch the videos.

Weeks to months before the exam:
The book is a good starter for those who are fresh graduates, or who have recently completed the CK exam. Otherwise, reviewing the CS topics in a medical textbook is strongly recommended. We advise a quick prerequisite review of the fundamentals of history-taking and clinical exam from your standard medical textbooks before starting the CS exam preparation using *CS for IMGs*. We have minimized redundancy and repetition of these specific basic concepts in an effort to make this book as concise as possible, and more exam-oriented.

Start by reading "The Basics" that includes history-taking questions, physical exam, and PN. Try to memorize the mnemonics. Learn how to quickly go through taking a general medical history. Practice the history-taking questions and the physical exam steps with a partner until you feel comfortable doing so, and they flow automatically.

Next, read the Communication and Interpersonal Skills (CIS) chapter. Once you feel that you have truly grasped its content, try to practice communication with a partner. It is vital to act "in character" and behave in a professional manner.

In each chapter, review the common line of questioning that should be asked for history, clinical exam technique, suggested diagnostic studies, and the commonly asked CIS questions. Prior to beginning your practice case, it is advised to read the discussion of PNs in each chapter.

When you begin reading *CS for IMGs*, explore the typical case presentations of each chapter. For example, in the Chest chapter, you will find cases such as sore throat, cough, chest pain, palpitation, etc. You may find it necessary to go back and review some of these topics from your medical textbooks in order to gain a full understanding. Then come back to *CS for IMGs* and continue.

Never practice without completing a PN for each case.

When you first begin practice cases, we advise you to stick to "The CS for IMGs method." Over time, and with practice, you will feel more comfortable with the format. You will be able to develop your own personal mnemonics and create your own method.

The online videos, which are available for this book, will help you grasp the concepts of this book more thoroughly, and this will help enhance your performance.

Few weeks before the exam:
Find a study partner whose exam is scheduled close to your exam date. In the beginning, do not choose random cases; instead, start practicing chapter by chapter. Within each chapter, choose the case first, and study it well before practicing.

Do not move on to another chapter until you finish the one in hand. Apply the same strategy for the entire book. Always practice with PN typing.

A couple of weeks before the exam:
Ask your study partner to select practice cases randomly from different chapters. This is an opportunity to find your areas of weakness so that you can address them before the exam day.

A full day of practicing cases may seem grueling, but you will find that this is a highly effective method of preparation. It is the only way to build stamina for the long hours of testing at the CS exam center. Try to practice at least six cases at a time (half a day) in a continuous manner. This will help simulate the rigors of the actual CS exam.

Stress only on analysis of each complaint and a possible differential diagnosis. Practice live for the physical exam and focus on typing the PN.

How to perform practice cases
Find a practice-partner who will assist you with role-play. The acting needs to be as realistic as possible; however, your partner does not necessarily have to be of the same gender as the particular practice case you are performing. Ask him/her to use a stopwatch or timer to help you manage time precisely. There are CS timer apps available for smartphones that can be downloaded from the Apple or Android app stores. Moreover, CS for IMGs timer is also available online.

While performing the "physician role" in your practice cases, ensure that you do NOT know what the SP will say. This will train you to think of appropriate replies to the SP's questions as well as appropriate actions to take. This kind of role-play is what will best prepare you for the real CS exam.

Make sure to take the role-play seriously and follow the CS exam protocol. Begin the encounter by reading the doorway information, knocking on the door, and addressing your practice-partner by the family name, as indicated on the doorway information sheet. At about 10 minutes, make sure an announcement of *"Five minutes remaining"* is made. End your encounter with a final announcement at 15 minutes.

Once the 15 minutes is up, you must proceed directly to writing the PN. Allow yourself only 10 minutes to complete it.

It is vital that you simulate the role-play as realistically as possible to the CS environment. Your practice-partner should act like a real SP. Signs and symptoms should be presented by simulating acute pain, lying supine on the exam table without movement, simulating photophobia, displaying the blunt affect of depression, acting anxious, etc. If your practice-partner is not a medical professional, he/she must learn how to simulate physical exam signs, such as rebound tenderness, muscle weakness, CVA tenderness, Rinne test, etc.

The use of patient gown, bedsheet, gloves, and other simple tools will help you recreate the CS environment more realistically. We have provided blank checklists for CIS and SEP. These can be copied for multiple use and utilized for all practice cases. For ICE, a customized checklist is provided at the end of each chapter. The checklist will improve your performance while practicing.

When you begin performing practice cases, initially you may feel that you are:

- Nervous and rushed during the encounter
- Short on time to finish the encounter and/or for closure and counseling
- Forgetting to ask important questions to the SP
- Missing important clinical exam steps
- Running short of time for PN documentation

Don't worry! This is typical and happens to all of us in the initial phases of practicing cases. Your performance will improve over time and with practice.

When you finish each encounter, ask your partner to grade you on three checklists (ICE, CIS, and SEP). If your partner is a medical student or graduate, he/she can grade the PN as well. If not, you will have to grade the PN yourself.

1–2 days before the exam:

Review the cream only—the disciplines for medical history, physical exam, and CIS. Review common cases expected on the CS exam like abdominal, chest, joint pain, and others. Review the differential diagnosis for all cases.

A day before the exam:

- If needed, review only the differential diagnoses quickly for each case.
- Prepare and iron your attire including your white coat. Make sure you have your stethoscope ready as well. Those tiny things may cause unnecessary delay on the exam day.
- Check that you have your identification such as your passport and your scheduling permit in order.
- In the late afternoon, stop reading any books or studying. Go outside and relax. Enjoy yourself at a park or spend time with your family and friends.
- Choose accommodations that are close by or within an easy commute to the exam center.
- Recheck the address of the exam center and arrange for transportation if needed.

On the exam day:

- Plan to arrive at the testing center no later than 7:30 a.m. (30 minutes before the exam time) as you may encounter delays. No one is allowed to enter the exam center after 8:30 a.m. You must monitor USMLE website for the latest information.
- Be sure that you have your identification and scheduling permit before leaving your hotel or home.
- The on-site video orientation session starts at 8:30 a.m. Afterward, there is an opportunity to preview a simulation room that looks exactly like one of the real exam rooms (on-site orientation). Try out all of the equipment (the exam table, the dimmer on the light switch, otoscope, ophthalmoscope, reflex hammer, instruments used to test for sensory exam, etc.). Getting acclimated at this point will help you avoid embarrassment once the real exam begins.
- You get three breaks during the exam: Ten minutes after case #3, 30 minutes after case #6 with a meal, and 10 minutes break after case #9.

- You may expect little stress in the first case, but this is the norm and will disappear in the second case and thereafter.
- Finally, be sure to bring your white coat and stethoscope with you to the center on exam day; other tools are usually provided for you.

Remember that each encounter is videotaped. This is done in order to ensure the SP's safety and for research purposes but is not used in grading.

Do not expect the real exam cases to be presented EXACTLY as they are in *CS for IMGs*. However, with your training from *CS for IMGs*, you will find yourself comfortable to handle most of the exam cases. Typically, you will find a few cases that present with vague, odd, or unique complaints. Many times, these cases have been added for research or experimental purposes.

When encountering an odd case, follow the same steps presented in the book. Write down the possible differential diagnoses, knock on the door, smile, ask the essential questions for history-taking, do a focused general and local exam, and do a simple closure and counseling. Do not forget to address the SP's questions and concerns. Write the PN and go on to the next case.

In the CS exam, you are not expected to be perfect in every encounter or in all three components. Mistakes happen for all of us; just try your best to keep them to a minimum. If a portion of a case goes wrong, let go of it before you move on to your next case.

After the exam:

Once you've finished the exam, **do not discuss the exam cases with other past or future examinees. Do not share cases online either.**

Try not to be overly anxious about the exam results. It is obviously preferable to pass the exam on your first attempt. But in case you do not, please realize that it is not the end of the world. Many brilliant and outstanding people throughout history have experienced failures before realizing great success in life.

This book is a result of my cumulative experience gained in three CS exam attempts, having had a scholarship in the United States, writing this book for more than three years, and teaching the CS to various IMGs. This book is sufficient to help you pass the CS exam in the first attempt with no need for other resources, if used correctly. However, you can take advantage of other exam preparation resources as well. In addition to any study resources, practicing is the key to pass this exam. Try to seek the advice and opinions and feedback of past examinees and those who practice in different medically oriented professions (students, nurses, attending physicians, and tutors).

Lastly, my advice to you is to take the exam only when you feel that you are truly prepared. If you are not truly ready in even one component, failure is quite likely. Do not take the exam unless you are confident that you can pass all three components with ease.

I do believe that this first edition of *CS for IMGs* will not be the last one. I will endeavor to continually improve this book. I encourage readers to please send me suggestions, comments, or criticisms at info@csshool.org.

Best of luck,
Mohamed M. Elawdy, MD

Acknowledgments

We would like to thank the following people for their generous contribution:

Ayman Abdelaziz, MD, MSc
Specialist
Department of Cardiology
Armed Forces Hospital
Riyadh, Saudi Arabia

Osama Abdelsalam, MD
Medical Student
Mansoura University
Mansoura, Egypt

Rasha Taha Abouelkheir, MSc, MD
Consultant
Department of Radiology
Urology and Nephrology Center
Mansoura University
Mansoura, Egypt

Mohini Abreo, MD, DGO
Consultant Obstetrics and Gynecology
National Institute of Laser and Endoscopic Surgery
    and Aakar IVF Centre
Mumbai, Maharashtra, India

Shafique Ahmed, MD
Senior Medical Officer
Emergency Department
Alama Iqbal Medical College
Lahore, Pakistan

Farida Mohsin Ambusaidi, MD
Specialist
Department of Radiology
Ibri Hospital
Ministry of Health
Ibri, Oman

Immad Attique, MD
Resident
Department of Internal Medicine
Maryland Medical Center Midtown Campus
Maryland, Baltimore, USA

Haythum M. Atya, MD, MSc
Specialist
Department of Orthopedics
Ministry of Health
Cairo, Egypt

Ameya Atul Chumble, MD
Medical Student
Virginia Commonwealth University School of Medicine
Richmond, Virginia, USA

Tarek Dabash, MD, MSc
Lecture of Cardiology
Department of Medicine
Al-Azhar University
Cairo, Egypt

Ahmad Emad Elawdy, MD
Medical Student
Mansoura University
Mansoura, Egypt

Abir S. Elshuhumi, MD
Medical Officer
Department of Family Medicine
Ibri Hospital
Ministry of Health
Ibri, Oman

Nishat Fatema, MD
Medical Officer
Department of Obstetrics and Gynecology
Ibri Hospital
Ministry of Health
Ibri, Oman

Mohammad Abdel Fattah, MD, MSc
Specialist
Department of Immunology and Rheumatology
Aswan Hospital
Cairo, Egypt

Alan T. Forstater, MD
Attending Physician
Department of Emergency Medicine
Thomas Jefferson University Hospitals
Philadelphia, Pennsylvania, USA

Oday Halhouli, MD
Medical Intern
Medicine School—The University of Jordan
Amman, Jordan

Hisham M. Ibrahim, MBBS, DCH, MRCPCH
Specialist
Department of Pediatrics
Ibri Hospital
Ministry of Health
Ibri, Oman

Ehab Elsyed Kakha, MD, MRCS
Lecturer
Department of Surgery
Al-Azhar University
Cairo, Egypt

Nagy Ismail, MD, MS
Specialist
Department of Pediatrics
Sohar Hospital
Ministry of Health
Sohar, Oman

Mohammad Khoujah, MD
Medical Intern
Medicine School—The University of Jordan
Amman, Jordan

Vijay Kumar Kolluri, MD
Medical Intern
Soochow University Medical College
Suzhou, China

Nermeen Mostafa, MD
Assistant Professor
Department of Medical Oncology
Ain Shamas University
Cairo, Egypt

Nermin Moufy, MD
Specialist
Department of Psychiatry
Ibri Hospital
Ministry of Health
Ibri, Oman

Mohamed Rajab, MD, MSc
Specialist
Department of Neurology
Saudi German Hospital
Riyadh, Saudi Arabia

Ahmad Samir, MD, MSc
Specialist
Department of Cardiology
Sohar Hospital
Ministry of Health
Sohar, Oman

Mahmoud Sharwer, MD, MSc
Specialist
Department of Orthopedics
Sohar Hospital
Ministry of Health
Sohar, Oman

Reda Sheta, MD, MSc
Specialist
Department of Orthopedics
Ibri Hospital
Ministry of Health
Ibri, Oman

Sreenivas A. V., MD
Senior Specialist
Department of Neurosurgery
Amrita Institute of Medical Sciences and Research Centre
Kochi, Kerala, India

Gerald P. Whelan, MD
Former President
American Board of Emergency Medicine;
Vice President
Clinical Skills Assessment Services
Educational Commission for Foreign Medical Graduates
Philadelphia, Pennsylvania, USA

Souzan Yahia, BS Pharm
Clinical Pharmacist
Ministry of Health
Egypt

Tamer Zaafrani, MD, MSc
Specialist
Department of Psychiatry
Ibri Hospital
Ministry of Health
Ibri, Oman

Language and English Editors
Chuck Miller
Dara B. Oken
Douglas Forbes
Rob Bignell
Sherrie Smith

1 The Basics, Component 1, Integrated Clinical Encounter

Keywords: integrated clinical encounter, medical history, physical examination, patient note

1.1 Introduction

The Clinical Skills exam has three parts: Integrated Clinical Encounter (ICE), Communication and Interpersonal Skills (CIS), and Spoken English Proficiency (SEP). Please read the U.S. Medical Licensing Examination (USMLE) Bulletin of Information at www.usmle.org to find out more about how the CS exam is scored.

The ICE focuses on how you apply basic medical knowledge rather than simply measuring the quantity of your medical knowledge. The ICE tests how you come up with a possible diagnosis through the history-taking and physical examination (PE). It also assesses your ability to convey data to another physician through a Patient Note (PN).

The CS exam is different from other USMLE Step 1 and Step 2 CK tests, which use multiple choice questions to test the prospective physician's medical knowledge and in which a high level of medical knowledge is required for a passing mark. The CS exam instead is an interactive exam, with an actor playing the role of a patient. Only basic medical knowledge about the most common diseases in the Emergency Room (ER) and the family medicine clinic is needed. Therefore, asking sophisticated questions and searching for rare differential diagnoses (DDs) will not help you pass the exam.

The clinical encounters on the CS exam strive to mimic reality. For example, the CS Exam Center has been built to resemble a large clinic. The patients have problems similar to what doctors frequently encounter. However, it is not quite real and different in a few aspects.

Each clinical encounter is limited to 15 minutes. This gives you only enough time to take a relevant history and to do a focused clinical exam, not a detailed one, as you would do in a real clinic.

The second difference is that the patients are healthy people, acting as if they were sick. They are called "SPs," which stands for Standardized Patients (SPs). The SPs complain of medical problems and conditions, but there are no physical manifestations (pallor, tachycardia, murmurs, edema in the lower limbs, high temperature, etc.). However, you are expected to act as if there were. At times, some of the SPs will have fabricated physical manifestations such as fake scars, ecchymosis, or erythema. Again, you are expected to behave as if these were real. Do NOT ignore them; treat these fake signs as real. After all, the encounter is a role-play to mimic a reality.

Each examinee will have 12 clinical encounters during the day of the exam. There are three subcomponents to each encounter of the ICE—the history and the PE that are graded by the SP, in addition to the PN that is graded by a physician.

1.2 Section A: Medical History

Taking the patient's history is an important part of the CS exam (▶Video 1.1). You should have already learned the fundamentals of history in medical school. The purpose of this book, therefore, is to help you learn the art of efficiently taking the patient history by tailoring your questions to fit well within the CS exam. This is because time is of the essence. You cannot afford to ask superfluous questions.

Passing this subcomponent requires you to know when to shorten or expand your investigation into the patient's complaint. Though you will not ask all the history questions to each SP, during the course of the exam you will likely spread the questions over the 12 SPs.

An example of tailoring your questions to fit a patient is when interviewing an SP who has **epigastric pain,** focusing on the symptoms that are related to the gastrointestinal (GI) system (nausea, vomiting, heartburn, bowel movements, dark stool, and vomiting of blood). You would not waste time asking questions about headaches, hearing loss, joint pain, etc.

In a case with a chief complaint (CC) of **ankle pain**, ask about symptoms that are relevant to the joint problem, such as about swelling, redness, hotness, and possible complications such as sensory or motor deficit and limb disabilities, which are areas of concern, rather than symptoms that are related to the chest, GI system, or a detailed obstetrics and gynecology (OB/Gyn). You need to focus on the task at hand (i.e., the cause of the CC).

A general OB/Gyn history is essential for all females in all cases, while a detailed one should be taken in OB/Gyn cases (suspected abortion, ectopic pregnancy, vaginal bleeding and amenorrhea, etc.).

For the purposes of the CS exam, the patient history can be divided into two main categories: history of present illness (HPI) and the past history and others.

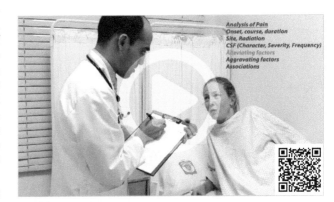

Video 1.1 This video will teach you how to tailor the medical history to satisfy CS requirements and time limitation. The emphasis is on the analysis of the most common complaints in the CS. https://www.thieme.de/de/q.htm?p=opn/cs/20/3/11453119-17a31cb2

1.2.1 History of Present Illness

This is the most important part of the history because it is:

- *Dynamic*: It changes. Each case and complaint is unique.
- *The SP's first impression of you as a doctor*: It breaks the ice of taking the history, a time when both patient and doctor may feel nervous and be uncomfortable.
- *Crucial*: You rely on the information you get from this part to arrive at a preliminary diagnosis.
- Upon seeing the Doorway Information before you enter the examination room, brainstorm three to four possible causes as a presumptive diagnosis. Jot them down on your scratch paper. It is highly recommended that you do this to increase your focus and concentration before starting the case. Make sure you start the HPI interview with open questions, such as *"What brings you in to the hospital today?"*

The HPI has two components: analysis of two subcomponents (CC and possible causes) and review of two systems (local system and general systems). Follow the order below (1–4) for taking the history and documenting it in the PN. For example, a case with a CC of **low back pain** is taken.

Analysis of the two subcomponents:

1. Analysis of CC (back pain as an example).
2. Analysis of the possible DD (muscle strain, fracture spine, disk herniation, etc.).

Review of two systems (local and general):

3. *Symptoms related to the local affected system*: these are the symptoms that have not been mentioned by the SP, but which could be linked to the same system (sensory and motor function, range of motion, urinary and bowel control, etc.).
4. Review of systems (**ROS**) including OB/Gyn history, sleep, appetite, weight, etc.

Analysis of Chief Complaint

Only the most frequent complaints will be discussed in this section; other complaints will be dealt with in their individual, case-specific chapters.

Pain is the most common complaint on the CS exam. Therefore, memorize and rehearse questions related to pain.

Use this mnemonic device to help you remember the categories that you should ask about: **LIQOR AAA**: It stands for **Location, Intensity, Quality, Onset** + course + duration, **Radiation, Aggravating factors, Alleviating factors, Associations.** Or

Onset, course, and duration

Location and Radiation

CSF (**C**haracter, **S**everity, and **F**requency):

Aggravating and Alleviating Factors

Associations

In ▶ **Table 1.1**, **Intensity** corresponds with **Severity**, and **Quality** corresponds with **Character** and **Frequency**. (More than one question may be given for each category.)

Other common complaints that SPs are likely to have are fever, nausea and vomiting, diarrhea, cough, or bleeding. The relevant questions to ask for each common complaint are:

Fever:

- *How long have you had a fever?*
- *Did you check your temperature at home?*
- *What was your temperature when you took it at home?*
- *Have you taken any medicine for the fever? If yes, what did you take?*
- *Has the fever come down since you took the medicine?*

Nausea and vomiting:

- *Do you feel nauseous?*
- *Have you been vomiting?/Are you able to keep things down?*
- *How many times a day do you vomit?*
- *Have you noticed any blood in the vomit?*
- *What is the color of the vomit?*

For any body fluids or excretions (vomit, diarrhea, sputum, etc.), *use the formula* **Onset + ABCD:**

A = **A**mount: *Could you estimate the amount of ...?*

B = **B**lood: *Have you noticed blood in your ...?*

C = **C**olor: *What color is it? Is it bright or dark red?*

D = o**D**our: *What does it smell like?*

Category	Sample questions
Onset, course, and duration	*How long have you had this pain?/When did the pain start?* *Did it come on suddenly?/Did it start hurting all of a sudden?* *Since the pain started, has it gotten worse, or has it stayed the same?*
Location and radiation	*Where is your pain?/Where does it hurt?/Could you point to where it hurts?* *Do you feel the pain anywhere else?/Does the pain travel to anywhere else?*
Character, Severity, Frequency (**CSF**)	*Could you describe the pain to me?/Tell me how it hurts?* *On a scale of 1 to 10, with 10 being the worst, how would you rate the pain?/How bad is your pain on a scale of...?* *Is it a constant pain, or does it come and go?* *If the pain comes and goes, ask, "When and how often does it occur?"*
Alleviating, Aggravating factors	*What makes it better?/Does anything make your pain better?* *What makes it worse?/Does anything make it worse?*
Associated symptoms	*Do you have any other symptoms besides pain?* *What were you doing when the pain first started?*

Table 1.1 Mnemonic for analysis of pain

Diarrhea:

- *Do you have diarrhea? If yes:*
- *How many times per day do you have diarrhea?*
- *Do you have diarrhea every time you go to the bathroom?*
- *Have you noticed any blood? Any mucous? Do you have any rectal pain?*

Cough:

- *Do you have a cough?/Have you been coughing lately? If yes:*
- *Is it worse in the daytime or at night?*
- *Does anything make your cough worse?*
- *Does anything make your cough better?*
- *Do you cough up any mucous?* If yes, ask **ABC**:
- **A** (A = Amount): *How much mucous comes up when you cough?*
- **B** (B = Blood): *Did you cough up any blood?*
- **C** (C = Color): *What is the color of the mucous?*

Bleeding disorders:

- For cases of hematemesis, rectal bleeding, hemoptysis, etc., use the ABCDE formula:
- **Amount** = *Could you estimate the Amount of the blood you bled? A teaspoon, tablespoon, or half cup?*
- **Blood thinner** = *Are you taking any Blood thinner meds?* (This question to estimate the amount: loss of too much blood causes dizziness.)
- **Color** = *Could you describe the Color of your blood?*
- **Dizzy** = *Do you feel Dizzy?*
- **Else** = *Do you bleed from anywhere else?* (To inquire about general [systemic] causes of bleeding.)

If you suspect infectious diseases, ask the following:

- *Have you been around any sick person recently?*
- *Are your shots up to date?*
- *Have you traveled outside the United States recently?*

For complaints that come in episodes, like, bronchial asthma (BA), transient ischemic attack, panic attack, palpitation, dizziness, hot flashes, start with:

- *How often do you have…?*
- *When was the last time?*
- *How long does/did it last?*
- *Does anything make it better?*
- *Does anything make it worse?*

Feeling sad/depression:

- *Do you feel sad?*
- *Do you feel depressed?*
- *Have you ever felt like life is not worth living?*

If the SP answers by yes, go through and ask the questions for depression in detail (see Chapter 9, Psychiatry).

Suggested open-ended questions for all complaints:

- *Do you have any other symptoms besides (pain, fever, vomiting, loss of weight, etc.)?*
- *Do you have any idea what might have caused that?*

Analysis of Possible Differential Diagnosis

Asking about possible causes is important not only in the documentation of the HPI section but also in the DD section of the PN. This is because the SP history will contain facts that could lead you to arrive at more than one diagnosis. When you take the CS exam, you will see that the PN has three blank spaces in the DD section. You are expected to give at least two DDs.

When you look at the doorway information, it is a good idea to think about diseases that could be possibly causing the CC. **Brainstorming three to four possible causes** before entering the room goes a long way in succeeding with this part.

The latest change to the USMLE after July 2012 included major changes in the PN documentation. The PN is no longer just an enumeration of the DDs as it used to be. Now you need to list supporting evidence for each possible cause from your history and the clinical exam. As true clinical signs are few and far between on the CS exam, the DD relies on the history in the majority of cases.

- *Example 1*: The doorway information said that the patient complains of a **headache**. You came up with three to four possible causes and jotted them down on a piece of scratch paper. After you finished your analysis of the CC (headache), you found that migraine was the most probable cause. The next step would be to ask about other possible causes, such as tension headache, cluster headache, or brain tumor.
- *Example 2*: In a case of **dizziness**, the analysis of the complaint points to benign paroxysmal positional vertigo. Asking about other possible causes (vasovagal attack, medication side effect, or arrhythmia) is necessary to complete the history and fill out the PN correctly (▶ Table 1.11).

> **Note:** Thyroid abnormalities frequently come up in the DD on the CS. The questions to ask are tabulated in ▶ Table 1.2.

Symptoms Related to the Affected Body System

After analyzing the CC and the possible causes, you should ask questions about other symptoms that are manifested in the same body system. For example, if the complaint is a **cough,** you should ask about the symptoms of the respiratory system.

In a case with a **headache**, passing out, or limb weakness as the CCs, the history should be completed by asking about symptoms of the neurological system. For **feeling sad** as a CC, **SIG E CAPS** questions should be asked (see Chapter 9, Psychiatry).

Table 1.2 Manifestations of thyroid abnormalities

Hypothyroidism	Hyperthyroidism
Are you intolerant to cold temperature?/Do you feel cold when others don't?	*Do you have intolerance to heat?/Do you feel hot when others don't?*
Do you feel constipated?	*Do you have diarrhea?*
Have you gained weight recently?	*Have you lost weight recently?*
Note: hypothyroidism should be one of the differential diagnosis (DD) for the following complaints: fatigue, depression, weight gain, constipation, and menstrual abnormalities (amenorrhea)	Note: hyperthyroidism should be one of the DDs for the following complaints: anxiety disorder, panic attack, weight loss, diarrhea, and menstrual abnormalities (polymenorrhea)

Review of Systems

We finish the HPI by making a general review of the patient's health. Ask about symptoms of other body systems that are **not** the ones affected by the CC.

> Here is a mnemonic device for remembering what to ask:
> - *For male patients:* **I SAW** 2 systems (**GI** system and **U**rinary system).
> - *For female patients:* **I SAW** 3 systems (**GI** system, **U**rinary and **G**enital systems; ▶ Table 1.3).

Table 1.3 Review of systems mnemonic with example questions

I	*I am going to ask you a few questions about your health in general.*
Sleep	*How is your sleep?/Have you been sleeping well?*
Appetite	*How is your appetite?/Have you been eating well?*
Weight	*Have you had any recent changes in your weight? If yes:*
	Have you lost or gained weight? How much? Over what period of time?
2 GI/GU(♂)	*Have you noticed any recent changes in your bowel movements?*
3 GI/GU/ Gyne (♀) (▶ Fig. 1.1)	*Have you had any problems in passing urine? In female, add the following: PPC + GPA*
Period	*When was your last menstrual Period?*
Pap	*Have you had a Pap smear done? If yes:*
	When? Was it normal?
Contraception	*Are you using any kind of Contraception?*
Gravidity	*Have you ever been Pregnant? If yes:*
	How many times?
Parity	*How many times have you given Birth?*
Abortion	*Have you ever had any Abortion or miscarriage?*

1.2.2 Past Medical History

This is the final part of the history. This includes the patient's medical history, the family medical history, the social history (SH), and perhaps the sexual history.

This part differs from the HPI, in that:

It is easier. You ask every SP the same questions. There is no tailoring of the questions to match the CC.

It takes less time. As this part is not as important as the HPI, you should not spend as much time on it.

It does not affect your grade as much. If you forget to ask about something in this part, it will not affect your overall performance on the exam, whereas omissions in the HPI will.

To maximize your performance, remember that the objectives of taking this part are not only to just make documentation in the history section of the PN but also to support your DD. So use this part to fill out the blank spaces in the DD section of the PN.

Many medical diseases are associated with well-known risk factors. For example, **heart attack** is associated with hypertension (HTN), diabetes mellitus (DM), hypercholesterolemia, and smoking. **Cerebral stroke** is associated with HTN and heart disease. **Chronic obstructive pulmonary disease (COPD)** and **lung cancer** are associated with smoking and some occupations. **Sexually transmitted diseases (STDs)** and **human immunodeficiency virus (HIV)** are associated with unprotected sex (▶ Table 1.4).

> There are eight categories of questions to ask about (▶ Table 1.4).
>
> That is a bit daunting, so here is a mnemonic device to help you remember them:
>
> **PDS** was used to suture **PDA** and resulted in **F**ast **S**urgery ± **S**car.
>
> The PDS is a surgical suture, and PDA stands for Patent Ductus Arteriosus.

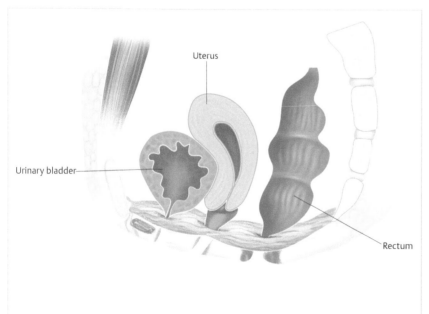

Fig. 1.1 The three systems as a reminder to the review of systems.

Uterus

Urinary bladder

Rectum

Table 1.4 Past medical history mnemonic with example questions

History	Sample questions
Past medical history	I'm going to ask you a few questions regarding your past medical history.
Diseases	Do you have any kind of medical diseases? If yes:
	What conditions or diseases do you have?
Surgical	Have you had any surgeries done? If yes:
	When did you have it done?
Previous episodes	Have you had a similar condition before? If yes:
	When was the last time?
	What medicine did you take when that happened?
Drugs (medications)	Are you taking any medicines on a daily basis? If yes:
	Do you remember what the dose is?
	How often do you take it?
Allergies	Do you have any allergies?
Family	Does anyone in your family have the same complaint?
	Does anyone in your family, especially your parents, have major medical problems?
Social (SODA): • Smoking • Occupation • Drugs • Alcohol	What do you do for a living?
	Do you smoke? If yes:
	How long have you been a smoker? How many cigarettes do you smoke per day?
	Do you drink?
	Do you use any street drugs?
	Who do you live with? (To assess home safety in some special cases.)
Sexual	Do you have any problems in your sexual life? See "Sex Life" in notes following

Diseases and Medical Conditions

Any medical disease is possible on the exam, but SPs commonly suffer from DM, HTN, and/or hypercholesterolemia. Remember that common complications for **DM** are vision problems (retinopathy), chronic epigastric pain (this may be a symptom of gastropathy), decreased sensation in the legs (peripheral neuropathy), and erectile dysfunction. For **HTN**, the complications include severe headache, cerebral stroke, and chest pain (heart attack). If there are complications to DM or HTN, or if the SP says he or she has not been taking his/her medication, **counseling is mandatory**. Ask these questions:
- Is your diabetes/blood pressure under control?
- Do you have regular checkup visits?
- When was the last one?/What was the last reading?

Surgical History

Appendectomy and lap cholecystectomy are among the most common surgeries you are likely to encounter, and the SP will likely sport a fake scar. However, most SPs have an irrelevant surgical history.

Previous Episodes

Some diseases are known to come in episodes. The SP usually remembers when an episode last occurred and what he or she took or did.

Diseases that commonly have previous episodes are the following:
- Migraine headache relieved by nonsteroidal anti-inflammatory disease (NSAID).
- Disk herniation (cervical or lumbar) relieved by rest and NSAID.
- Peptic ulcer relieved by antacids (Tums).
- Angina relieved by nitrates.
- Sinusitis relieved by antihistamines.
- Any allergy (BA relieved by albuterol inhaler).

Drugs (Medication)

If the SP is taking a medication, he or she may call it by the generic or pharmaceutical name, so you should be familiar with both. Both of the names are listed in Chapter 13, Appendix. Also, be familiar with the side effects of the most common medications. This is important because it is sometimes a part of the DD (see Chapter 13, Appendix, 13.4 Common Medications in CS Exam Scenarios.).

Most SPs, when they give the name of the medication, also say the dosage and concentration. If they do not mention this, you should ask for it, just for the purposes of documentation.

In the cases where the SP has a chronic disease (e.g., DM, HTN, or hypercholesterolemia), ask them if they have been compliant with their medications: *"Have you been taking your medication regularly?"* If the SP has not been compliant, remember that you **must** counsel the SP at the end of the encounter.

Allergies

The questions in the chart above are usually sufficient for most SPs. However, in some cases (those who have an allergy or are hypersensitive [BA, sinusitis with allergic rhinitis, or skin rash]), you need to investigate further. Ask the following:
- Are you allergic to any food?
- Do you have allergies to pollen or molds?
- Any allergies to medicine such as penicillin?
- Are you allergic to pets such as cats? What about bee stings?

If yes for any allergens, ask, What usually happens when you come into contact with… (say the allergen)?

Family History

This is a very important part of the history, as it can be a key to a possible diagnosis. Family history (FH) plays a great role in infectious diseases, diseases that have genetic backgrounds, and cancer (▶Fig. 1.2).

Infectious diseases that may include common cold, upper respiratory tract infections, pneumonia, meningitis, and gastroenteritis. Ask if any of the SP's family members have the same condition, as it may be the key to the diagnosis.

Diseases that have **genetic backgrounds** include DM, HTN, hypercholesterolemia, allergies, kidney/gall stones, and heart diseases.

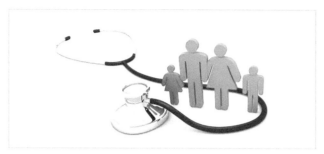

Fig. 1.2 Family history.

Finally, the history of **cancer** in the family is important for the DD and for the screening: Knowing the type of cancer, such as prostate or colon cancer, will guide you about if the SP is at risk and should be tested. If the SP informs you that a family member died of cancer (or anything else, for that matter), show sympathy by saying, *"I'm sorry to hear that, my condolences."* If the SP does not offer the cause of death, make sure you ask what it was. Do not ask if anyone in the SP's family is alive or dead. It isn't necessary for the purposes of the exam and it may evoke negative emotions. In the end, the point of asking about the family is to discover the diseases that (have) run in the family, not if the members are alive or dead.

Social History

Be aware that the SP's work may have a connection to the complaint (▶**Fig. 1.3**). There are certain occupations that are well known to predispose workers to certain diseases. **Stressful jobs** cause anxiety, panic attacks, and sleep disorders. Jobs (such as **mining or asbestos removal**) that require proximity to or handling of carcinogens or pollution cause risk for lung cancer. **Production workers** often suffer hearing loss due to being around extremely loud machinery. **College students** are at risk for psychiatric disorders (anxiety and sleep disorder), drug abuse, and STDs. In the CS exam, those are the most commonly encountered.

Many SPs admit to smoking. If you have a smoker, write that down so you remember to provide counseling at the end of the encounter. See Chapter 2, The Basics, Component 2, Communication and Interpersonal Skills, to find out how you should best provide counseling for smoking.

Likewise, most SPs will tell you that they drink socially. If that is the case, do not ask more and document that SP drinks alcohol socially. However, for heavy alcohol users (rare in CS histories), you should use the CAGE questionnaire (see Chapter 2, The Basics, Component 2, Communication and Interpersonal Skills). The definition of a heavy alcohol user is a man who drinks more than two drinks per day and a woman who drinks more than one. For those who engage in binge drinking, you should ask them about the type of alcoholic beverage they usually drink (beer, wine, liquor).

Though SPs do not commonly admit to using illegal drugs, if they do, then cocaine and marijuana are the ones usually used. A few of the common street names for recreational drugs are speed (amphetamine), crack (a form of cocaine), and angel dust (phencyclidine).

Sexual History

A detailed sexual history is not usually required for cases such as chest pain, severe headache, or ankle pain, etc. (▶**Fig. 1.4**). But if you feel you need to take this history, start like this:

"We're almost finished. I just have a few questions about your sex life. Everything that you tell me will be kept confidential. Do you have any problems in your sexual life or any concerns?"

It is a good open-ended question and according to the response of SPs, you may need to go through a detailed history. You need to take a detailed sexual history in the following cases:

When it is the CC (weak penile erection/erectile dysfunction).

Urogenital cases (BPH [benign prostatic hyperplasia], urethral discharge, vaginal discharge, HIV, vaginal bleeding, etc.).

If the sexual functions are affected or compromised by a disease (e.g., uncontrolled DM or HTN) or medications (beta-blockers, SSRIs [selective serotonin reuptake inhibitors]).

Sample Questions for Detailed Sexual History:
- *Are you sexually active?*
- *How many sexual partners have you had in the last year?*
- *Are you sexually attracted to men, women, or both?*
- *Have you had an HIV test done?*
- *Have you had any sexually transmitted diseases?*

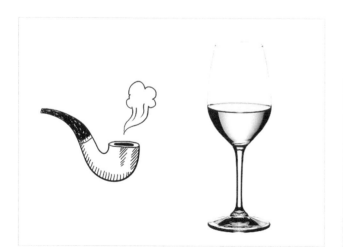

Fig. 1.3 Social history.

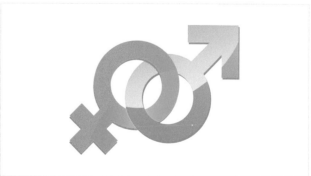

Fig. 1.4 Sexual history.

1.3 Section B: Physical (Clinical) Examination

1.3.1 Foundation

This section is not going to teach you the fundamentals of doing a PE (▶Video 1.2). Those are best learned from one of the many other medical textbooks. The objective of this chapter is to teach you how to **apply** your skills in clinical exam in order to pass the CS exam.

You will not do every step of a PE in one encounter, but you will most probably go through all the steps during the course of the exam day, seeing 12 SPs. Therefore, it is important to know which PE steps to focus on doing in each encounter. For example, in the case of a **headache**, the head, neck, and the neurological exam should be done in detail, but there is no need for an abdominal exam.

Meanwhile, the abdominal exam is an essential part in a case of **right lower quadrant (RLQ) or left lower quadrant (LLQ) pain**. Similarly, the upper limb and the shoulder joint exams are areas of concern in the case of **shoulder pain**, while the lower limb and the ankle joint are the areas of concern in an **ankle pain** case.

The PE on the CS exam differs from a real clinical exam in a few ways. First, you are expected to complete your general and local exam in 5 minutes or less. In a real clinical setting, you may need more time to accomplish this task, which is not possible on the CS exam. Though the short time limit is a major challenge, it is, in fact, a reasonable length of time if you are prepared well. You can overcome the time obstacle in each case by doing only the relevant PE on the affected system. The CC will guide you in deciding what to do and what not to do.

The USMLE CS uses SPs who grade your performance. They will observe how you use the tools of the trade, such as the ophthalmoscope and stethoscope. They will watch you go about abdominal, chest, thyroid, and other steps of PE. They will see if you conduct tests such as Murphy's sign, psoas sign, and costovertebral angle (CVA) tenderness with the appropriate steps.

They also evaluate your clinical exam procedural skills. Did you remember to wash your hands before beginning an examination? Did you draw back the patient's gown to examine an affected area, or did you examine the affected area while it was covered by the gown? If you drew the gown back, did you use correct draping techniques when uncovering the affected area? Did you repeat maneuvers that caused them pain? At all times, the SP will be evaluating your technique to see if you are completing the steps and following standard operating procedures.

The SPs are not professional actors, but they have been trained to act like a real patient and they become experts at playing the role. They not only alter their behavior and complain of nonexistent physical conditions, but also have cosmetic scars, rashes, and bruises.

Expect most of the SPs to have normal physical signs. Do not waste time looking for unusual findings such as a congested neck vein, carotid bruit, lung crepitation, or murmurs. Move swiftly from one step to the next; do not waste time performing unnecessary steps. The goal of the PE is to do the required steps,

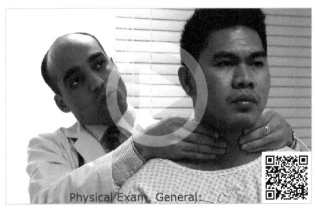

Video 1.2 This video gives a realistic approach to perform the physical exam within the allocated time on the CS exam. https://www.thieme.de/de/q.htm?p=opn/cs/20/3/11453120-da084477

to do them correctly, and to do them in a reasonable amount of time.

Their altered behavior includes acting as if they were:
- Undergoing severe, agonizing pain.
- Expressing difficulty breathing (dyspnea).
- Feeling extreme anxiety and being easily irritated.
- Suffering from depression.
- Having photophobia.
- Experiencing an altered mental status or disorientation.

Nonexistent physical signs may include the following:
- Tenderness (in sinuses, joints, or abdomen).
- Rebound tenderness.
- Neurological conditions (loss of sensation, reduced muscle power, poor reflexes).

Positive physical maneuvers or tests:
- SPs can simulate positive drop arm test, Murphy's sign, Brudzinski's sign, Romberg's sign, and others.

Cosmetics:
Fake scars can be created with makeup. They are most often found on the abdomen, as if from appendectomies.

They can be used to portray **local problems** such as erythema (redness), which indicates inflammation, local rash, or recent trauma, and ecchymosis (bruises), which often will be blue, green, or black. They may be evidence of domestic violence or old trauma.

Cosmetics also can indicate a **general problem** that is systemic. An example is skin rash or bleeding disorder. For this situation, the makeup will appear in multiple locations on the SP.

How do you deal with these induced or faked clinical signs? For the purposes of the exam, you must pretend that they are real and work around them. You can neither remove them nor mention that they do not seem real.

Of course, there are some things that cannot be faked by acting or with cosmetics. For example, in a case of fever and cough, you may suspect pneumonia as a DD. However, you will not detect lung crepitation. So, you will probably find the SP's lungs to be normal, and you should document them as such. Similarly, hyperthyroidism will not be accompanied by an enlarged thyroid. Other similar physical signs in this category include pupil size and papilledema, lung and heart sounds, swollen thyroid and lymph nodes (LNs), carotid bruit, congestion and postnasal drip, erythema of the throat, and jugular venous distention (JVD).

In addition, there are vital signs, which are usually given in the doorway information. These include high temperatures, tachycardia, and high blood pressure. There is no need to check them again; accept the doorway information as fact.

Remember that on the CS exam, you do not do breast, genital, rectal, pelvic exams, nor the corneal reflex; you can often also omit the gag reflex. If they are indicated, tell the patient you would like to do them sometime to get a better understanding of disease, and also make sure to document the need for these exams in your PN.

1.3.2 Strategy for Physical Examination

There are two parts to the PE: the **general examination** and the **local examination**. Do the general exam first for several reasons. First, it is a good icebreaker between you and the SP. Second, it is simple and does not take too much time, so you are likely to succeed at it; doing something well at the beginning may bolster your confidence and put you at ease. Finally, it fits in well with the organization of the SP checklist.

Do the general exam exactly as you would do it in a clinic. Have the SP sit on the bed, unless he or she is lying down when you walk in. In that case, do the exam while the SP is lying down. It is better to start from the head and work your way down to the foot (head and neck, chest, heart, upper limb, and finish with the lower leg). Note the SP's appearance and position (decubitus) before you start the exam. Document this in the PN afterward. Always tell the patient what you are going to do, for example, *"Let's start with the general examination of*

your body," "I am going to feel your pulse," "I am going to listen to your heart."

Here is a mnemonic device to help you remember the items you need to check, the order in which they should be checked, and also the order in which to document them in the PN (▶ Table 1.5):

*Vital signs may change hormones (**ADH + NE + LH**) that are given by local shots.*

- *Fundus examination*: If the SP is diabetic or hypertensive, it is important to do a **fundus** examination (▶ Fig. 1.5). It is also indicated in neurology cases (headache, syncope, dizziness, etc.). Tell the SP that you will examine the back of the eyes, and then dim the light. Test the ophthalmoscope on your hand. Examine the right eye while holding the ophthalmoscope in your right hand and standing on the SP's right. Then repeat on the left side while holding the ophthalmoscope in your left hand and standing on the SP's left side. If the SP is lying on the bed and cannot sit up, do it while the SP is lying down. Again, do not wait too long to see the pupil reaction. Move on to the next step.
- *Mouth*: Use a tongue depressor (▶ Fig. 1.6) if the SP has a sore throat and for upper respiratory infection (URI) cases. Ask the SP to open his mouth and say, *"Ahh."* As at the end of every step, you should say something like, *"Your throat looks healthy."*
- *Neck exam (carotid bruit and JVD)*: See cardiac exam in Chapter 4, Chest (Cardiology and Respiratory).
- *Lung and heart (LH) exam*: For better time management, LH exam can be tailored accordingly. A focused LH exam is recommended only for all cases where the systems in question—lung and heart—are not affected (abdominal,

---

Table 1.5 Physical examination mnemonic

General exam	Notes
Vital signs	Look at the doorway information for vital statistics, and note them on the blue sheet.
Appearance Decubitus (position)	Look at the patient's appearance and position, so you don't forget to put them in the PN. Please see Patient Note section.
Head	HEENT: Head, eyes, ears, nose, throat
	Eyes: Ask the SP to look up and then down without moving his head. Use an otoscope (light source) to examine the eyes.
	Mouth: *Ask the SP to open his mouth and say, "Ahh."*
Neck: • LNs • Thyroid	Stand behind the SP and put your fingers on the anterior border of the sternomastoid, palpate the LNs from above and move downwards, feeling for any swelling of the glands. Next, examine the thyroid gland. Gently feel it and then ask the SP to swallow.
Extremities	Start with the hands. Look at the SP's palm, dorsum, and fingernails. Check the radial pulse for about 10s. Check the legs for edema; ask the SP if his legs have been swollen.
Lungs	Tell the SP you will untie the gown. Warm the stethoscope in your hand before touching it to the chest. Put it on the back of the chest away from the scapula. Ask him or her to take a deep breath. Move the stethoscope to the other side and repeat.
Heart	Tell the SP you need him or her to lower his or her gown as you need to listen to his or her heart. Listen to the aortic and the mitral areas. Retie the gown to cover the patient up after you finish.
Local exam	This includes detailed lung and heart, abdomen, joints, and neurological system.
	See the corresponding chapter for details.
Special test	This includes the CVA, Murphy's, psoas, Rovsing's, and Romberg's signs, rebound tenderness, drop arm, Rinne's tests, etc.

Abbreviations: CVA, costovertebral angle; LNs, lymph nodes; PN, patient note; SP, standardized patient.

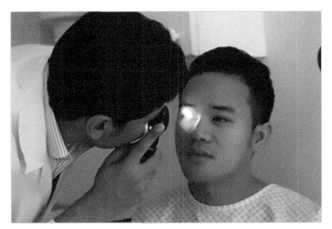

Fig. 1.5 Fundoscopic exam of the eyes.

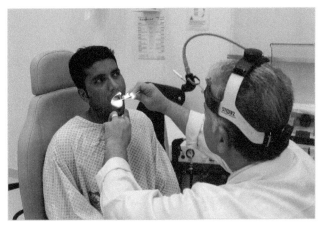

Fig. 1.6 Throat exam.

gynecology, musculoskeletal cases, etc.); in these cases, auscultation is enough. A detailed LH exam is needed only for chest cases. See Chapter 4, Chest (Cardiology and Respiratory), for more details. When the complaint is far from chest and heart and you feel rushed, you can cancel the LH exam completely and focus on the local exam (happens usually in long neurological cases).

From my experience, most of the CS cases do not need a detailed lower limb or foot exam. Thus for the best time management, I recommend, in a general exam for CS, starting with examining the head, hands, and then legs. Those can be done while you are in front of the SP. Then go to the back, do a neck exam, and then examine the chest (LH). With this method, it is enough to look at the legs while asking the SP: *Have you had any swelling in your legs?*

However, on rare occasions you need to examine the feet (if there are ankle problems). Wait until you finish the exam, so that the feet are the last thing you touch in the exam. Some people might object to having you touch their feet and then their chest.

> Role-play different types of cases so you can practice eliminating irrelevant steps and focus on the relevant ones.
>
> The general exam can be adapted to better fit the case and the time constraints. Be flexible!

1.3.3 Suggested Dialogue for Physical Examination

For best results, practice this with a friend who will agree to play the role of SP. Have him/her hold this dialogue. You go over it, and if you forget what to say next, have him/her remind you by saying the next sentence.

"I'm going to do a general exam first to see what's going on.

Let's start with your eyes. Please look up without moving your head.

Now look down. Your eyes look moist; that's good. Okay, now I will shine a light in your eyes.

Please open your mouth. Your throat looks healthy.

I'm going to examine your hand; let's take your pulse. Relax. Your pulse is regular.

Have you had any swelling in your legs? I will take a look just to check them out.

I am going to examine your neck from behind. I am feeling for any swollen glands. Now I'll check your thyroid. Could you swallow, please? How about a sip of water now?

I need to examine your lungs. May I untie your gown? Let me first warm my stethoscope.

Take a deep breath in and out, again in and out. Thank you.

Okay, almost done. The last thing I need to do is to listen to your heart. Would you please lower your gown? Thank you. Now, allow me to re-tie your gown."

For a fundus exam of the eye: "Now, I want to examine the inside of your eyes. Excuse me, I'm going to dim the light. Thanks."

1.4 Section C: Patient Note

The PN is the only component of the CS exam that is graded by physicians (▶Video 1.3). It has four sections: history, PE, DD, and the Diagnostic Studies (workup).

After you finish examining an SP, you are given 10 minutes to type the PN. **There will be two bell** sounds during the PN documentation time. The first one comes 2 minutes before the end; the final one signals that time is up. You have to stop typing at the second bell and click "Submit." Tailoring the documentation for each SP is the key to completing the PN in the time given, and therefore, one of the keys to passing the CS exam. Another key is time management; allocate 5 minutes for completing the history and 5 minutes for the other sections.

There are several ways to go about typing up the PN. The first is to type from "Top to Bottom." Type the information in the same order you conduct the clinical encounter. Start with the patient's history, then list the PE results, give the DD, and finish with the Workup. This is a good way to go

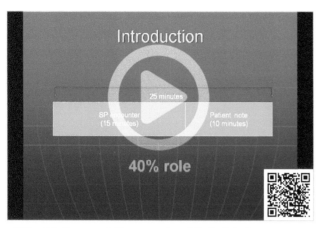

Video 1.3 The current CS resources have failed to introduce a universal system for PN typing. This video was prepared to help the candidate to document PN effectively. https://www.thieme.de/de/q.htm?p=opn/cs/20/3/11453141-6ebdbae4

about it because you are less likely to forget anything. Moreover, you can use the copy-and-paste function to pick out the evidence from the history and PE to support your DD.

Another way is the "Reverse Order" method, in which you start with the Workup, then do the DD and the PE, and finish with the history. Why use for this method? Well, test-takers tend to be stressed out and in a rush during the last 2 minutes of the exam (after the first bell). If you are shaking like a leaf or running around like a beheaded chicken, you should opt for the Reverse Order method because the lion's share of the PN grade is the DD and Workup. Therefore, if time is called and you have not completed the PN (and such a scenario has been known to happen), at least you will have earned more points than if the history is finished but not the DD.

The total time for the clinical encounter and the PN documentation is 25 minutes. If you finish the clinical encounter early, you can start typing up the PN early, and have more than 10 minutes to complete it.

However, we advise against leaving the exam room early to give more time to PN, as you can always use clinical encounter time to do counseling and closure. Ten minutes is usually sufficient for typing up the PN. By the way, in the cases where the patient is not present (e.g., pediatrics cases—there are no child SPs), you usually finish the clinical encounter early.

You will be given 12 sheets of blank paper to be used for scratch paper over the whole day, and you will be instructed to discard the used paper after each encounter. It is difficult to write everything that the SP tells you on your scratch paper, but try to write down as much as you can while speaking with the SP. **Remember to keep eye contact**. Note possible DD before you enter the exam room and focus on things that are easily forgotten after leaving the room like medications, allergies, and numbers (age, dates, dose, etc.).

It is advisable to use colloquial (informal) terms when speaking with the SP, but use medical terminology for conditions in the PN. Remember the PN is used to convey information to other doctors and medical personnel, and you will be graded on how appropriately you communicate (▶ Table 1.6).

Table 1.6 Colloquial terms with corresponding medical terms

Colloquial term	Medical term
Pounding or racing heart	Palpitation
Difficulty breathing	Dyspnea
Breathing difficulties while lying down	Orthopnea
Burning urination	Dysuria
Coughing up blood	Hemoptysis
Redness	Erythema
Swelling in the lower limbs	Edema

1.4.1 Sample of a Complete Patient Note

Here is a sample of a complete PN for a patient who complained of a cough (refer to the doorway information and the SP's role, case 3).

History

35 yo M c/o cough for 3 days, gradual in onset, present all the time, worse at night, and better with OTC meds. Started as dry cough, then associated with little whitish-yellow thin mucous with no blood, mild sore throat, post-nasal drip, and tender sinuses. Has mild chest pain while coughing. Denies any voice change, difficulty breathing, heartburn, orthopnea, recent travel, exposure to T.B pt, or use of new medication. He had a common cold and rhinorrhea last week. ROS: Normal sleep and appetite, no change in weight and no urinary or bowel habit problems. PH: bronchial asthma, sinusitis. Meds: albuterol MDI, loratadine. ALL: pets and pollen. FH: father with asthma. SH: tobacco use half ppd/10 years, drinks socially. Irrelevant sexual history.

Examination

VS: WNL apart from fever (100.4° F). Alert and conscious with no acute distress. HEENT: tender sinus, no enlargement of LNs, ears have normal TM, nose is w/o rhinorrhea, noncongested nasal turbinates, throat w/o erythema. Extremities: no pallor or cyanosis. Chest: no chest deformities, normal Tactile Vocal Fremituss (TVF), no air or fluid per percussion, CTA, B/L no wheezes nor crepitation, normal S1 and S2, no murmurs or gallop.

Differential Disgnosis (▶ Table 1.7) and Diagnostic Studies (▶ Table 1.8)

As you notice, we have started with an analysis of a cough as a complaint (onset, course, what makes it better and worse, and sputum), then the possible causes were analyzed (upper/lower respiratory tract infections, medication side effects, gastroesophageal reflux disease). Symptoms of the respiratory tract (involved system) were asked, and finally the ROS was done. Past history, family, social, and others were then documented.

In the clinical exam section, the fever, the ENT, and chest exam were documented in detail.

According to the history and the clinical exam findings, acute bronchitis and sinusitis were mentioned as the most possible

Table 1.7 Differential diagnosis of cough

History finding(s)	Physical exam finding(s)
1. Acute bronchitis	
Dry cough that turned productive	
Feels feverish	Fever (100.4°F)
History of common cold	
2. Acute sinusitis	
Dry cough that turned productive	
Feels feverish	Fever (100.4°F)
Post nasal drip	Sinus tenderness
History of common cold and sinusitis	
3. Pleurisy	
Diffuse chest pain	
Pain increases with deep inspiration	

DD. The support for each diagnosis was written beneath the history and PE column.

Finally, the necessary workup such as chest X-ray is mentioned.

1.4.2 Tips for History-taking Documentation

The documentation of the SP's history is the lengthiest component of the PN, and the part most likely to vary between cases. However, take no more than 5 minutes for typing it up, lest you find yourself without enough time for the PE and the DD. To meet the 5-minute limit, mention only the data relevant to the SP's CC.

Follow a routine when writing the PN up. Organize your History documentation by following the framework of the History. Start with the HPI (CC followed by the possible causes). Then write the Symptoms Related to the Affected System. Finish with the ROS. This routine structure will be efficient and make you less likely to forget anything.

When writing the PMH, follow the mnemonic device framework: **"PDS for PDA results in Fast Surgery ± Scar"** so that you do not forget anything and so that you can type quickly, knowing what you will talk about next. To cut down on your documentation time, use abbreviations listed by the USMLE (see Appendix at end of book). Avoid non–USMLE approved abbreviations!

History of Present Illness Documentation

This documentation is written for the purpose of training. For doorway information and case scenarios, look at their individual chapters.

Practice Case 1

Doorway information: The patient is a 55-year-old woman who complains of dizziness. Her VSs are normal.

We assume you wrote the **Possible Diagnoses.** You should do this before you enter the exam room. Possible diagnoses would be the following:

- Benign paroxysmal positional vertigo and ear diseases (Meniere's disease and vestibular neuritis).

Table 1.8 Diagnostic studies for cough

Sputum culture

Chest X-ray

- Cardiac causes (arrhythmia) and neurological causes (acoustic neuroma).
- Vasovagal attack and medication side effects.

What is the first thing that you should write in the HPI? What is the next thing you should write? What is the third step? Think about these three questions before you proceed. Then give an answer. Continue reading, and compare your answers with the ones in the next paragraph.

The first thing to document is the **Analysis of the Chief Complaint.** Below is a sample:

55 yo female c/o dizziness, started 1 month ago. It was infrequent. Now it occurs 2–3 times/day. The last time was this morning. It lasted less than a minute. Feels like the room is spinning around her. It increases w/sudden change of position, no warning signs beforehand.

Now, since the complaint most probably refers to benign paroxysmal positional vertigo, the next step is to ask about the **other possible causes:**

No hearing problem or recent URI. Mild chest pain in the left side with palpitation at the time of the episodes; no headache, vomiting, or blurry vision; normal gait and never passed out; not associated with new medication use; sometimes she has lightheadedness.

Now you have specific data and have eliminated other DDs; it is likely that the CC is either *benign paroxysmal positional vertigo* or *cardiac arrhythmia* (pounding heart).

Here is the documentation of the **Symptoms of the Affected System** (chest/neuro): *No dyspnea, orthopnea, or peripheral edema; no headache or blurry vision.*

The last part of the documentation is the **ROS.**

ROS: Normal sleep and appetite. No recent changes in weight. No urinary problems or change in bowel movements. Postmenopausal 3 years ago.

That is a complete form. If you are short of time, you could abbreviate the report as below. Note: you could say "irrelevant" for "N/A."

ROS: N/A. Postmenopausal 3 years ago.

Practice Case 2

Doorway information: A 60-year-old woman came to the ER with back pain. VS: WNL (▶**Table 1.9**).

Possible diagnoses would be the following:
- *Muscle:* muscle strain.
- *Bone:* fracture spine and osteoporosis.
- *Intervertebral disk:* degenerative arthritis, herniated disk.

Past Medical History Documentation

Example 1: In a case of chest pain with possible myocardial infarction (MI), here is an example:
Past medical history (PMH): HTN 20y, DM 10y and hypercholesterolemia 15y, history of similar attack 1 month ago, relieved

Table 1.9 Documentation of practice case 2

Analysis of the chief complaint (pain)	60 y old female came to ER w/severe low back pain radiating to Rt leg. It came on suddenly 2 d ago while lifting heavy furniture at home. The pain is progressive—it is like an electric shock (4/10 at rest, 9/10 w/movement). It is constant, partially relieved with Aleve and rest and increases when doing work. It is associated w/numbness in Rt leg.
Possible causes	The pain was not preceded by any back trauma or accident; it does not change with position. She takes calcium tablets. No history of cancer.
Symptoms related to affected system	She has numbness in the Rt leg and is unable to walk. Normal urine and bowel control.
Review of system	Normal sleep and appetite, no recent change in weight, urinary problems, no bowel change. Postmenopausal for 9 y.

Abbreviations: ER, emergency room; Rt, right; w/, with; yo, year old.

by sublingual nitrate, Meds: propranolol, metformin, and simvastatin. No known drug allergy (NKDA), FH: father died of MI. Works as paramedic, smoker 1 ppd/20y, drinks socially.

Example 2: In a case of headache with possible subarachnoid hemorrhage, here is an example:
PMH: no medical diseases or similar episodes. NKDA. FH: mother has migraine headaches, father has cystic renal disease. SH: accountant, smokes 1 PPD/10y. Drinks 1 beer/d and more on the weekend, uses cocaine, multiple sexual partners, no history of STDS, nor tested for HIV.

Example 3: In a case of cough and sinusitis as the DD, here is an example:
PMH: Two similar episodes last year. Meds: loratadine. ALL: pets and pollens. FH: brother with BA. SH: college student, denies smoking and alcohol consumption.

Notice: What is given in the previous example models for PN documentation to learn how the history is tailored and can be changed between cases.

1.4.3 Physical Examination Documentation

This part is considered much easier than the history documentation, as the SPs do not have many abnormal physical signs. As with the other parts of the PN, ensure your notes follow the organization given in the mnemonic devices.

> For the PE, remember:
>
> "*V*ital *S*igns *m*ay *c*hange *h*ormones (**ADH + NE + LH**) that are given by *l*ocal *S*hots."

Therefore, start the PE section with the **VSs**. They are listed on the doorway information and also on the computer screen next to the PN. If they are normal as per the doorway information, write "WNL," which means "within normal limit." If you have a patient who complains only of fever (and only one VS is abnormal), you can document it in two different ways:

VS: Temp: 101°F (38.3°C), PR: 80/min, RR: 16/min, BP: 120/80
Or VS: Temp: 101°F (38.3°C), all others WNL.

Do not forget to mention the patient's **appearance**. It is an important part of the documentation. If the patient has no acute distress, write: "Patient with no acute distress." This will

be for the majority of the SPs. However, there will always be some who are *in pain*, in *acute distress (dyspnea)*, who suffer from *photophobia* (do not forget to dim the lights), or who are visibly *depressed*. Rarely, the SP will have chronological and spatial disorientation. Document what you see and hear!

The **decubitus**, or patient position, is often ignored when writing up the PE. Following the mnemonic device should remind you to remember it. It only needs to be documented if the SP is **not** sitting on the bed. Fortunately, in most of the cases, the SPs will always be sitting on the bed when you walk in. Positions sometimes can be a clue as to the underlying problem, for example, a *restless SP moving around the room* may be suffering from renal colic. In addition, if the SP is *lying back on the bed in pain* when you walk in, take the history and do as much of the exam as you can without asking the SP to change position.

Here is documentation for PE in normal finding:

Head: Head has five parts (**HEENT**):
- **Head: NC** (normocephalic), **AT** (atraumatic), **NT** (nontender).
- **Eye: PERRLA** (pupils equal, round, reactive to light and accommodation), **EOMI** (external ocular muscle intact). **Fundus** exam: intact red reflex.
- **Ear: TMs** (tympanic membranes) are normal or showed the cone of light bilaterally. In a case of hearing loss, describe the ear exam in detail.
- **Nose** without rhinorrhea.
- **Throat** without erythema.

Neck: Supple, no palpable cervical LNs, normal thyroid exam, no JVD, or carotid bruit.

Extremities: Palpable peripheral pulsation, no peripheral edema, cyanosis, or clubbing.

Lung and Heart: For nonchest cases, the following is sufficient: Chest: CTA/BL (clear to auscultation bilaterally). Heart: Normal S1 and S2 with no murmurs, or gallop.

Local exam: See corresponding chapter for documenting chest, abdominal, and neurological exams.

Special signs: Document the finding of the special signs as CVA, Murphy's, psoas, Rovsing's, and Romberg's signs, rebound tenderness, drop arm, Rinne's test, etc.

Here you need to be flexible with your documentation of the clinical exam items; tailor it to fit the individual case and SP. This will save your time and draw your focus to the CC. Here are some examples of how the **head and neck exams** would be affected (and therefore, documented) by different cases.

In a case of **headache where Subarachnoid Hemorrhage** (SAH) is a possibility, the fundus eye exam is an important item; it is not mandatory in other cases. Document the HEENT as follows: *AT, NC, and NT. PERRLA. No papilledema. Neck is stiff with positive Brudzinski's signs, no tenderness over the sinuses. Mouth: good dentition.*

Documentation of local exam for **a hearing loss case** would be as follows:

HEENT: PERRLA, EOMI, no papilledema. Nontender ear pinna, clear external ear with no cerumen, TMs with light reflex, nose is without rhinorrhea, throat without erythema. Rinne's test is … and Weber's test is ….

In a case of cough with **URI**, the HEENT notes would then be as follows: *Tenderness over the maxillary sinuses. Ear: normal TMs bilaterally. Noncongested nasal turbinates, throat without erythema. Neck: no lymphadenopathy.*

As you have noticed, while an ear exam is described in detail in a case of hearing loss, it is just briefly mentioned in a case of upper respiratory tract infection and does not need to be mentioned in abdominal, musculoskeletal, and OBS/Gyn cases, as it is unrelated to the CC. Likewise, nose, throat, sinuses, and LNs should all be mentioned in detail in cases of upper respiratory tract infection, though they should be mentioned only briefly in other cases.

When describing the SP's condition, avoid using the word "normal" too much. Using more descriptive words can earn you a higher score on the PN portion of the exam. See ▶ Table 1.10 for examples.

Do not forget to write down all the positive signs and special tests on the clinical exam for Murphy's sign, psoas sign, Rovsing's sign, rebound tenderness, Rinne's test, drop arm test, etc. Mention them in both the PE section and the DD of the PN.

1.4.4 Differential Diagnoses Documentation

The CS exam does not expect you to give a single, final conclusive diagnosis. Rather, you should list several possible DDs because you have only a little evidence to go on—information that came mainly from the history and to a lesser extent from a few physical signs.

Here are some guidelines to follow in writing up the DD:

- List at least **two** possible diagnoses; put the most probable one first. Under each diagnosis, write the details from the history and PE that support it.

- If you have a third DD, write it down even if you lack supporting details.
- Always write the CC (cough, headache, chest pain, dizziness, etc.) in the first line in the history column.
- Support for the **DD** does not necessarily have to be positive or already existing symptoms/signs; you can also list nonexisting items—this will help fill in all the spaces.

Example Differential Diagnoses

Here are two examples for dizziness (▶ Table 1.11) and back pain (▶ Table 1.12). As no PE was conducted in these example cases, the information here is just provided as a model.

- **Practice Case 1 (Dizziness; ▶ Table 1.11).**
- **Practice Case 2 (Back pain; ▶ Table 1.12).**

Documenting closely related DDs: Some items support multiple DDs, which are closely related. You may need to do a little editing (copy and paste). This will save you time while covering all the bases. Here are some examples:

Table 1.11 Differential diagnosis of dizziness with supporting history and physical examination findings

History finding(s)	Physical exam finding(s)
1. Benign paroxysmal position vertigo	
Dizziness	Free neurological exam
Room spins around	No facial weakness
Brief episode increase in getting up suddenly	Normal Rinne's and Weber's tests
No hearing loss	
2. Cardiac arrhythmia	
Dizziness	Free neurological exam
Palpitation	
Mild chest pain	

Table 1.12 Differential diagnosis of back pain with supporting history and physical examination findings

History finding(s)	Physical exam finding(s)
1. Herniated lumbar disk	
Low back pain, like electric shock, radiates to right leg	Tenderness over the lumbar spine
Came after lifting heavy object	She has numbness in the right leg and is unable to walk
Pain relieved by Aleve and rest	+ straight leg raising test
2. Osteoporosis	
Low back pain	Tenderness over the lumbar spine
Postmenopausal for 9 y	
Taking calcium	
3. Muscle strain	
Low back pain	Tenderness over the paraspinal muscles
Pain increases with movement	

Table 1.10 Recommended descriptions for different normal findings

Not recommended	Recommended
Normal sensation	Intact for fine touch and pinprick sensation
Normal reflexes	Deep tendon reflexes: +2
Normal throat	Throat without erythema
Normal heart sounds	Normal S1 and S2 w/o murmurs or gallop

Table 1.13 Differential Diagnosis of LLQ pain and vaginal spotting

History finding(s)	Physical exam finding(s)
1. Ectopic pregnancy	
Acute LLQ pain	Tenderness over the LLQ
Vaginal spotting	Tachycardia
Missed her LMP	Low blood pressure: 90/60
Sexually active, no contraceptive use	
2. Abortion	
Vaginal spotting	Tenderness over the LLQ
Abdominal pain	Tachycardia
Missed her LMP	
Sexually active, no contraceptive use	

Abbreviations: LLQ, left lower quadrant; LMP, last menstrual period.

Example A: The patient is a 25-year-old woman with acute LLQ pain and vaginal spotting. In view of her having missed last menstrual period (LMP), you suspect the chief cause is either ectopic pregnancy or spontaneous abortion. There are two DDs. After you write up the first DD (ectopic pregnancy; ▶ **Table 1.13**), just copy and paste the history and clinical exam items for the second DD, abortion (▶ **Table 1.13**).

Do little modification to better fit the second diagnosis.

Example B: The patient complains of shoulder pain after trauma. There are three DDs: shoulder dislocation (▶ Table 1.14), fractured humerus (▶ Table 1.14), and rotator cuff tear (▶ Table 1.14).

Copy and paste the history and PE items for your second DD (▶ **Table 1.14**).

For the third DD, rotator cuff tear (▶ **Table 1.14**), simply copy and paste the history and PE items from the previous DD. However, you will need to add and modify information (see below):

You can apply the same idea (copy and paste) with little modification to related DDs:

- In a case of hemoptysis, you can use the same data for **COPD** as you use in a case of **lung cancer**.
- **Gastritis** and **peptic ulcer** in case of epigastric pain and hematemesis.
- **Acute cholecystitis** and **biliary colic** in case of RUQ (right upper quadrant) pain.
- **Unstable angina** and **myocardial infarction** in case of acute chest pain that refers to acute coronary syndrome.

The data that support the history can be used to support the clinical exam, though you may need to modify the language.

You can use the same information that is mentioned in the history column for the PE beneath each DD. "Pain," as a symptom in History, can be noted as "tenderness" in the PE. This will help you to fill up most of the spaces, which is a very important part of the PN.

Some examples are given in ▶ Table 1.15.

Table 1.14 Differential diagnosis of shoulder pain

History finding(s)	Physical exam finding(s)
1. Shoulder dislocation	
Right shoulder pain	Tenderness over right shoulder
History of falling and landing on right arm	
History of shoulder swelling, redness, and inability to move right arm	Erythema over right shoulder, restricted range of motion (abduction, adduction, flexion)
2. Fractured humerus	
Right shoulder pain	Tenderness over right shoulder
History of falling and landing on right arm	
History of shoulder swelling, redness, and inability to move right arm	Erythema over right shoulder, restricted range of motion (abduction, adduction, flexion)
3. Rotator cuff tear	
Right shoulder pain	Tenderness over right shoulder
History of falling and landing on right arm	
History of shoulder swelling, redness, and inability to move right arm	Erythema over right shoulder, restricted range of motion (abduction, adduction, flexion)
Inability to abduct the right arm	Positive drop arm test

Table 1.15 Examples of symptoms with the corresponding physical examination findings

History finding(s)	Physical exam finding(s)
Pain	Tenderness ....
Fatigue, weight loss	loss = ...lbs
Vital signs:	
• Feels warm (feverish)	Temperature...
• Palpitation	Pulse...
• Dyspnea	RR...
Neurology exam:	
• Forgetfulness, impaired memory	MMSE is....
• Decreased sensation	Impaired sensation to pinprick and fine touch
• Muscle weakness	Muscle power 3/5
• Appeared sad/depressed	Blunt affect
Musculoskeletal exam:	
• Redness	Erythema
• Inability to move	Restricted range of movement (flexion, extension, etc.)

Abbreviations: MMSE, mini mental status exam; RR, respiratory rate.

1.4.5 Diagnostic Studies (Workup)

When you write down the Workup, follow this order to avoid missing important items:

- Prohibited clinical exams (especially pelvic exams in abdominal and genitourinary cases).
- Laboratory tests (urine, blood, etc.).
- Imaging/radiology (X-ray, CT, MRI, etc.).
- Intervention and others (endoscopy, biopsy, ECG, etc.).

1.4.6 Patient Note Typing Skills

Although this book is not about learning typing skills, we intend to put a special stress on its great importance. As mentioned, PN, as a component of ICE, is the only component to be graded by a physician.

It is going to be sad if you put great efforts on all CS components but you fail in ICE due to bad PN quality with a subsequent "overall failure."

Remember, touch typing cannot be mastered in a few weeks or months. It takes years. So START EARLY in mastering typing before the exam.

Step-by-Step Strategy for Typing Skills for CS Exam

As a beginner, start training in touch typing with the help of specialized programs. Many are available on the web. Start from how to put your fingers on the keyboard in the standard way.

Continue typing general and nonmedical words, typing common words (the, is, are, he, she, and, etc.) and continue your training until you reach at least 30 WPM (word per minute).

Type the given PNs many times until you find yourself familiar with medical terminology. I strongly recommend putting the most effort in words that are commonly repeated in the PN (patient, chest, heart, abdomen, thyroid, fever, urinary,

bowel, etc.). Then, do more training on difficult and long words (dyspnea, rhinorrhea, arrhythmia, hemoptysis, gastroenteritis, costochondritis, etc.).

It is fine if you finish the PN in 12 to 13 minutes in the beginning; with practice, you will be able to master completing it within 10 minutes. One note of caution—the day of the exam is very stressful, and you have tons of information on your blank sheet to be typed up within 10 minutes, so try to do extensive training to learn to finish the PN within 9 minutes.

A common mistake is practicing CS encounters, taking medical histories, doing PEs, etc. and leaving the PN blank. Always type the PN as soon as you finish practicing a role-play with your partner.

I strongly recommend reviewing your PN as soon as you finish and to have it reviewed by your partner if he or she is a doctor. If using the USMLE Web PN, you can use screenshots emailed to your study partner. Moreover, www.csshool.org offers a PN that can be printed, saved, and emailed instantly. Always compare your PN to a standard one.

On the CS exam and while typing the PN, relax and do not rush. As you sit down, take a deep breath and start typing. Repeat this maneuver whenever you find yourself stressed.

2 The Basics, Component 2, Communication and Interpersonal Skills

Keywords: communication and interpersonal skills for USMLE CS, counseling, closure

2.1 The Basics of Communication and Interpersonal Skills for CS Exam

Communication and Interpersonal Skills (CIS) assess many different types of skills simultaneously:
- *Professional knowledge*: providing information and counseling patients in making decisions.
- *Personal appearance*: attire and grooming.
- *Interpersonal skills*: fostering a friendly yet professional relationship, maintaining an appropriate bedside manner, and giving emotional support.

You should practice for the CIS part of the Clinical Skills (CS) exam until the skills above come instinctively, naturally, and effortlessly. You can easily achieve this by constantly practicing and honing your skills at every opportunity. For example, when you are doing your clinical rotations, give a tissue to the patient if he coughs. Wash your hands before examining a patient. End each visit with a review, preliminary diagnosis, and plan for the next step.

If you are not meeting patients, have friends or family members role-play with you.

It is preferable to practice with native English speakers (or persons who have a good command of English), as that is what the standardized patients (SPs) are during the test.

2.2 Components of Clinical Encounter

The components of a clinical encounter can be divided into three parts:
- The beginning of the clinical encounter.
- During the encounter.
- The end of the encounter (closure).

These classifications are useful because they are easily mastered and ensure you will not miss anything.

2.2.1 The Beginning

Knock audibly on the door:
Do not wait for the patient to say, "Come in" (▶ Audio 2.1).

While entering the room, address the SP **using a title and surname**, for example, *"Mr. Smith" or "Ms. Jones."*

Greet the SP:
"Good morning/afternoon/evening."

Introduce yourself:
"My name is Dr. X, one of the attending physicians (or medical students). I'll be taking care of you today. It's nice to meet you." (Introducing yourself as you enter the room before starting with the history is very important, as it makes a good initial impression on the SP.)

Shake hands and smile while maintaining eye contact:
Skip this step if the SP is lying on the bed in pain, or if holding an elbow (as in the case of shoulder trauma). In such situations, speak and act accordingly (minimize your smile, adopt an appropriate tone of voice, and gently pat the SP's shoulder). Remember to be proactive in dealing with the SPs. Always take their emotional and physical conditions into account.

Ask for permission to examine the patient:
"I'd like to ask you a few questions regarding your medical history, and then, I'd like to do a physical exam. Is that Okay with you?"

Here is a sample monologue that you can use to practice:

> *"Good morning, Ms. Jones. I'm Dr. X, one of the medical students; I'll be taking care of you today. It's nice to meet you. I'd like to ask you a few questions about your medical history, and then, I'd like to perform a physical exam. Is that okay?"*

Dealing with special situations:
Sad/depressed SPs: After knocking and introducing yourself, you can say, "It seems to me that you may be sad Ms. X. Is there something troubling you?/Would you mind sharing your trouble with me?"/"Is there anything in particular that is bothering you?"

SPs in pain: "I'm sorry to see you in pain Mr. X. Could you tell me a little bit more about your pain?"

Telephone encounter: *"Hello Mr./Ms. ..., I'm Dr. X. I was informed that your child (father, etc.) has a fever (shortness of breath, etc.). Could you tell me a little bit more?/Could you fill me in on the details?"*

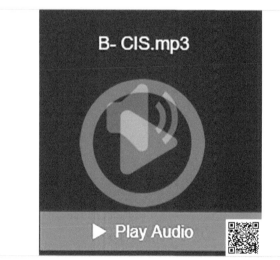

Audio 2.1 The audio contains the core of the CIS and can be used as a quick review before the exam. https://www.thieme.de/de/q.htm?p=opn/cs/20/3/11453142-02f99082&t=audio

2.2.2 During the Encounter

Communication and Interpersonal Skills Components

Visual—Eye contact:
- Your eyes have an important role in establishing a good relationship with your patient; try to keep proper eye contact throughout the history.
- You can write your notes rapidly, and then return to look at your patient.
- A common mistake is to focus on your paper throughout the encounter and to keep writing and not make proper eye contact.
- Nodding with eye contact gives an impression to the SP that you are concerned with his or her condition and you are paying attention to him or her.

Verbal—Tone of voice:
- Keep your speech loud, clear, and slow.
- Change your tone according to the patient's situation. Express sadness in the following cases: severe pain, depression, domestic violence.

Do not:
- Speak too quickly. The SP may not be able to follow you, and it gives the impression that you are in a rush. Avoid slang.
- Be monotonous, but try to be reactive and natural with a rising and falling tone. This is an integral part of CS assessment.

Body language:
- Body language is a kind of nonverbal communication where thoughts, intentions, or feelings are expressed by physical behaviors, such as facial expressions, body posture, gestures, movement, and touch. Proper use of body language is a good way to communicate. It presents a better understanding of your speaking and keeps the SP more focused on your interaction. Avoid being rigid or stiff.
- Facial expression is integral when expressing emotions with the body. Combinations of eye, eyebrow, lips, nose, and cheek movements help form different moods of an individual (e.g., happy, sad, depressed, angry, etc.).

Emotions:
- Be calm and do not lose your temper. During the encounter, you may be provoked by some SP to assess your reaction, for example, an angry SP or extremely anxious one.
- It is advisable to sit down and relax in the chair while taking the history; this alleviates your stress.
- *If the SP is in pain or lies back on the bed*, it is preferable to stand for a while in the begging of the patient encounter; that shows more concern about his pain.
- *Overall,* **maintain a pleasant smile** on your face throughout the encounter, unless the patient is expressing sadness or grief; in that case, you should show empathy.

Do not be:
- Distracted, nervous, or irritable.
- Sad or angry.
- Focused only on your paper and looking at it throughout the encounter.

Conversation Skills during the Encounter

Start with open-ended questions:
This gives a chance for the patient to express himself or herself. You can say: *"What brings you to the hospital today?/What brought you here today?/How can I help you?/I saw from the nurse's notes that you have…. Can you tell me a little bit more about?"*

Ask only one question at a time:
"Pause" means to wait for a while till the SP responds.

Example 1

Wrong: How bad is your pain, and is your pain constant?

Correct: How bad is your pain? (Pause) Is it constant?

Example 2

Wrong: Do you smoke or drink?

Correct: Do you smoke? (Pause) Do you drink?

Do not ask a leading question:

Example 1

You never used street drugs, right? (Wrong)

Do you use any street drugs? (Right)

Example 2

You don't have multiple sexual partners, do you? (Wrong)

How many sexual partners do you have in the last year? (Right)

Use proper English with correct grammar and word order.

Example 1

Are you have a similar condition before? (Wrong)

The correct form is: *"Have you had a similar condition before?/Did you have a similar condition before?"*

Example 2

How long you have had a fever? (Wrong)

The correct form is: "How long have you had a fever?"

Emphasize the important words (Content Words):
No one can focus on what you are speaking about all the time, so stressing important words catches the SP's attention.
- *Do you* **smoke?**
- *Do you have any* **allergies?**
- *Have you had a* **pap smear done?**

Use simple language and make sure not to use medical jargon when interviewing patients.

Example 1

Do you feel any palpitation? Not recommended.

Correct: *Do you feel a racing heart?/Do you feel irregular beats in your chest?*

Example 2

Have you noticed any erythema on your shoulder? Not recommended.

Correct: *Have you noticed any redness on your shoulder?*

Note: Sometimes you may unintentionally say a medical term; if that happens, just stop and try to explain it in a simple way.

Doctor: It could be pleurisy; pleurisy means inflammation in the membranes that surround the lung.

Do Not Be Judgmental:

Example 1

SP: I'm not compliant with my medicine.

Doctor: That's bad. (Wrong)

Why you are not compliant with your medicine? (Correct)/How can I help you with this?/Is there anything in particular that makes you incompliant with your medicine?

In this way, you can figure out any reasons (bad taste, side effects, financial problems) and then you can work on them.

Example 2

SP: I have more than one sexual partner.

Doctor: That is unhealthy. (Wrong)

But you can say: *I just want to remind you to take precautions by using condoms. This is to protect yourself from sexually transmitted diseases and to avoid any unwanted pregnancies."* (Correct)

Do Not Give False Reassurance:

Example 1

An SP who has ankle sprain asks: *Do you think I can play soccer again?*

Doctor: Sure, you can play again. (Inappropriate)

Correct: *It's hard to say right now, but after doing X-rays first for your ankle.*

Example 2

An SP who has a heart attack or subarachnoid hemorrhage (SA Hge) asks: *Is it serious? Am I going to die?*

Doctor: Don't worry, you will be fine. (Inappropriate)

Correct: *Sounds hard for you, but rest assured that you have here a professional team in the hospital and we are going to do everything possible to make you feel better.*

Do Not Interrupt the SP:

The SP usually gives short answers, but still remember not to interrupt while the SP speaks.

On rare occasions, the SP may be overtalkative (see later how you should respond).

Finally, use **transition phrases** while taking the history and inform the SP of the next step of the physical exam:

- Before the past history: *"I am going to ask you a few questions regarding your past medical history."* Now pause because usually the SP says, *"That's fine."*
- Before the social history: *"I am going to ask you a few questions regarding your lifestyle."*
- Before the lung exam: *"I am going to listen to your lungs."*

Note: By using transition phrases, the SP is prepared for the next step.

2.2.3 Closure (after Finishing the Clinical Exam)

Use the following guidelines while making closure (▶ Video 2.1):

Provide Information about:
- Patient history and exam (a summary).
- The preliminary diagnosis and workup needed.
- Possible treatment options.

Assure the SP that:
- You will see/meet/sit with him or her again to tell the results of the diagnostic studies.
- You will be accessible at any time to him or her.

Address Any Questions and Concerns:
- Ask: *Do you have any other questions or concerns?* Finally, shake hands with the SP, and say goodbye.

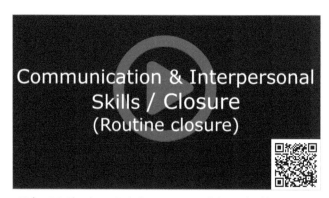

Video 2.1 The closure includes a summary of the medical history, physical exam, preliminary diagnosis and more. This video explores these components, and includes a live demo of different types of closure. https://www.thieme.de/de/q.htm?p=opn/cs/20/3/11450541-9c79fa53

Example of a Suggested Closure:

Provide information: "*Mr./Mrs...., let's review your case. I need to be sure that I've understood it correctly. You just told me that you have...and..., and also you told me that..., ..., ... You do not have... Is that right? Based on your history and my clinical exam, I have a preliminary diagnosis. It could be ... or ..., but I can't eliminate the other possible causes of your illness.*

I need to run some blood tests and some X-rays/imaging of..... When the results come back, I will meet with you again to tell you the final diagnosis, the treatment options, and I'm going to help you to take the next step."

- **N.B.:**
  When providing information, try to give a summary rather than reflecting on all the information that you heard from the SP.

Assure:
Say to the SP that: "*Until then if anything comes up, don't hesitate to call us any time. We are available 24/7.*"

Address Any Questions or Concerns:
"*Do you have any questions? Do you have any other concerns?*"

- **Finally, Dismissal:** "*Thank you for your time. Have a good day.*"
  Shake hands, keep eye contact, and maintain a nice smile.

- **Do Not Leave the Room Early:**
  Leaving the room without doing proper counseling is a great mistake that will compromise your CIS subcomponent.

  Ten minutes is enough time to document the important data in patient notes for an average typist, so try to spend the maximum time with the SP.

- **Do Not Leave the Room until Addressing All the SP's Questions and Concerns:**
  After you finish counseling and closure, always ask the SP: *Do you have any questions?*

  After the SP finishes, ask more: *Do you have any other concerns?/Did I address your concern?*

- **If the Time Finishes while You Are Still Speaking with the Patient, How You Can Respond:**
  Stop talking and say, "*I'm sorry, there is a page from the ER, so I have to go now. I will be back as soon as I'm done.*"

Provide More Information:

You may provide a general idea to the SP regarding what you think is a preliminary diagnosis.

Examples:

In an ankle sprain case:

"*As you know, when the bones come together, the joint forms, and besides that there are some ligaments that keep bones tight together and allow for movement. As a result of the twisted ankle, most probably there is an injury in one or more of these ligaments; I need to order an X-ray to see what is going on.*"

In a case of rheumatoid arthritis:

"*As you know, we have the immune system in our body that guards against any foreign body invasion. Sometimes this immune system forms antibodies by mistake that attack parts of our body like joints, as in your case, and cause inflammation.*"

In the same way, you can introduce a small piece of information about other diseases (Handout).

Say to the SP: "*I have here some handouts regarding (diabetes mellitus [DM], hypertension [HTN], bronchial asthma [BA], etc.). Please read them and write down any questions. Next time, I'll be happy to address your concerns.*"

Emergency cases:

If you encounter a case that is considered as an emergency, inform the SP that the workup will be done immediately, and you should assure the SP that you will return to him or her as soon as possible. In serious cases (severe chest pain or abdominal pain, etc.), inform the SP that admission is strongly advised in such situations. Sometimes, the SP insists to go home for social reasons, health insurance issues, etc. Try hard to convince him or her; figure out and solve the problem and inform him or her that this is for the best interest of his or her health.

Example

"*Mr....you have told me that you have ...,....,... and...,....,.... I am going to run some blood work. I will order an ECG (which is...) and chest X-rays. They will be done as soon as possible. Because your condition is serious and I'm very concerned about your health, I strongly recommend that you be admitted to the hospital to be kept under observation so that if anything develops we can deal with it immediately. How does that sound?*"

Cases That Need a Pelvic or Rectal Exam (Prohibited in the CS):

In cases like vaginal bleeding, bleeding from the rectum, or urinary problems, tell the patient the following:

"*Mr./Miss..., I need to do a pelvic/rectal/vaginal exam; would you mind if I ask the nurse-in-charge to prepare you for this exam?*"

Do not forget to write it down in your workup.

Telephone Encounter and Nonattendant Patient:

In such cases, you will take only the history, without an exam, and when you finish, do closure like: "*Mrs....You told me that...and ... and... As you know, I can't rely on the history alone. I need to see your child right now. I'm going to do a physical exam, I will examine..., I will order for........ Can you bring him/her to the hospital now?*"

Special Kinds of Patients—Patient Who is Worried about His or Her Disease:

Example 1

Doc, I can't sleep from.../Doc, I will lose my job if.../Doc, I am so worried about...

Answer: "*I understand your concern; we are going to do everything possible to make you feel better.*"

Example 2

SP: *Am I going to die?*

Doc: Ask him first: "*Why are you feeling this way?*"

If he or she is scared of something in particular, address that for him or her. If he or she is silent, continue like: "*The hospital has a professional medical team and we are going to do our best in treating you.*"

Angry/Noncompliant Patient:

Example 1

SP: *I have only…Why are you asking me all these questions?*

Doc: *"I understand your concern. Although your… is your concern, your whole health is my concern, too. I need to ask just a few questions to be sure that everything fine. Is that OK?"*

In overlay talkative SPs, you can say: *"I understand your concern, but please let us focus on the task at hand"*

Example 2

After finishing a telephone encounter with a mother whose child has a serious problem, and who you asked to immediately come to the hospital to do a physical exam, she may say: *"Doc, I don't have a car. How can I go to the hospital? What am I going to do?"*

Response: *"Please, it's serious. Your child is sick, and I need to see him as early as possible. Call 911 right now, please."*

Example 3

SP: *"I have been here for a long time waiting for you!"*

Doc: *"I apologize. I was in the ER and I encountered unexpected delays there. I am very sorry. Anyhow, I'm now available to you. Could you tell me what is going on?"*

2.3 Counseling

It is advisable to do counseling for chronic disease (HTN and DM) in all patients, but it is a mandatory if the disease is uncontrolled, complicated, or the patient is not complaint to the medications. Complications of the DM are peripheral neuropathy, retinopathy, gastropathy, and others. For HTN, the complications are severe headache, chest pain, or with erectile dysfunction…, etc.

Ask the Following:
- *Is your diabetes/or blood pressure well controlled?*
- *Do you usually do a regular checkup visits for…?*
- *When was the last checkup visit?/When was the last reading?*

You can use the following in most situations: **Triple 2 rule**:
- **Do 2** (exercise and diet).
- **Quit 2** (smoking and alcohol).
- **Be compliant with 2** (medicine and checkup visits).

Suggested counseling: *"Mrs. …, I have recommendations for you for better control of… (DM, HTN). Please exercise regularly at least 20 minutes per day, 5 days a week and please watch your diet. I usually advise my patients to stop smoking and drinking alcohol. As you know, smoking is … and alcohol is … I also recommend that you become compliant with your medicine and please stick to your checkup visits."*

2.3.1 Smoking

You may not find enough time to do counseling for smoking in every case, but it is mandatory in heavy smokers or if the complaint is directly related to smoking (▶ **Fig. 2.1**). Examples

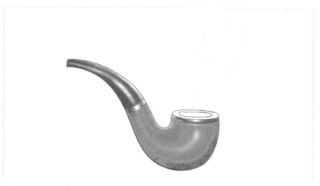

Fig. 2.1 Smoking.

include hemoptysis, chronic cough, chronic obstructive pulmonary disease, dyspnea, stroke, etc.

Say to the SP: *"As you know, smoking is a leading cause of many diseases like high blood pressure, heart disease, and lung cancer. Also, it has a direct relation to your complaint. I usually encourage my patients to quit smoking. Do you have the interest to quit smoking right now?"*
- If the SP says yes, reply: *"I'm glad to help you; what about scheduling an appointment next week? I am going to offer you the programs that will help you to quit smoking. Also, we have support groups that you can join."*
- If the SP says no, say: *"No problem. Take your time and when you have the interest, give me a call."*

2.3.2 Alcohol

Most of the SPs on the CS exam drink socially and there is no need to counsel for alcohol in every patient. On rare occasions, if you have an SP who is a heavy drinker (more than TWO drinks per day in males and ONE drink per day in females) or if the problem is directly related to alcohol (epigastric pain in heavy drinker with a possibility of pancreatitis) do counseling (▶ **Fig. 2.2**):

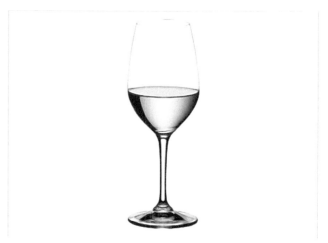

Fig. 2.2 Alcohol.

"As you may know, drinking is a leading cause of liver and stomach diseases; it may also make you bleed easily. In addition, it may affect your memory in the future. Are you interested in cutting down or quitting?"

CAGE questionnaire: To be asked for heavy drinkers only.
- **C:** *Have you ever tried to cut down drinking alcohol?*
- **A:** *Have you ever been annoyed by people's criticism regarding your drinking?*
- **G:** *Have you ever felt guilty about your drinking?*
- **E:** *Do you drink alcohol first early in the morning?*

2.3.3 Safe Sex Recommendations

In the cases that report multiple sexual partners without condom use, counseling should be done about safe sex precautions:

"As you told me, you have many sexual partners with occasional use of condoms; I do recommend condom use any time you have sex to protect yourself from STDs and to avoid unwanted pregnancies."

2.3.4 Drug Abuse

It is not a common case on the CS, but just in case you have a case with drug abuse (cocaine, marijuana, etc.), do minor counseling like (▶ Fig. 2.3):

"As you know, using these kind of drugs cause serious physical and emotional harm to you and also your loved ones. Do you interest now in quitting?"

"I have wonderful programs as well as support groups. Do you have the interest right now?"

Go ahead in the same way mentioned in smoking (according to the SP response).

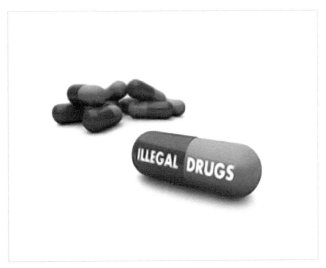

Fig. 2.3 Drug.

2.3.5 Psychiatric Cases or Cases that Need Assessment of Home Safety

In cases of Depression, Alzheimer's, or violence, assessment of the patient's home safety and home situation is very important and an integral part of counseling and case evaluation (see the corresponding cases).

2.4 Communication Skills for Physical Examination

Tips for clinical exam are integral part of your scoring by the SP; you may know how to do the physical exam steps well, but you may be underscored because of **improper command** (forgetting hand-washing and examining over the gown, improper draping technique, repeating painful maneuvers, etc.).

Always remember that USMLE expects you to be within a certain standard deviation (SD) in all components rather than to be smart or extremely positive on one component and bad or extremely negative on the others.

Follow the following rules while doing the physical examination (PE).

Before starting the PE:
Always **wash your hands** before starting the PE. Do whatever you prefer to remind yourself such as drawing a hand at the bottom of your blank paper. Still, you can use gloves.

Inform the SP that you are going to **start the physical exam:** *"Mr./ Mrs. …. Now I'm going to do a physical exam on you. Is that OK?"*

Draping and SP's positioning:
Never examine over the gown.

Use proper draping technique and limit the area that is exposed while doing the exam. For example, ask the SP to untie the gown exposing only the back while examining the chest from the back, then ask the SP to lower his or her gown to examine lungs from the front and to examine the heart. To do abdominal examination, tie the gown first, then ask the SP to lie back, drag a white/ blue sheet up to cover his or her legs and then drag the gown up.

Avoid asking the SP to change position many times during the encounter. Do not tell the SP: *"Please lie down. Now please sit up. Lie down again."*

In using medical tools and equipment:
Warm your stethoscope before examination. Use a new disposable tool such as an ear speculum for otoscope or tongue depressor (rarely needed).

Be familiar with the medical devices in the examination room (how to recline and extend the bed, where you can dim the light, how to use the otoscope, etc.). They seem to be fine tricks, but mistakes may make you look awkward in front of the SP.

Throughout the encounter, be:
Gentle—Remember, the SPs are exposed to repeated exams the entire day. Do not repeat painful maneuvers; instead say to the SP, *"I'm sorry, I won't do it again."*

Interactive while doing the exam. Inform the SP about what you are doing and what you will do. For example: *"I'm going to examine your neck from behind"* and *"I need to listen to your heart"* and *"I'll check your muscle power."* After doing the test, inform the SP of the findings (*"Your throat looks fine."* *"Your heart sounds are normal,"* *"There is erythema on your ankle"*).

Remember: As you know from the USMLE instructions, rectal, pelvic, breast, and inguinal LNs exams are not allowed on the CS exam. Those can be added on the patient note.

2.5 Communication Skills Questions

Almost all the SPs will ask you one or more questions, usually to assess your response and interpersonal skills.

After reading the following questions and topics, you will have a good background to answer most of the questions on the CS exam as most of the questions on the exam are around them.

2.5.1 General Rules

- If you are asked something that you cannot answer, stay calm and say, *"Well, I understand your concern. It's hard for me to tell you for sure at this moment. I'm going to figure out...and I will address that on your next visit (or I'm going to give you a call)."*
- Saying that you understand the SP's concerns gives you time to think of the answer.
- When you finish your answer, always ask the SP: *"Have I addressed your concern?"* Then ask, *"Do you have any other questions?"*
- Be interactive in your facial expressions and voice tone according to the situation and the nature of the question. For example, show sadness in replying to the SP who says: *"Doc, I am living alone/my husband beats me."*

The Questions Can Be Categorized into:
- Questions around the disease or the diagnosis.
- Questions around the diagnostic studies (workup).
- Questions around the treatment options.
- Other concerns.

2.5.2 Questions around the Disease or the Diagnosis

Examples of common questions during the clinical encounter:
The SP asks: *Do you think that I have cancer, heart attack, stroke, etc.?/What do you think about my disease?*

If the SP asks while you are taking the history or during the clinical exam, respond:

"I understand your concern. Please give me a few minutes to finish taking your medical history and doing clinical exam first. I'll write your questions down here and I am going to answer you when I'm done. Is that OK?"

Do not answer even if you know the answer.

If the SP asks at the end of the encounter, it depends on the impression that you got from the complaint, the history, or/ and the positive signs of the exam.

If it is not a possibility, say, *"Well, I understand your concern. Based on your medical history and what you told me, you don't have...and...From my clinical exam, I didn't find...or...so I would say it's a remote possibility."*

If it is a possibility, say, *"Well, I understand your concern. Based on your medical history and what you told me, you have...and... From my clinical exam, there is...and...So I would say there is a possibility that you have...."*

In both situations, say, *"But I could not eliminate the other possible causes. To be sure, I need to run some...and...Next visit I will be in a good place to answer this question. Have I addressed your concern?"*

Example 1

A young patient who has a dry cough and chest pain that started after a common cold; the pain is mild, 4/10, and worse with taking a deep breath.

The SP: *"Doc, do I have something serious in my heart?"*

Doctor: *"Mrs. ....., as you told me, you have chest pain and that it is mild and all over your chest. It increases when you take a deep breath and you had common cold few weeks ago."*

"Based on your history and my exam, it's a remote possibility to have something serious in your heart. You are young, healthy, and you don't have risk factors for that."

"I would say you probably have inflammation of the membranes around your lungs; however, I could not eliminate the other possible causes, so to be sure I will do...and...Next visit I am going to tell you the final diagnosis. Have I addressed your concern?"

Example 2

An old patient, who is a heavy smoker, comes with hemoptysis and loss of weight.

Patient: *"Do I have lung cancer?"*

Doctor: *"Well, I understand your concern. As you told me, you have been coughing for ... years, you coughed blood yesterday and lost ...lb. Being a smoker for many years puts you at risk for lung cancer, but it could be something else. To be sure, I need to do...Next visit I am going to tell you the diagnosis. Did I address your concern?"*

Note: If you have not got any conclusion, don't worry. Spread your answer out and don't give any conclusion. **Just say:** *"It's difficult to tell you for sure at this moment. I need to run...and... Next visit when the results come back I'll be in a better situation to address you concerns, sound good?"*

2.5.3 Questions around Diagnostic Tools (Workup)

The SP may ask you: "*What is the meaning of <any diagnostic tool>?*"

Here are some simple definitions of commonly used diagnostic tools:
ECG: It is a machine that monitors and records the electrical activity of your heart.

CT scan: It is a high-resolution X-ray machine. It takes pictures that get analyzed by a computer and gives us clear images of your (brain, chest, etc.).

MRI: It is an imaging machine that uses a magnetic field to create detailed pictures of the body organs.

Endoscopy: An endoscope is a thin tube with a built-in camera at its end. It allows us to visualize your (stomach, colon, etc.).

Biopsy: In this technique, we collect small pieces of tissue to be examined under the microscope for better diagnosis for your disease.

Culture: It is a sample of your mucus, discharge. We put it in a special media to search for any bacteria or any harmful bugs and to figure out the most appropriate antibiotics.

2.5.4 Questions around Treatment Options

Medications
Example 1: SP asks: "*Doc, can you give me any medicine for this pain?*"

Answer: "*I understand your concern, but giving any medicine now may change the quality of your pain and make it difficult for us to diagnose the underlying cause. I need first to do…,….. As soon as I have a final diagnosis, I'm going to give you the proper medicine. We are going to do that as soon as possible. How does that sound to you?*"

Example 2: SP asks: "*Doc, can you give me antibiotics?*"
Doc: "*I understand your concern, but as you may know, antibiotics are only for bacterial infections. I need to run some blood tests first to see what's going on. If it's a bacterial infection, antibiotics work. If it's a viral or anything else, antibiotics will be useless or even harmful*"

Example 2: SP asks:
1. "*Doc, what do you think about steroid injections for my knees?*"
2. "*Should you prescribe hormone replacement therapy?*"

Please write your answers and see the suggested answers at the end of the chapter.

Nonpharmaceutical Medicine
SP asks: "*What about herbal medicine?*"

Doc: "*As you know, there are many names of herbal medicines on the market, some of them are FDA approved, others not; please give me the name and I'll figure research it and I going to give you a call.*"
   3. SP: "*Can I try acupuncture?*" (See the suggested answers.)

Surgery
Example 1: SP: *Do I need surgery?*
Doc: "*It's hard for me to tell you for sure at this moment: As you know, some diseases can be treated with pills; in others, surgery is the only option. I need to do…,…and…When the results come back, we are going to work together to choose the best option for you?*"
   4. *Do I need a cast for my fracture?* (See the suggested answer at end of this chapter.)

2.5.5 Others (Nonmedical Concerns)

Health Insurance or Social Problems:

> **Example 1:** SP: *I have no health insurance.*
>
> Doc: "*I understand your concern. If you do not have health insurance, it does not mean that you will not be given the proper medical care. We have social workers here, would you mind if I contact one of them to assist you in this issue?*"

Try to answer the following questions:
5. *I have left my kids at home. I have to leave the hospital right now.*
6. *When will I be able to go home?*
7. *Are you going to admit me to the hospital?*
8. *Can you give me some days off work?*

Suggested Answers for Practice CS Questions

Question 1.	*Doc, what do you think about steroid injections for my knees?*
Answer:	"*It is difficult to tell you for sure right now if steroid injections will work for your knees; I need to do X-rays of your knees and we may need an MRI, which is…. Next time, when I have a final diagnosis, I will be in a better position to answer you. Have I addressed your concern?*"
Question 2.	*Should you prescribe hormone replacement therapy (HRT)?*
Answer:	You can answer as previously; however, if the chief complaint is hot flashes and there are not any contraindications for HRT, you can answer as follows:
	"*HRT has its advantages and disadvantages. It works for your hot flashes, as well as helping with your sex life. However, there may be some side effects. It can increase the risk of breast cancer and heart disease. So, I can prescribe the lowest dosage for the minimum amount of time to avoid the side effects.*"

The situation is different if the chief complaint is vaginal bleeding in a postmenopausal woman. The answer could be: "*Well, I understand your concern. Unfortunately, vaginal bleeding is one of the contraindications for HRT, so I can't prescribe it for you now. Let us first figure out your problem. I need to do... (Proceed as routine).*"

Question 3. *Can I try acupuncture?*
Answer: "*Although acupuncture as a part of the treatment is effective in alleviating pain in many diseases, I'm not sure if it will work in your case. I'm going to figure it out and give you a call.*"

Question 4. *Do I need a cast for my fracture?*
Answer: "*At this moment, I'm not sure if you have a fracture. Please let me first take some pictures of your..., then we are going to decide if a cast is needed. Have I addressed your concern?*"

Question 5. *I have left my kids at home. I have to leave the hospital right now.*
Answer: If the condition requires hospital admission, answer as follows: "*I understand your concern. We have social workers in the hospital, and they have good experience with these issues. They are going to take care of your kids. Would you mind if I contact one of them to figure out this issue for you?*"

Question 6. *When will I be able to go home?*
Answer: "*It is difficult for me at this moment to tell how long you will stay in the hospital. We haven't made a final diagnosis yet. If there is anything in particular that you are concerned about at home, please let me know.*"

Question 7. *Are you going to admit me to the hospital?*
Answer: The answer to this question depends on the nature of the case. If the case is emergent (acute chest pain, suspected appendicitis or ectopic pregnancy, stroke, etc.) say, "*Mr...., I'm so concerned about your health, so I do recommend that you be admitted to the hospital to be kept under observation so that if anything develops we can deal with it immediately. How does that sound?*"

Question 8. *Can you give me some days off work?*
Answer: The answer depends on if the condition needs sick leave and rest at home. If it warrants sick leave, say: "*I understand your concern. I believe that your condition needs rest at home; however, it's difficult for me to recommend that at the current time. I need to do...and.... When the results come back, I'll be in a better position to write for you a sick leave certificate. We are here for helping you.*"

If you see that the condition does not need sick leave and feel the SP is malingering, say, "*I under-stand your concern; unfortunately, I can't recommend a sick leave at the current time for you. I haven't made a final diagnosis yet. We need to do...and.... When the results come back, I'll figure out this issue for you. Do you have any questions for me?*"

Remember

During the whole encounter:
- Keep calm. Never get angry or be judgmental.
- Maintain a pleasant smile and keep eye contact.
- Be gentle and humble with the SPs.

Before the PE:
- Do not forget to wash your hands before PE.

At the end:
- Address any concerns for the SPs in an intelligent and professional way.
- Do not give a final diagnosis; try to explain it with possibilities.

Finally, practice and practice what you have learned in this chapter many times. This is the key to mastering the CIS for this exam.

2.6 Appendix: Delivering Bad News

The scenario can be divided into three parts: before, during, and after. Before delivering the bad news, you need to prepare the patient to receive the information. Next, you deliver the information. Finally, you have to support and address the patient's emotions.

Before (Preparing the patient):

Did you come alone?/Do you have someone to attend with you?

What is your understanding about the procedure we performed? (name the procedure.)

What do you expect the results will be?

How would you like me to give the information about...?

During (Delivering the bad news):

"*Mr./Ms. ..., I wish the news were better, but the biopsy result came back and it shows cancer. I reviewed the results again with the laboratory team, and they confirmed the diagnosis. I am so sorry to tell you this news.*"

After (Supporting the patient):

"*Mr./Ms. ..., I want to assure you that there are many options in treating cancer; surgery, chemotherapy, and radiotherapy. The hospital has experts in treating cancers. Please don't hesitate to call me anytime. I am available 24/7, and will be here when you need help.*"

If you notice sad emotions from the patient, you can put your hands on his shoulder to comfort him, or hold his hand.

3 The Basics, Component 3, English Proficiency

Dara B. Oken and Mohamed M. Elawdy

Keywords: spoken English Proficiency, SEP, English pronunciation, American English accent

3.1 Introduction

Spoken English Proficiency (SEP) is one of the three components of the United States Medical Licensing Exam (USMLE) Step 2 Clinical Skills (CS). Many International Medical Graduates (IMGs) pass the Integrated Clinical Encounter (ICE) and Communication and Interpersonal Skills (CIS) components, only to fail in SEP. The difference in passing rate is significant: 98% of native English speakers pass on their first attempt, while the passing rate among IMGs is 79% (http://www.ecfmg.org/resources/data-performance.html and http://www.usmle.org/performance-data/default.aspx).

The lower performance of IMGS on the CS exam may be due to a variety of factors, including the difficulty in knowing how to self-assess English-speaking skills. Although there are many programs available to study English, very few of them focus on the patient encounter, none directly related to the USMLE CS exam and the needs of IMGs. The central objective of this chapter and video course is to assist the IMGs in passing the USMLE CS exam on their first attempt.

3.1.1 Contents

The following chapter components address the concepts behind clear speech in English and the mechanics, or movements, behind creating clear American English sounds. The Initial Assessment (**Speech Sample**) is your tool to capture a pretraining baseline recording, as well as a posttraining recording for comparison to highlight improvements.

Each of the following sections addresses different aspects integral to clear speech and communication. All of the examples used are relevant to the exam candidate's preparation for the patient interview. The **Word Concepts** section includes syllables, stress, and unstressed syllables, and provides an explanation as to why words in English often sound differently than they are spelled. The Consonants and Vowels Section addresses several of the sounds that are difficult to pronounce for many non-native English speakers. This section should be individualized to your specific speaking needs. Use the "Minimal Pair Sound Discrimination" exercise to help determine your needs. The **Grammar Question Patterns** section details verb tenses and meanings for questions frequently used in the patient encounter, as well as the two prescribed forms for question intonation.

The SEP Checklist is intended for self- and peer-assessment of communicative skills, similar to the one used by the SPs while scoring candidates during the exam. It is useful to note that CS candidates will be scored not only on speaking, but on listening skills as well.

This foundational resource is not exhaustive, but instead is an introductory approach to word-level and sound-level pronunciation features, as well as grammatical features. An advanced-level resource in development will address pronunciation concepts of connected speech.

3.1.2 How to Study?

Individualization is one of the tenets of effective learning, and exam candidates vary in the ease or difficulty they have with spoken English. The optimal study approach will depend on your specific language needs, your background knowledge of pronunciation concepts, and your preferred learning modality.

The book and complementary videos provide a basic overview of SEP concepts. The www.csschool.org program includes additional videos and small group course options. The one-on-one training option integrates the above components with guided, personalized coaching and individualized feedback.

3.1.3 Patterns of Spoken English

Many American English sounds and speech patterns may not exist in your first language. Your language may contain the same sounds, but patterns in connected speech may make it sound completely different in context. The process of adapting to American English pronunciation involves rethinking how speech *should* sound and learning new concepts that allow for English to flow smoothly and clearly. Adapting pronunciation involves reconceptualizing the sounds of speech and extensively practicing with this new framework.

It is important to learn how to "read sounds." Once you develop an understanding for the "sound code" of spoken English, clearer pronunciation will follow. English has borrowed words from many languages, and as a result, clear phonological rules do not apply. In many instances, spellings do not directly correspond with sounds. This lack of correspondence makes pronouncing words in English particularly challenging.

Our 26-letter alphabet is not sufficient to represent all 40 sounds in the English language. Different sounds may be represented by the same letter. For example, the vowel letter "o" has a different pronunciation in each of the following: hot, look, color, both, and office. Sometimes different letters are used to spell the same sound, such as /f/: half, graph, and staff. In addition, there are silent letters in words such as "know," "caught," "benign," and "strength." We must learn the spelling of these words for written communication; however, we must not rely on the spelling patterns when it comes to speaking clearly. The key to improving English pronunciation is to think in sounds, not letters.

3.1.4 Guide for Independent Practice

Adapting pronunciation takes dedication and persistence. Speaking is a motor skill and adapting speech patterns can be broken down into four phases:

1. Decoding and replacing the old pattern.
2. Gaining awareness of the new pattern.
3. Training through repetition with the new pattern.
4. Demonstrating instinctive and automatic facility with the new pattern.

To maximize the benefit of your training, do not try to memorize the material. Memorizing will not aid in the transference of newly learned speech patterns to different contexts. In order to be able to apply new sound patterns flexibly and naturally, you will need to develop a deeper understanding to bypass the autopilot, that is, your mouth speaking as you would in speaking your native language.

To achieve this deeper understanding and ultimate carry over, there are several steps to be aware of in your practice. First, focus your attention on the concept being introduced, not the words, but the concept. Second, be consciously aware of what you are physically doing to create this new sound or pattern. This step is most important if the sounds or patterns feel new or unusual to you. *What is mechanically happening in your mouth?* Third, recognize the critical differences between your native language (the default) and spoken English patterns. *Does a particular vowel exist in your native language? What is the closest sound? How is it different?* Finally and most importantly, bring your new awareness of the concept, the mechanics and the critical differences, out into the real world. Listen for the sounds and patterns in conversation or when watching a movie. In sum, make your practice meaningful in your daily speaking and listening encounters. The result will be lasting changes.

Each week plan to work with one to three target sounds and/or speech patterns as appropriate to you, based on your Comprehensive Speech Analysis or self-assessed need. Plan to devote a minimum of 10 minutes twice daily to practice in order to effectively make speech changes. Some learners are able to create significant change in their speech patterns with less practice, but the more you practice, the faster you will be able to develop your new speech habits.

Facility with new grammatical patterns can be approached in phases as well. First, decode the question form, the prescribed words, and word order that signify a specific verb tense. Develop awareness of the function of that verb tense, and through training and repetition, focus your attention on the contexts in which that verb tense is used. In time and with practice, these new patterns will become automatic.

3.1.5 Speech Sample

Purpose: To be used for Comprehensive Speech Analysis (if you are working with a professional pronunciation trainer) or informal pre/post comparison.

The following words have been selected for their **consonant** and **vowel** combinations. They are grouped logically to assist you in spontaneous speech.
1. Read each of the words within a word block.
2. Say each word within a spontaneous sentence that you make up (▶ Table 3.1).

Sounds in Connected Speech

Read and record the following patient notes while speaking naturally:

Mr. Smith is a 33-year-old Caucasian man who presented in the Emergency Room after experiencing chest pain and dizziness for 12 hours. The patient was in his usual state of health until approximately 1 day ago.

Mrs. Jones, a 49-year-old woman, presents to the clinic complaining of headache for 2 hours. It is on the right side of the head, nonradiating, sharp pain, 7/10, constant, increases by light, noise, and cold, decreases in dark, rest, and NSAID (nonsteroidal anti-inflammatory disease) accompanied by nausea, a sharp, jabbing sensation in her anterior scalp and recurrent headaches. She has been referred by her primary care physician.

A 12-day-old newborn presents to Urgent Care at 3:15 p.m. Monday with parents stating that the neonate has had episodes of vomiting and cannot keep down fluids. The last wet diaper was approximately 11:00 p.m. Sunday.

3.2 Word Concepts

3.2.1 Syllables

Each syllable is the "beat," or letters that combine to make one melded sound (▶ Video 3.1). A single syllable can have a variety of sounds, but only one vowel sound. To determine the number of syllables, an experiential method is helpful. When pronouncing a particular word, pay attention to the number of "jaw movements" within the word. In each of the words "no," "note," and "notes," the jaw moves only one time, regardless of the additional letters. However, if we change the word to "noted" or "noting," we add a second jaw movement, a second syllable.

Look at the examples of words in the same word family. With each additional component, there is an additional jaw movement, and an additional syllable (▶ Table 3.2).

Table 3.1 Speech assessment

Time/amount words		Body words		Other descriptive words	
Four	Some	Blood	Leg	Big	Right
Hour	Time	Bone	Mouth	Clear	Safe
Most	Third	Foot	Skin	This	Sore
Next	Twelve	Hair	Teeth	Where	Strong
Now	Year	Heart	Valve	Late	Worse
Actions		**Other nouns**			
Breathe	Learn	Cause	Lump		
Catch	Sting	Choice	Plans		
Choose	Think	Drug	Stage		
Fall	Wash	Fire	Wife		
Help	Should	Job	Zinc		

Spoken English Proficiency

For

USMLE Step 2 CS

Word Concepts

Video. 3.1 This video helps the speaker pronounce individual words clearly with the concepts of syllables, stress, and unstressed syllables. https://www.thieme.de/de/q.htm?p=opn/cs/20/3/11450513-e08ce34d

How many syllables are in each of the following words?

Remember: Pay attention to jaw movements to determine how many vowel sounds are in the word. The number of vowel sounds is the number of syllables.

Examples: change—1 syllable; patient—2 syllables; services—3 syllables (▶ Table 3.3).

Answers: function (2 syllables), tests (1 syllable), advanced (2 syllables), treat (1 syllable), units (2 syllables), gain (1 syllable), conditions (3 syllables), and decision (3 syllables).

The same words are divided into syllables. Notice how the number of **letters** in each word does **not** correspond with the number of **syllables**. Again, each syllable contains one jaw movement, which is one vowel sound. These words are "sounded out" as they are really pronounced with an American English accent (▶ Table 3.4).

3.2.2 Word Stress

In English, stress is one of the main tools used to convey meaning. Understanding the stress system is essential to speak intelligibly. Key in this concept is that word stress follows distinct patterns. You may be accustomed to the concept of stress from your home language, but those stress patterns often differ from those in English.

As a generality, the stressed syllable in a word is pronounced higher, louder, and longer than the other syllables in the word. It is pronounced with a full vowel sound. The stress in a word is predetermined and may fall on any syllable in the word. The stress falls on the first syllable in "hospital," the second syllable in "prescription," and the third syllable in "personnel" (▶ Table 3.5).

Table 3.2 Syllables in words

1-syllable word	2-syllable word	3-syllable word
Help (HELP)	Helpful (HELP ful)	Helpfully (HELP ful ee)
Stand (STAND)	Withstand (with STAND)	Withstanding (with STAND ing)
New (NOO)	Renewed (re NOOD)	Renewing (re NOO wing)

Table 3.4 Words separated into syllables and sounded out

Function	*funk shun*	Units	*yoo nits*
Tests	*tess*	Gain	*geyn*
Advanced	*ad vanst*	Conditions	*kun dih shinz*
Treat	*treet*	Decision	*duh sih shjin*

Table 3.6 Practice identifying the stress in words

Function	Units
Tests	Gain
Advanced	Conditions
Treat	Decision

Word stress patterns are not always predictable. A good strategy is to rely on your ear, and to look up particularly challenging words in the dictionary. Once you confirm the correct pronunciation, keep a running list of your "challenge words," both spelled accurately and sounded out for future reference.

Which syllable is the stress or strong part in each of the following words?

Remember: The stress sounds usually higher, louder, or longer than the other syllables in the word. **Tip:** If you are unsure of how to say a word, try saying the word with all the stress pattern possibilities. *Which one sounds right?* Underline the stress. In one-syllable words, the stress will be the whole word. Do not look at the answers below.

Examples: **change**—one syllable; **pa**tient—two syllables; **ser**vices—three syllables (▶ Table 3.6).

Answers: **func**tion, **tests**, ad**vanced**, **treat**, **units**, **gain**, conditions, and de**ci**sion.

The same words are divided into syllables with word stress in CAPITAL LETTERS. Notice how the stressed syllable falls in different places within a word. Stress patterns vary, but a clue to identify the stress is to think of a word with the same suffix, or word ending, such as -ion (*condition/decision*). The stress pattern often matches. These words are "sounded out" as they are pronounced with an American English accent (▶ Table 3.7).

Table 3.3 Practice identifying the number of syllables in words

Function _____	Units _____
Tests _____	Gain _____
Advanced _____	Conditions _____
Treat _____	Decision _____

Table 3.5 Stress in words (separated into syllables and sounded out)

3-syllable words	1	2	3
Hospital	HOS	pih	tuhl
Pre**scrip**tion	pruh	SKRIP	shun
Perso**nnel**	PER	suh	NEL

Table 3.7 Exercise words with stress identified, separated into syllables and sounded out

function	*FUNK shun*
tests	*TESS*
advanced	*ad VANST*
treat	*TREET*
units	*YOO nits*
gain	*GEYN*
conditions	*kun DIH shinz*
decision	*duh SIH shjin*

3.2.3 Unstressed Syllables

The additional syllables in a word, which are unstressed, are shortened, or reduced, often with a neutral vowel sound. In many cases, regardless of the vowel(s) that make up the "spelling" of the word, the unstressed syllable is pronounced as "uh" or "ih." For example, the word "medical" has three syllables (three jaw movements). The stress is on the first syllable. The second syllable is reduced to "ih" and the third is reduced to "uh": medical (MEH dih kuhl).

The differences between stressed and unstressed syllables are more pronounced in English than in many other languages. Becoming familiar with word stress, and its function within words, is essential. The way consonants and vowels are pronounced in English is influenced by this central aspect of speech. Look at the following examples of two- and three-syllable words. Each word has one stress, and the other syllables (underlined) are unstressed (▶ Table 3.8).

Which Syllables are Unstressed in Each of the Following Words?

Remember: these syllables often sound like "uh" or "ih," which are quick sounds with little mouth movement. **Tip:** For neutral vowel sounds, make the vowel very brief, or imagine there is no vowel and pronounce the consonant sound to consonant sound. The neutral vowel will take care of itself, for example, "s-t" for "sit."

Underline the unstressed syllables in the following exercise. (**Note:** one-syllable words are stressed, so you will underline nothing in these words.)

Examples: change—one syllable; patient—two syllables; services—three syllables (▶ Table 3.9).

Answers: function, tests, advanced, treat, units, gain, conditions, and decision.

The same words are divided into syllables with unstressed syllables in lower case letters. Notice how many of the unstressed syllables are pronounced as "uh" or "ih," regardless of the vowels written (see red color). Other unstressed syllables are pronounced with a full vowel, but with a weaker sound than the stress. These words are "sounded out" as they are really pronounced with an American English accent (▶ Table 3.10).

3.2.4 Word Concepts Review

Practice with Syllables

How many syllables are in each of the following words?

Remember: Pay attention to "jaw shifts" to determine how many vowel sounds are in the word. The number of vowel sounds is the number of syllables.

Examples: change—one syllable; patient—two syllables; services—three syllables (▶ Table 3.11).

Answers: change (1), patient (2), services (3), treat (1), daily (2), approved (2), accurate (3), injuries (3), choice (1), types (1), function (2), qualified (3), units (2), gain (1), conditions (3), nights (1), decision (3), plans (1), advanced (2), strong (1), tests (1), internal (3), provider (3), and increase (2).

Practice with Syllables and Stress: Sounded out

The two- and three-syllable words from the Review exercise: syllables are "sounded out" as they are really pronounced with an American English accent. Notice how the English spelling differs from the actual sounds. Also, notice how the number of **letters** in each word does **not** correspond with the number of **syllables**. Again, each syllable contains one "jaw shift," which is one vowel sound.

Can You Identify the Stressed Syllable in Each Word?

Remember: The stress sounds usually higher, louder, or longer than the other syllables in the word. **Technique:** If you are unsure of how to say a word, try saying the word with all the stress pattern possibilities. *Which one sounds right?* **Notes:** One-syllable words are not included here because the entire

Table 3.8 Words with unstressed (and stressed) syllable identified and sounded out

Word	Sounded out
complaint	(kum PLAIYNT)
medicine	(MED uh sin)
condition	(kun DIH shun)

Table 3.10 Exercise words with unstressed (and stressed) syllable identified and sounded out

function	FUNK shuhn
tests	TESS
advanced	ad VANST
treat	TREET
units	YOO nihts
gain	GEYN
conditions	kuhn DIH shihnz
decision	duh SIH shjihn

Table 3.9 Practice identifying the unstressed syllable in words

Function	Units
tests	gain
advanced	conditions
treat	decision

Table 3.11 Review exercise: syllables

change—Number of syllable(s): **one**	units _____
patient—Number of syllable(s): **two**	gain _____
services—Number of syllable(s): **three**	conditions _____
treat _____	nights _____
daily _____	decision _____
approved _____	plans _____
accurate _____	advanced _____
injuries _____	strong _____
choice _____	tests _____
types _____	internal _____
function _____	provider _____
qualified _____	increase _____

word is stressed. The noun and verb form or two-syllable words often have opposite stress (▶ Table 3.12 and ▶ Table 3.13).

3.3 Consonants

All consonants are produced by a particular "touch and hold or release" involving the lips and/or the tongue in contact with different parts of the mouth. In the following sections, particularly challenging consonants will be introduced. Not all consonant sounds used in English will be addressed (▶ Video 3.2).

3.3.1 Differences between Consonants

There are 25 distinct consonant sounds. There are more sounds than consonants in the alphabet, so we have additional symbols to describe particular sounds made by letter combinations, such as /tʃ/ for the "ch" sound. There are also letters that are sound combinations, such as the letter Q, which is a combination of /k/+/w/.

Where Is the sound made? How is the airflow affected?

The place of articulation involves where the lips, teeth, and/or tongue come into contact with a part of the mouth. For example,

the tongue must touch the gum ridge, the bump just behind the upper teeth, to produce either a /d/ or /t/ sound. The manner of articulation affects how the air is obstructed and directed. For example, when producing a /v/ sound, the air is forced through a narrow passageway between the upper teeth and lower lip.

Voiced and unvoiced pairs

There are several *voiced* and *unvoiced* pairs. Where and how these sound pairs are made is identical, but the difference is whether or not there is vibration in the vocal cords. For example, /b/ and /p/ are both produced by putting the lips together and temporarily stopping the airflow. When producing /b/, the sound is voiced with a vibration in the vocal cords. When producing /p/, the sound is unvoiced with only a small burst of air. Notice your voice when pronouncing the /b/ in "bat" and the absence of voice when pronouncing the /p/ in "pat." When the consonant is at the end of the word, it affects the vowel length. The /æ/ in "cab" will sound longer than the /æ/ in "cap" (▶ Table 3.14).

Stops and continuants

Some consonants are *stop* sounds, in which the airflow is temporarily stopped, such as /t/. Other sounds are *continuants* in which the airflow continues throughout the sound, such as /s/. Notice the stop in "but" and the continuant in "bus." Words ending in a stop sound have a shorter vowel than words ending with a continuant.

Released and unreleased

The position of a consonant in a word has an effect on how it is pronounced. The initial /t/ in "top" will have an "explosive" sound, and an aspirated burst of air is released. The same consonant /t/ will sound quite different at the end of a word, such as "pot" in which the /t/ is unreleased, without aspiration.

Table 3.12 Review exercise: stressed syllables

patient	*pey shint*
services	*ser vis iz*
daily	*dey lee*
approved	*uh proovd*
accurate	*ak yer it*
injuries	*in jer eez*
function	*funk shun*
qualified	*kwal ih faiyd*
units	*yoo nits*
conditions	*kun dih shinz*
decision	*duh sih shjin*
advanced	*ad vanst*
internal	*in ter nuhl*
provider	*pruh vaiy der*
increase	*in krees (NOUN)*
increase	*in krees (VERB)*

Table 3.13 Review exercise: stressed syllables (answers)

patient - **pey** shint	units - **yoo** nits
services - **ser** vis iz	conditions - kun **dih** shinz
daily - **dey** lee	decision - duh **sih** shjin
approved - uh **proovd**	advanced - ad **vanst**
accurate - **ak** yer it	internal - in **ter** nuhl
injuries - **in** jer eez	provider - pruh **vaiy** der
function - **funk** shun	increase - **in** krees (NOUN)
qualified - **kwal** ih faiyd	increase - in **krees** (VERB)

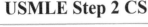
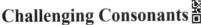

Spoken English Proficiency

For

USMLE Step 2 CS

Challenging Consonants

Video. 3.2 This video helps the speaker differentiate between similar consonants sounds and provides tips to avoid common errors. https://www.thieme.de/de/q.htm?p=opn/cs/20/3/11450514-e1e06d74

Table 3.14 Voiceless and voiced consonant pairs

Consonant pairs	Unvoiced	Voiced
θ/ð	thought, breath	though, breathe
p/b	pin, nap	bin, nab
k/g	call, back	goal, bag
t/d	time, white	dime, wide
s/z	sink, advice	zinc, advise
f/v	file, half	vile, have
ch/j	chest, each	jest, age

3.3.2 Challenging Consonants

The following are consonants that present particular challenge to speakers of other languages. Not every consonant is covered, and less frequently occurring consonants are not addressed. Please refer to the associated videos for articulation techniques to more accurately pronounce specific sounds.

Consonants: Minimal Pair Sound Discrimination Diagnostic

Which English consonants do you already pronounce accurately? Which do you need to spend time working on? Although the following communicative assessment is not an accurate speech diagnostic evaluation, it provides you with some concrete examples of where communication can break down due to individual sound differences.

Work with a partner, preferably a native English speaker, or someone who can easily hear the differences between the words. Read at random one of the two/three words (or nonwords) for each sound comparison (read across, not down). *Can your partner accurately determine which word you are saying—1, 2, or 3? If not, which sound are you substituting?* Read at random from the second example to confirm your findings, and repeat for further confirmation (▶Table 3.15).

The root cause of miscommunication can vary from the speaker's pronunciation to the listener's ability to hear and understand, but this simple exercise will provide you with valuable information. If you are trying to pronounce a particular word, and your partner hears a different word than the one you intended to say, this consonant sound requires attention. If you question the results, do the same exercise with a different partner. In the end, the goal is to identify your Personal Target Sounds, the consonants that you will focus on in the following sections, to improve your pronunciation and clarity.

List the target consonant sounds you will focus on.

3.3.3 Target Consonant Sounds

/ð/ and /θ/ Consonants

Articulation: Put your tongue between your teeth; blow air between your tongue and top teeth for /θ/ and use your voice for /ð/. Both are continuous sounds (▶Video. 3.3).

- **Beginning /θ/:** throat, thyroid, thank.
- **Beginning /ð/:** they, this, that, those.
- **Medial /θ/:** nothing, healthy, something.
- **Medial /ð/:** bother, other, father, mother.
- **Final /θ/:** growth, breath, length, mouth.
- **Final /ð/:** breathe, smooth, bathe, teethe.

/θ/:
- Now I'll check your **th**yroid.
- Could you open your mou**th**?
- Does any**th**ing make your pain better?

/ð/:
- Please brea**the** normally.
- Have you ever had difficulty brea**th**ing?
- Have you traveled outside **the** country recently?

/θ/ and /ð/:
- Is **th**ere any**th**ing in particular **th**at is bo**th**ering you?
- Al**th**ough your…is your concern, your whole heal**th** is my concern, too.

Note: The "th" sounds can be mispronounced by stopping the airflow between the tongue and upper teeth. The goal is to push the air gently through. **Tip:** If you can extend the sound, then it is a continuant. Another reason for mispronunciation is due to tongue placement, behind instead of between the teeth.

Compare /ð/ with /d/ and /θ/ with /t/

/ð/ and /θ/ are continuants and are pronounced with air flowing over the tongue, while the tongue is frontal between the teeth. /t/ and /d/ are stop sounds are pronounced by a momentary stop of airflow as the tongue touches behind the front teeth.

Table 3.15 Consonant minimal pair diagnostic

/θ/ (unvoiced "th"), /t/, and /s/	/ð/ (voiced "th"), /t/, and /s/
1 2 3	1 2 3
thank tank sank	then den zen
mouth mout* mouse	breathe breed breeze
/r/ and /l/	/v/, /f/, and /w/
1 2 3	1 2 3
rung lung	versed first worst
fear feel feeo*	have half
/z/ and /s/	/ʃ/, /tʃ/, /dʒ/
1 2	1 2 3
zinc sink	share chair jair*
eyes ice	aish* H age
/h/ an no consonant	/p/ and /b/
1 2	1 2
habit abbot	pest best
reheat reeat*	cope cobe*
/ŋ/, /m/, and /n/	
1 2 3	
fang fam* fan	

Spoken English Proficiency

For

USMLE Step 2 CS

Consonants /ð/ and /θ/

Video. 3.3 The two consonants spelled with 'th', voiced and unvoiced sounds, are described and practiced with words and sentences/questions. https://www.thieme.de/de/q.htm?p=opn/cs/20/3/11450515-d598f761

Voiced "th" and /d/: practice the transition: ðð d ðð d.

(Level 6) Word Comparison: Initial Sounds
Both words in the pair begin with a voiced consonant. Notice that the difference between the word pairs below is that the first word begins with a continuant, airflow, and the second word begins with a stop sound.

(Level 6) Word Comparison: Middle or Final Sounds
Both words in the pair end with a voiced consonant. Notice that the vowel in the first word, the continuant, is longer than the vowel in the second word, the stop (▶ Table 3.16).

Unvoiced "th" and /t/: practice the transition: θθθ t θθθ t.

(Level 6) Word Comparison: Initial Sounds
Both words in each pair begin with an unvoiced consonant. Notice that the difference between the word pairs below is that the first word begins with a continuant, airflow, and the second word begins with a stop sound.

(Level 6) Word Comparison: Middle or Final Sounds
Both words in the pair end with an unvoiced consonant sound. Notice that the vowel is the first word, the continuant, is longer than the vowel in the second word, the stop sound (▶ Table 3.17).

Compare /ð/ with /z/ and /θ/ with /s/
/ð/ and /θ/ are produced with the tongue between the teeth, while /z/ and /s/ are pronounced with the tongue behind the upper teeth.

Voiced "th" and /z/: practice the transition: ðð zzz ðð zzz.

(Level 6) Word Comparison: Initial Sounds
Both words in the pair begin with a continuous consonant. Notice that the difference is that the first word begins with the tongue between the teeth, and the second word begins with the tongue just behind the teeth.

(Level 6) Word Comparison: Middle or Final Sounds
Both words in the pair end with a continuant consonant. Notice that the difference is that the first word ends with the tongue between the teeth, and the second word ends with the tongue just behind the teeth (▶ Table 3.18).

Unvoiced "th" and /s/: practice the transition: θθθ sss θθθ sss.

(Level 6) Word Comparison: Initial Sounds
Both words in the pair begin with a continuous consonant. Notice that the difference is that the first word begins with the tongue between the teeth, and the second word begins with the tongue just behind the teeth.

(Level 6) Word Comparison: Middle or Final Sounds
Both words in the pair end with a continuant consonant. Notice that the difference is that the first word ends with the tongue between the teeth, and the second word ends with the tongue just behind the teeth (▶ Table 3.19).

Exercises: Consonants /ð/ and /θ/
As with the Minimal Pair Diagnostic, work with a partner. Listen as your partner reads one word from the pair. Which word do you hear? Then, practice the sounds in words in context.
(▶ Table 3.20)

/r/ Consonant

Articulation: Retract your tongue so the sides touch your back teeth. The tip of your tongue should be turned up without touching the roof of your mouth.

Beginning /r/: reason, rapid, range, wrong.

Medial /r/: serum, occurrence, measuring.
- *Do you feel a racing heart?*
- *Have you traveled outside the United States recently?*
- *Have you been around any sick person recently?*

Table 3.17 Compare /θ/ with /t/

initial /θ/	initial /t/	medial/final /θ/	medial / final /t/
thought	taught	math	mat
thank	tank	other	utter

Table 3.16 Compare /ð/ with /d/

initial /ð/	initial /d/	medial/final /ð/	medial/final /d/
those	dose	breathe	breed
they	day	lather	ladder

Table 3.18 Compare /ð/ with /z/

initial /ð/	initial /z/	medial/final /ð/	medial/final /z/
they	zey	soothe	sues
this	dis	father	fazzer

Table 3.19 Compare /θ/ with /s/

initial /θ/	initial /s/	final /θ/	final /s/
thank	sank	mouth	mouse
thought	sought	tenth	tense

Table 3.20 Exercises: consonants /ð/ and /θ/

Listening discrimination	Practice in context
Quiz yourself: Choose a word from each pair to read aloud to a partner. Ask your partner which word you read.	*Read each word first. Then, read it smoothly and clearly in the sentence/question.*
Compare /ð/ with /d/ *Which word do you hear?* 1. those/dose 2. they/day 3. bathe/bade	breathe Please _____ normally. breathing *Have you ever had difficulty _____?* the *Have you traveled outside _____ country recently?*
Compare /ð/ with /z/ *Which word do you hear?* 1. those/zose 2. breathe/breeze 3. them/zem	
Compare /θ/ with /t/ *Which word do you hear?* 1. thought/taught 2. thank/tank 3. health/healt	thyroid Now I'll check your _____. mouth *Could you open your _____?* anything *Does _____ make your pain better?*
Compare /θ/ with /s/ *Which word do you hear?* 1. thank/sank 2. mouth/mouse 3. math/mass	

Note: The /r/ sound is particularly challenging to speakers of Indian languages, among others. **Tip:** To prevent /r/ (a continuant) from sounding like /d/ (a stop), be sure the tip of the tongue does not touch anywhere on the roof of the mouth.

/l/ Consonant

Articulation: Raise and tense the back of the tongue. Press the tongue tip against the gum ridge.

Beginning /l/: lungs, lab, level, lower.

Medial /l/: hollow, swallow, balance, believe.

Final /l/: normal, oral, well, general.
- *How can I help you?*
- *Let's take your pulse.*
- *How long does it last?*

Note: The /l/ sound, in the end of words, is particularly challenging for Chinese and Slavic language speakers. For Japanese speakers, /l/ is problematic anywhere within words. **Tip:** To prevent /l/ from sounding like vocalic-r or /o/, keep lips horizontal, without rounding, and tense the tongue farther back. The /l/ at the end of words emanates from the back of the mouth, near the throat.

Compare /r/ with /l/ (▶ Table 3.21).
/r/ and /l/ are both continuants pronounced with the lips in a similar position. The difference between the two sounds is in the positioning of the tongue. In pronouncing /r/, the tongue is retracted so the sides touch the upper back teeth. In pronouncing /l/, the midpart of the tongue is tensed, while the front of the tongue is flat against the gum ridge.

/r/ **and** /l/: practice the transition: rrr lll rrr lll.

(Level 6) Word Comparison: Initial Sounds
Both words in the pair begin with a voiced consonant. Notice that the difference between the word pairs below is the tongue positioning and lip movement.

(Level 6) Word Comparison: Final Sounds
Both words in the pair end with a voiced sound. Notice again that the difference in lip rounding between /l/ and /o/.

Compare Final /l/ with /o/ Vowel
/l/ and the vowel /o/ (like all vowels) are both continuants. In pronouncing /l/, the lips are stretched horizontally, with the mid-section of the tongue tensed. In pronouncing the vowel /o/, the lips are rounded, and the tongue is low.

/l/ **and no consonant:** practice the transition: lll ou lll ou.

(Level 6) Word Comparison: Final Sounds
The word and nonword in the pair both end with a voiced sound. Notice that the tongue is engaged for /l/, and tongue is neutral with lips slightly rounded for /o/ or /u/ (▶ Table 3.22).

/v/ Consonant

Articulation: Gently bite lower lip and use voice (a vibration in the vocal chords). This is a continuous sound.

Beginning /v/: very, value, voice, and various.

Medial /v/: fever, deliver, level, every.

Final /v/: move, of, relieve, have.
- *Have you been vomiting?*
- *What do you do for a living?*
- *How long have you had a fever?*

/f/ Consonant

Articulation: Gently bite lower lip and release a stream of air. This sound is like a whisper, with no voice, and is a continuous sound.

Beginning /f/: pharmacy, first, factor, fracture.

Medial /f/: coughing, often, effect, rougher.

Final /f/: relief, safe, life, chief.
- Do you feel nauseous?
- Let me first warm my stethoscope.
- Have you ever felt like life is not worth living?

/w/ Consonant

Articulation: Place the lips in a tight circle. Use voice while unrounding the lips.

Beginning /w/: with, work, weaken, wash.

Medial /w/: growing, shower, away, anyway.
- *What makes it worse?*
- *What were you doing when the pain first started?*
- *I'd like to ask you a few questions regarding your medical history.*

Note: Speakers of many Indian languages confuse /v/ and /w/. Arabic speakers may replace /v/ with the unvoiced counterpart /f/. Mandarin speakers tend to replace /v/ with /w/ or /f/. **Tip:** For a clear /v/, be sure the upper teeth touch the inner lower lip, upper teeth are visible, and use your voice. For the /w/ sound, imagine "oo" before /w/ to achieve appropriate lip rounding, that is, work = ooWERK.

Compare /v/ with /w/
Both /v/ and /w/ are voiced continuants. In /w/, the airflow is not obstructed, and lips move from rounded to unrounded. In /v/, the airflow is obstructed with upper teeth and lower lip, without lip rounding.

/v/ **and** /w/: practice the transition: www vvv www vvv.

(Level 6) Word Comparison: Initial Sounds
Both /v/ and /w/ are voiced. Notice that the words beginning with /w/ are slightly longer than the words beginning with /v/.

(Level 6) Word Comparison: Middle Sounds
Both the word and nonword in the pair contain a voiced consonant. Notice the positioning of upper teeth on lower lip for /v/ and rounded lips for /w/ (▶ Table 3.23).

Table 3.21 Compare /r/ with /l/

initial /r/	initial /l/	final (vocalic) /r/	final /l/
ray	lay	fear	feel
right	light	sore	sole

Table 3.22 Compare /l/ with no consonant

final /l/	no consonant
call	kao
stool	stew

Compare /v/ with /f/

Both /v/ and /f/ are continuants, which are produced with air flowing between the upper teeth and lower lip. /v/ is voiced and /f/ is unvoiced.

/v/ and /f/: practice the transition: vvv fff vvv fff.

(Level 6) Word Comparison: Initial Sounds

Both /v/ and /f/ are pronounced with the same mouth positioning and same airflow. Notice that the difference is the first word begins with the voiced /v/ and the second word begins with an unvoiced /f/.

(Level 6) Word Comparison: Middle or Final Sounds

Both words in the pair end with a voiced continuant. Notice that the vowel in the first word, followed by the voiced consonant, is longer than the vowel in the second word, the unvoiced consonant (▶ Table 3.24).

/z/ Consonant

Articulation: Begin with lips slightly spread. Press the sides of the tongue lightly against the gum ridge. Do not let the tip of the tongue touch the gum ridge. Use voice. This is a continuous sound.

Beginning /z/: zinc, zero, zoom, Z.

Medial /z/: razor, sizing, causes, isn't.

Final /z/: eyes, phase, these, because.
- *Do you feel dizzy?*
- *Please exercise regularly, 5 days a week.*
- *Is it a constant pain, or does it come and go?*

Note: Speakers of many languages mispronounce the letter "s" in the end of words, assuming it sounds like an unvoiced "s," when it is often pronounced as /z/. **Tip:** To keep the voice in this final sound, imagine a very subtle "uh" sound at the end of the word, that is, eyes = AIYZ(uh).

/s/ Consonant

Articulation: Begin with the lips slightly spread. Touch the sides of the tongue to the side the teeth. Do not let the tip of the tongue touch the roof of the mouth. Force air out over the tip of the tongue. This is a continuous sound.

Beginning /s/: skull, sprain, smoke, sick.
- I'm sorry to see you in pain.
- *Have you been sleeping well?*
- *How many cigarettes do you smoke per day?*

Table 3.23 Compare /v/ with /w/

initial /v/	initial /w/	middle /v/	middle /w/
verse	worse	private	*priwate*
vain	wane	cover	cower

Table 3.24 Compare /v/ with /f/

initial /v/	initial /f/	middle/final /v/	middle/final /f/
versed	first	have	half
vial	file	fever	*feefer*

Note: Spanish and Portuguese speakers often insert an /ə/, schwa sound before /s/ in the beginning of words. **Tip:** To prevent this, extent the /s/ sound briefly, that is, skull = ssskull. It is particularly important not to omit the -s at the end of words because it often carries grammar information (plural -s and third person -s).

Compare /z/ with /s/ Consonants

/z/ and /s/ are continuants and are pronounced with air flowing through the space between the tongue and the back of the front teeth. /z/ is voiced and /s/ is unvoiced. The most common challenge with /z/ relates to spelling: knowing when to voice the letter "s" as "z." There are no clear rules, so you must learn on a word-by-word basis.

/z/ and /s/: practice the transition: zzz sss zzz sss.

(Level 6) Word Comparison: Initial Sounds

Both /z/ and /s/ are continuants. Notice that the difference in the word pair below is that the first word begins with a voiced consonant and the second word begins with an unvoiced consonant.

(Level 6) Word Comparison: Final Sounds

Both words in the pair below end in a continuant. The first word ends with a voiced consonant and the second word ends with an unvoiced consonant. Notice that the vowel is the first word, with the voiced ending, is longer than the vowel in the second word, with the unvoiced ending (▶ Table 3.25).

/tʃ/ Consonant

Articulation: Round your lips and push them forward. Raise the tongue, and the sides of the tongue should touch the teeth. There should be very little space between the top and bottom teeth. Release a stream of air with this continuous sound.

Beginning /ʃ/: shadow, sharp, shift, sure.

Medial /ʃ/: session, information, tissue, tension.

Final /ʃ/: fresh, push, brush, wish.
- *Do you feel nauseous?*
- *Have you had a similar condition before?*
- *Do you have to rush to the bathroom to urinate?*

Note: A challenge with this sound is to recognize it with its different spellings (sh, s, and t). Also, Spanish speakers often pronounce /ʃ/ as /s/. **Tip:** It can be helpful to purse the lips forward and pull tongue back a little from /s/ for /ʃ/.

/tʃ/ Consonant

Articulation: This sound is a combination of the sounds /t/ and /ʃ/. Press the tip of the tongue against the gum ridge. As you move to the /ʃ/ sound, use a burst of air while quickly releasing the tongue.

Table 3.25 Compare /z/ with /s/

initial /z/	initial /s/	final /z/	final /s/
zinc	sink	eyes	ice
zero	see row	close (not open)	close (not far)

Beginning /tʃ/: choose, challenge, change, chest.

Medial /tʃ/: temperature, catches, matching, natural.

Final /tʃ/: watch, switch, such, itch.
- Do you have regular **ch**eckups?
- I'm going to examine your **ch**est.
- Please wa**tch** your diet.

Note: A challenge with this sound, similar to /ʃ/, is to recognize it with its different spellings (ch, tch, and t). Also, it is a stop sound, with the air briefly blocked.

/dʒ/ Consonant

Articulation: This sound is a combination of the voiced /ʃ/ sound, /ʒ/, and /d/. Press the tip of the tongue against the gum ridge. Begin with /d/ and add voice and air while quickly releasing tongue.

Beginning /dʒ/: joint, general, gene, germ.

Medial /dʒ/: urgent, larger, oxygen, danger.

Final /dʒ/: urge, age, surge, edge.
- Do you have any aller**g**ies?
- Have you had any sur**g**eries done?
- I'm going to do a **g**eneral exam first to see what's going on.

Note: Many Portuguese speakers, as well as speakers of other languages, mispronounce this sound as a continuant. To create the /dʒ/ sound, the air must be briefly blocked.

Compare /ʃ/ with /tʃ/ Consonants
Both /ʃ/ and /tʃ/ are unvoiced, but /ʃ/ is a continuant and /tʃ/ is a stop sound. In both sounds, lips are pushed forward. To produce /ʃ/, the tongue is raised and air flows over it. To produce /tʃ/ the tongue is raised to touch gum ridge before releasing a burst of air.

"sh" and "ch": practice the transition: ʃʃ tʃʃʃ tʃ.

(Level 6) Word Comparison: Initial Sounds
Notice that the difference between the word pair is that the first word begins with a continuant, airflow, and the second word begins with a stop sound.

(Level 6) Word Comparison: Final Sounds
Both words in each pair end with an unvoiced consonant. Notice that the vowel in the first word, followed by a continuant, is longer than the vowel in the second word, followed by a stop sound (▶ **Table 3.26**).

Compare /tʃ/ with /dʒ/ Consonants
Both /tʃ/ and /dʒ/ are produced with the lips forward, the tongue on the gum ridge, and by releasing a burst of air. /tʃ/ is unvoiced, and /dʒ/ is voiced.

"ch" and "dj": practice the transition: tʃ dʒ tʃ dʒ.

(Level 6) Word Comparison: Initial Sounds
Notice that the difference in the word pair below is that the first word begins with an unvoiced consonant and the second word begins with a voiced consonant.

(Level 6) Word Comparison: Final Sounds
Notice that the vowel in the first word, with the unvoiced ending, is shorter than the vowel in the second word, with the voiced ending (▶ **Table 3.27**).

/h/ Consonant

Articulation: Begin with mouth slightly open. Keep the tongue in a relaxed position. Release a stream of air. This is a continuous sound.

Beginning /h/: habit, history, health, who.

Medial /h/: reheat, inhibit, enhance, perhaps.
- *How long have you had this pain?*
- *It's hard for me to tell you for sure at this moment.*
- *If you don't have health insurance, it does not mean that you will not be given the proper medical care.*

Note: French and Portuguese speakers, along with some Slavic and Indian language speakers omit the /h/ consonant. **Tip:** It can be helpful to conceptualize "noisy air" coming from the throat to produce this sound.

Compare /h/ with No Consonants
The difference between /h/ and no consonant (a vowel sound) is that /h/ is produced with "noisy air" from the back of the throat.

(Level 6) Word Comparison: Initial Sounds
The first word begins with "noisy air" coming from the back of the throat. The second word begins with a full vowel sound (▶ **Table 3.28**).

/p/ Consonant

Articulation: Press the lips together. Use a burst of air while quickly releasing the lips.

Beginning /p/: pain, part, period, put.

Medial /p/: simple, people, bypass, appetite.

Final /p/: cope, keep, map, help.
- *How is your appetite?*
- *When was your last menstrual period?*
- *Have you had any problems in passing urine?*

Note: Many Slavic and African language speakers, as well as Arabic speakers mispronounce /p/ at the beginning of words, by

Table 3.27 Compare /tʃ/ with /dʒ/

initial /tʃ/	initial /dʒ/	final /tʃ/	final /dʒ/
choke	joke	"H"	age
chest	jest	etch	edge

Table 3.26 Compare /ʃ/ with /tʃ/

initial /ʃ/	initial /tʃ/	middle/final /ʃ/	middle/final /tʃ/
Share	chair	wash	watch
shoes	chews	cashing	catching

Table 3.28 Compare /h/ with no consonant

/h/	no consonant
hear	ear
head	Ed

adding voice. **Tip:** Try to think of it as a "popping" sound in the initial position.

Compare /b/ with /p/ Consonants

/b/ and /p/ are stop sounds and are pronounced with the lips together. The first is voiced and the second is unvoiced.

/b/ and /p/: practice the transition: b p b p.

(Level 6) Word Comparison: Initial Sounds

Notice that the difference between the word pairs below is that the initial consonant in the first word (or *nonword*) is voiced and the initial consonant in the second is unvoiced and a puff of air is released when it is pronounced (▶Table 3.29).

/ŋ/ Consonant

Articulation: Press the back of your tongue against the entire soft palate. Using your voice, allow the sound to come through your nose. This is a continuous sound.

Final /ŋ/: long, hurting, young, saving.
- I am goi**ng** to listen to your lu**ng**s.
- *Does he have any difficulty swallowi**ng**?*
- *I am goi**ng** to ask you a few questions regardi**ng** your lifestyle.*

Note: /ŋ/ is often mispronounced as voiceless /k/ or /n/. Similar to /l/, imagine the sound emanating from the back of the mouth, near the throat. Keep it voiced by imagining an "uh" sound at the end of the word, that is, strong = STRAWNG(uh).

/m/ Consonant

Articulation: Press the lips together. Using your voice, allow the sound to come through your nose. This is a continuous sound.

Final /m/: them, time, am, aim.
- *I am going to examine your muscles.*
- *Based on your history and my clinical exam, I have a preliminary diagnosis.*
- *When the results come back, we'll work together to choose the best option.*

/n/ Consonant

Articulation: Press the tongue against the entire gum ridge. Using your voice, allow the sound to come through your nose. This is a continuous sound.

Final /n/: pain, brown, ten, gain.
- *May I untie your gown?*
- *Do you have joint pain?*
- *Did I address your concern?*

Table 3.29 Compare /b/ with /p/

/b/	/p/
bay	pay
batient	patient

Table 3.30 Compare /ŋ/with /nk/

middle/final /ŋ/	middle/final /nk/
sing	sink
angle	ankle

Note: Speakers of some languages omit final consonants altogether. Slavic language speakers often add a /k/ to /ŋ/. **Tip:** Be sure to finish off the final sound in English words.

Compare /ŋ/ with /nk/

/ŋ/ and /nk/: Practice the transition: ŋ nk ŋ nk.

(Level 6) Word Comparison: Final Sounds

The first word ends with a voiced, continuant sound. The second word ends with an unvoiced, stop sound (▶Table 3.30).

Compare /m/ with /n/ Consonant

/m/ and /n/ are voiced continuants. /m/ is produced with the lips together, and /n/ is produced with the lips slightly apart, and the tongue on the gum ridge.

/m/ and /n/: practice the transition: m n m n.

(Level 6) Word Comparison: Final Sounds

Both words in each pair end with a voiced continuant consonant. There is no difference in vowel length. The key is to be sure not to omit the ending sound after the vowel (▶Table 3.31).

3.4 Vowels

All vowels are produced by a particular movement and/or positioning of the lips, tongue, and jaw (▶Video. 3.4). All vowels are voiced, meaning there is vibration in the vocal cords, and the air is not blocked in any way.

Differences between Vowels:

A, e, i, o, u, and sometimes y, are the English vowels, but there are actually 14 different vowel *sounds* in English. This is a big difference from many other languages that have only five to eight vowels. There are vowels with one mouth movement ("ih" in "sit"). There are vowels with a "y" sound ("ee(y)" in "tea"), and a vowel with a "w" sound ("oo(w)" in "two"). Beyond the 14 vowels, vowels with /r/ are called /ɚ/, or vocalic-r.

Five of the vowel sounds, known as "long vowels," are pronounced identically to vowel letter names. Each of these long

Table 3.31 Compare /m/with /n/

final /m/	final /n/
time	tine
seem	seen

Spoken English Proficiency

For

USMLE Step 2 CS

Vowel Sounds

Video. 3.4 This video helps the speaker differentiate between similar vowel sounds and provides tips to avoid common errors. https://www.thieme.de/de/q.htm?p=opn/cs/20/3/11450516-d74c5fae

vowels has a "short vowel" counterpart, produced by relaxing the jaw a little lower than each long vowel. Be aware that this is an oversimplification. Not all vowels make the same sound in all words, and vowel pronunciation is actually determined by where the sound is located in the word. However, the following chart is a good place to start. The long and short vowel pairs explain 10 of the 14 American English vowel sounds, not including the vocalic-r vowels (▶ Table 3.32).

Spelling and Sounds:

A spelling rule can be helpful in determining pronunciation of long and short vowel sounds: When one-syllable words have a vowel in the middle, the vowel usually has a short sound. When two vowels are next to each other, the first vowel is usually long, and sounds the same as the letter. Also, when a word ends in vowel, consonant, and -e, then the first vowel is usually long with a silent "e" (▶ Table 3.33).

Positioning:

Vowels can be grouped by lip positioning: *rounded*, such as "oo" in "boot," *neutral*, such as "uh" in "but," and *stretched*, such as "ey" in "bait." Rounded and stretched vowels are described as *tense*, with tension in the muscles. More neutral vowels are described as *lax*, with more relaxed muscles. Some vowels are *high*, with the jaw almost closed, such as "ee" in "heat." Other vowels are *low*, with a dropped jaw and open mouth, such as "ah" in "hot."

Vowel Length:

Vowel length varies. Generally, tense vowels are longer and lax vowels are shorter. Vowel length also depends of the sound that follows. If the consonant that follows is *voiced*, then the vowel will be longer. If the consonant that follows is *unvoiced*, the vowel sound will be shorter.

Challenging Vowels and Tips:

The following are vowels that present particular challenge to speakers of other languages. Not every vowel is covered, and less frequently occurring vowels are not addressed.

Vowels: Minimal Pair Sound Discrimination Diagnostic:

Which English vowels do you already pronounce accurately? Which do you need to spend time working on? Although this communicative assessment is similar to the one used for consonants, it is not an accurate speech diagnostic evaluation; it will provide you with some concrete examples of where communication can break down due to individual sound differences.

Work with a partner, preferably a native English speaker, or someone who can easily hear the differences between the words. Read at random one of the two/three words (or non-words*) for each sound comparison (read across, not down). *Can your partner accurately determine which word you are saying—1, 2, or 3? If not, which sound are you substituting?* Read at random from the second example to confirm your findings and repeat for further confirmation (▶ Table 3.34).

The root cause of miscommunication can vary from the speaker's pronunciation to the listener's ability to hear and understand, but this simple exercise will provide you with valuable information.

If you are trying to pronounce a particular word, and your partner hears a different word than the one you intended to say, this consonant sound requires attention. If you question the results, do the same exercise with a different partner. In the end, the goal is to identify your Personal Target Sounds, the vowels that you will focus on in the following sections, to improve your pronunciation and clarity.

List the target vowel sounds you will focus on.

3.4.1 Target Vowels

Long A: /e/ Vowel

Articulation: Stretch the lips in a horizontal position and drop your jaw slightly. Move the jaw up slightly, ending with /i/ positioning.

Beginning /e/: ache, age, able, aim.

Medial /e/: today, same, pain.
- *Does anything make your pain better?*
- *Are you taking any medicines on a daily basis?*
- *On a scale of 1 to 10, with 10 being the worst, how would you rate the pain?*

Note: Many Mandarin and Vietnamese speakers have trouble differentiating the /e/ vowel from /i/. **Tip:** Be aware that /e/ is a "moving vowel"; begin with "eh" and transition to "ee" in one continuous syllable.

Table 3.32 Long and short vowels

Vowels	Long	Short
Letter A	/ei/ male	/ae/ at
Letter E	/i/ meet	/eh/ met
Letter I	/ai/ ice	/ih/ is
Letter O	/o/ own	/ah/ on
Letter U	/u/ cute	/uh/ cut

Table 3.33 Long and short vowel spelling rules

Long vowel sound (two vowels)	Short vowel sound (one vowel)
seat	sat
hear	her
Long vowel sound (vowel + consonant + "e")	Short vowel sound (vowel + consonant)
same	Sam
take	tack

Table 3.34 Vowel minimal pair diagnostic

/e/ /ɛ/ /æ/ 1 2 3	/i/ /ɛ/ /ɪ/ 1 2 3
pain pen pan	cheek check chick
made med mad	feel fell fill
chased chest chaste	reach wretch rich

/æ/ /ɑ/ /ɛ/ 1 2 3	/ai/ /æ/ /ɪ/ 1 2 3
sad sod said	fight fat fit
gnat not net	eyes as is
lag log leg	signed sand sinned

/o/ /ɑ/ /ɔ/ 1 2 3	/ə/ /ɚ/ /oɚ/ 1 2 3
coat cot caught	shut shirt short
goes gahz* gauze	fussed first forced
low la* law	cuss curse course

Short A: /æ/ Vowel

Articulation: Stretch the lips in a horizontal position, dropping the jaw lower than when making the sound /e/ (▶Video. 3.5). Keep the tongue at the floor of the mouth.

Beginning /æ/: answer, after, analyze, ask.

Medial /æ/: plan, fast, manage, have.
- *Has he ever passed out?*
- *I am going to answer you when I'm done.*
- *I'd like to ask you a few questions about your medical history.*

Note: Many English speakers, who first learned British English, as well as Spanish speakers, pronounce the American /æ/ sound as /ɑ/. **Tip:** Tense the cheek muscles slightly outward and downward.

Exercises: Vowels /e/ and /æ/

Exercises for vowels /e/ and /æ/ are presented in ▶Table 3.35.

Long E: /i/ Vowel

Articulation: Stretch your lips in a horizontal position; drop your jaw very little. Move your tongue up slightly as you make this sound.

Beginning /i/: each, either, even, E.

Medial /i/: team, breath, clear, reach.
- *Do you feel sad?*
- *How is your sleep?*
- *Take a deep breath.*

Note: This sound is not commonly problematic and is often overused in place of /ɪ/.

Short E: /ɛ/ Vowel

Articulation: Keep mouth in a relaxed position without stretching the lips. The jaw drops slightly more than when making the sound /e/.

Beginning /ɛ/: every, elevate, enter, evident.

Medial /ɛ/: said, rest, check, heavy.
- *Let's take one step at a time.*
- *Can you tell me a little bit more?*
- *Does anything make your cough better?*

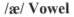

Spoken English Proficiency
For
USMLE Step 2 CS

/æ/ Vowel

Video. 3.5 The "short A" vowel sound is described and practiced with words and sentences/questions. https://www.thieme.de/de/q. htm?p=opn/cs/20/3/11450517-71861c91

Note: Many Slavic language speakers, as well as Spanish speakers, are challenged by neutral vowels, such as /ɛ/. **Tip:** To prevent /ɛ/ from sounding like /i/, make it a very short sound and slightly drop the jaw.

Long I: /ai/ Vowel

Articulation: In this two-part sound, glide from /a/ to /i/. Your lips should move from an open circle, with the jaw low, to a horizontal position, with the jaw almost closed.

Beginning /ai/: I, eye, ice, isolate.

Medial /ai/: sign, nice, try, light.
- *Do you have diarrhea?*
- *How long have you had diabetes?*
- *I need to examine your belly right now.*

Note: Many Mandarin and Vietnamese speakers have trouble differentiating the /ai/ vowel from /a/. **Tip:** Remember to end with the "y" horizontal stretch in this two-part "moving" sound.

Short I: /ɪ/ Vowel

Articulation: Keep the mouth in a relaxed position without spreading the lips. Drop the jaw a little more than when making the sound /i/. Do not spread the lips horizontally.

Beginning /ɪ/: it, issue, imply, interest.

Medial /ɪ/: history, women, cyst, shift.
- *Did it come on suddenly?*
- *It makes you an addict and it will be very hard for you to quit.*
- *Did your child have any yellowish or bluish skin discoloration at birth?*

Note: Many Spanish and Portuguese speakers are challenged by neutral vowels, such as /ɪ/. **Tip:** To prevent /ɪ/ from sounding like /i/, make it a very short sound. Many Slavic language speakers have the inverse challenge, pronouncing /i/ as /ɪ/. **Tip:** Spread the lips more.

Table 3.35 Exercises: vowels /æ/ and /ɑ/

Listening discrimination	Practice in context
Compare /e/ with /i/ Which word do you hear? 1. same/seem 2. raid/read 3. rate/reet	Vowel /e/ make/pain Does anything _____ your _____ better? taking/daily/basis Are you _____ any medicines on a _____ _____? scale/rate/pain On a _____ of 1 to 10, with 10 being the worst, how would you _____ the _____?
Compare /æ/ with /ɑ/ Which word do you hear? 1. add/odd 2. tap/top 3. lack/lock	Vowel /æ/ has/passed _____ he ever _____ out? am/ answer I _____ going to _____ you shortly. ask I'd like to _____ you a few questions about your medical history.
Quiz yourself: Choose a word from each pair to read aloud to a partner. Ask your partner which word you read.	*Read each word first. Then, read it smoothly and clearly in the sentence/question.*

Long O: /o/ Vowel

Articulation: This two-part sound begins with the mouth relaxed and open. Move your lips into a tight circle. This should be done as one smooth motion.

Beginning /o/: over, own, only, obese.

Medial /o/: know, show, almost, whole.
- *Do you have a runny nose?*
- *Do you feel cold when others don't?*
- *As you know smoking is a leading cause of many diseases.*

Note: Many Slavic language speakers mispronounce /o/ as /u/. **Tip:** It is pronounced as the letter "O." Remember this is a two-part "moving" sound, which rounds, a reverse /w/.

Short O: /ɑ/ Vowel

Articulation: Drop the jaw without stretching your lips horizontally. The tongue is low, and your mouth should be opened wide.

Beginning /ɑ/: on, operate, ocular, onset.

Medial /ɑ/: problem, shock, stop, block.
- *It is a possibility.*
- *When did you first notice the problem?*
- *Have you had any severe abdominal pain?*

Note: Many speakers of other languages confuse /ɑ/ with /o/ because it is often spelled with the letter "O."

"U" Sound: Long U

y + /u/ Vowel

Articulation: Begin with /y/ sound, with the tongue up and back. Push your lips forward into a circle.

Beginning y+/u/: usual, you, use, unique.

Medial y+/u/: unusual, regular, continue, particular.
- *Do you cough up any mucous?*
- *Are you using any kind of contraception?*
- *Is there anything in particular that you are concerned about?*

Note: Many language speakers are not aware of the "hidden-y" sound in many words spelled with the letter "u."

Short U: /ə/ Vowel

Articulation: Keep the mouth in a relaxed position. Do not stretch the lips. The jaw and tongue should be slightly lower than when making the sound /ɪ/.

Beginning /ə/: unsure, up, above, under.

Medial /ə/: was, roughly, does, blood.
- *When and how often does it occur?*
- *Is your blood pressure under control?*
- *Do you have any other symptoms besides pain?*

Note: The /ə/ (schwa) vowel is challenging to speakers of many languages. Many Spanish and Asian language speakers mispronounce the sound as /ɑ/ or /ʌ/. **Tip:** To prevent this, make it a short, quick sound, with the tongue neutral in the mouth. It can be helpful to imagine that there is no vowel at all. Allow the mouth to shift from one consonant to the next, and the schwa vowel will take care of itself.

/ɔ/ Vowel

Articulation: Begin with the jaw dropped and lips rounded in an oval shape. Keep the tongue at the floor of the mouth.

Beginning /ɔ/: also, awful, ought, all.

Medial /ɔ/: cauterize, nausea, saw, thought.
- *Can your child crawl?*
- *Have you been coughing lately?*
- *Would you mind if I call my nurse to get you ready?*

Note: Many Japanese and Slavic language speakers have trouble differentiating the /ɔ/ vowel from /o/ or /au/ "ow." **Tip:** Remember that it is a one-part sound without movement. Also, be aware that the sound emanates from the central part of the mouth, not the back.

Vocalic-r: /□/ Vowel

Articulation: Begin with the mouth slightly open. Raise and pull back the tongue (▶ **Video. 3.6**). Sides of the tongue should slightly touch the upper teeth. Purse your lips. Tip of the tongue should not touch any part of the mouth.

Medial /ɚ/: turn, further, heard, worsen.

Final /ɚ/: later, doctor, occur, were.
- *Do you have any other concerns?*
- *Let me first warm my stethoscope.*
- *Does it burn while you are urinating?*

Note: Speakers of many languages mispronounce the very American /ɚ/ vowel because the sound does not exist in those languages, and it is pronounced very differently in British English.

/□/ Dipthongs

Articulation: Begin with the first vowel. Glide smoothly into the "rr" sound by raising and pulling back the tongue. Sides of the tongue should slightly touch the upper teeth. Purse lips. The tip of the tongue should not touch any part of the mouth.

Medial /ɚ/: repairable, fears, starting, information.

Spoken English Proficiency

For

USMLE Step 2 CS

Vocalic-r /ɚ/ Vowel

Video. 3.6 The "vocalic-r" vowel is described and practiced with words and sentences/questions. https://www.thieme.de/de/q.htm?p=opn/cs/20/3/11450518-20053a22

Final /ɚ/: here, chart, retire, more.
- *When did the pain start?*
- *Could you point to where it hurts?*
- *Did you have a similar condition before?*

Note: Speakers of many languages mispronounce the /ɚ/ vowel, as /ə/ (schwa). The key difference between the sounds is tensing and pulling back the tongue for /ɚ/.

Vowel Comparisons: Tense and Lax

Compare /i/ with /ɪ/ Vowels
/i/ is tense and stretched, while /ɪ/ is relaxed and neutral. Imagine stretching a rubber band for the /i/ sound and releasing the rubber band for /ɪ/.

Practice the transition: iii ɪɪɪ iii ɪɪɪ.

(Level 6) Word Comparison
Notice that the vowel in the first word is tense, or stretched, and is longer than the vowel in the second word, which contains a short, more neutral vowel (▶ Table 3.36).

Compare /e/ with /ɛ/ Vowels
/e/ is tense and stretched, while /ɛ/ is relaxed and neutral. Imagine stretching a rubber band for the /e/ sound and releasing the rubber band for /ɛ/. Both /e/ and /ɛ/ are pronounced with the tongue and jaw slightly lower than when pronouncing /i/ and /ɪ/.

Practice the transition: eee ɛɛɛ eee ɛɛɛ.

(Level 6) Word Comparison
Notice that the vowel in the first word is tense, or stretched, and is longer than the vowel in the second word, which contains a short, more neutral vowel (▶ Table 3.37).

Compare /æ/ with /ɑ/ Vowels
/æ/ is a tense, horizontal stretch, while /ɑ/ is vertical with the jaw wide. Imagine stretching a rubber band for the /æ/ sound and releasing the rubber band and dropping the jaw for /ɑ/. Both /æ/ and /ɑ/ are pronounced with the tongue and jaw slightly lower than when pronouncing /e/ and /ɛ/.

Practice the transition: æææ ɑɑɑ æææ ɑɑɑ.

(Level 6) Word Comparison
Both words contain vowels with the jaw low. The vowel in the first word is a tense, horizontal stretch. The vowel in the second word has no horizontal stretch, and the jaw is dropped lower (▶ Table 3.38).

Vowel Comparisons: Two- and One-Part Sounds

Compare /e/ with /i/ Vowels
Both /e/ and /i/ are tense and stretched, while /e/ is produced by first slightly dropping the jaw before raising the jaw and stretching horizontally to produce /i/. /i/ is a one-part sound with a higher jaw.

Practice the transition: eee iii eee iii.

(Level 6) Word Comparison
Notice in the first word that the jaw shifts from "eh" to "ee" in one smooth movement, beginning with the jaw slightly dropped for "eh." In the second word, the mouth remains in the tense "ee" position (▶ Table 3.39).

Compare /e/ with /æ/ Vowels
Both /e/ and /æ/ are tense and stretched, while /æ/ is produced by first slightly dropping the jaw before raising the jaw and stretching horizontally to produce /i/. /æ/ is a one-part sound with a lower jaw.

Practice the transition: eee æææ eee æææ.

(Level 6) Word Comparison
Notice in the first word that the jaw shifts from "eh" to "ee" in one smooth movement, beginning with the jaw slightly dropped for "eh." In the second word, the jaw remains lower with lips spread (▶ Table 3.40).

Compare /o/ with /ɔ/ Vowels
Both /o/ and /ɔ/ are tense and rounded, while /o/ shifts with one smooth movement from relaxed into a tight circle. /ɔ/ is produced with the jaw lower and lips in an oval shape.

Practice the transition: ooo ɔɔɔ ooo ɔɔɔ.

(Level 6) Word Comparison
The vowel in the first word is oval shaped with the jaw low. The vowel in the second word begins neutral, and lips move to a very rounded position (▶ Table 3.41).

Vocalic-r and Combinations

Compare /ɚ/ with /☐/ Vowels
/ɚ/ is produced with the tongue retracted to the upper back teeth, with the jaw almost closed. In contrast, /ə/ is a relaxed and neutral sound, with the jaw slightly open, very little mouth movement.

Table 3.36 Compare /i/ with /ɪ/

/i/	/ɪ/
sleep	slip

Table 3.37 Compare /e/ with /ɛ/

/e/	/ɛ/
pain	pen

Table 3.38 Compare /e/ with /ɛ/

/æ/	/ɑ/
add	odd

Table 3.39 Compare /e/ with /i/

/e/	/i/
say	see

Table 3.40 Compare /e/ with /æ/

/e/	/æ/
pain	pan

Table 3.41 Compare /o/ with /ɔ/

/o/	/ɔ/
cold	called

Practice the transition: əəəɑɑɑəəəɑɑɑ.

(Level 6) Word Comparison

The vowel in the first word is very neutral and short. The vowel in the second word is very tense, with the tongue in a retracted position (▶Table 3.42).

Compare /ɚ/ with /oɚ/ Vowels

/ɚ/ is produced with the tongue retracted to the upper back teeth, with the jaw almost closed. In contrast, /oɚ/ is a two-part vowel beginning with /o/ and gliding into /ɚ/.

Practice the transition: ɚɚɚ oɚɚɚɚ oɚ.

(Level 6) Word Comparison

The vowel in the first word is tense with jaw nearly closed. The vowel in the second word is longer, with a transition between the sounds (▶Table 3.43).

Compare /ɚ/ with /ɑɚ/ Vowels

/ɚ/ is produced with the tongue retracted to the upper back teeth, with the jaw almost closed. In contrast, /ɑɚ/ is a two-part vowel beginning with /ɑ/ and gliding into /ɚ/.

Practice the transition: ɚɚɚɑɚɚɚɚɑɚ.

(Level 6) Word Comparison

The vowel in the first word is tense with the jaw nearly closed. The vowel in the second word is longer, with a transition between the sounds (▶Table 3.44).

Grammar Question Patterns: Patient Interview

There are many ways to form questions; however, in the CS exam, it is recommended to use simple, short, and direct questions rather than using long and complicated questions (▶Video. 3.7). Grammatical forms are prescribed, so question patterns can be memorized. In the following examples, "be" verb forms are contrasted with other verbs in the present and past tenses. In the continuous tense examples, present and past are contrasted. The remaining tenses are presented individually. Explanations of the meaning of each tense are outlined below:

Table 3.43 Compare /ɚ/ with /oɚ/	
/ɚ/	/oɚ/
turn	torn

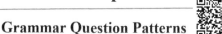

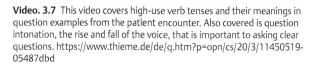

Video. 3.7 This video covers high-use verb tenses and their meanings in question examples from the patient encounter. Also covered is question intonation, the rise and fall of the voice, that is important to asking clear questions. https://www.thieme.de/de/q.htm?p=opn/cs/20/3/11450519-05487dbd

- **Past tense:** completed action.
- **Present tense:** repeated action, or fact.
- **Past continuous tense:** ongoing action in the past.
- **Present continuous tense:** ongoing action in the present.
- **Present perfect tense: action began in past, and was recently completed**, or continues into the present.
- **Present perfect continuous tense:** actions began in past, and continued until recently.
- **Modal tense:** implies likelihood, ability, permission, or obligation, depending on the verb.

3.4.2 Chart Abbreviations

- **S:** Subject
- **O/C:** object or complement (plus indirect object in some cases).
- **AUX:** auxiliary, or helping verb.
- **BV:** base, or main verb.
- **Wh:** who, what, when, where, why, how, how many, which kind....
- **V+ing:** base verb plus -ing ending.
- **PP:** past participle.

3.4.3 Intonation and Structure

Intonation includes the rise and fall of the voice, the melody. Within the spoken language framework, the sounds in focus will be the ones that preserve the intonation patterns.

Questions have two intonation patterns, rising and falling, depending on the question structure. As a rule, information questions (wh- questions) end with a falling voice. Yes/no questions (all non-wh- questions) end with a rising voice (▶Table 3.45).

Table 3.42 Compare /ə/ with /ɚ/	
/ə/	/ɚ/
shut	shirt

Table 3.44 Compare /ɚ/ with /ɑɚ/	
/ɚ/	/ɑɚ/
hurt	heart

Table 3.45 Question intonation	
Questions starting with	**Falling intonation**
WHEN	When do you... /When does she... When did you
HOW OFTEN (etc.)	How often do you... / How often does he...How often did you
Questions starting with	**Rising intonation**
BE	Are you... /Is he...
DO	Do you... /Does she... Did you...
HAVE	Have you noticed... /Has he ever... Had you taken...
CAN COULD MAY (etc.)	Can you manage... Could he walk... May I examine...

- *Does it hurt right here? (rising).*
- *How long have you been feeling this way? (falling).*
- *Did it come on suddenly? (rising).*

Question Intonation Practice

Which questions below end in a **rising** intonation? Which questions end in a **falling** intonation? **Remember:** yes/no questions rise at the end, and information questions fall.

Example: *Did it come on suddenly?* ___rising___ (▶ **Table 3.46**).

Answers: 1. Rising; 2. Falling; 3. Rising; 4. Falling; 5. Falling; 6. Rising; 7. Rising; 8. Falling; 9. Falling; 10. Rising.

3.4.4 Common Question Patterns

Past Tense Yes/No Questions

The following yes/no questions have a rising intonation (▶ Table 3.47).

Past Tense Wh- Questions The following information questions have a falling intonation (▶ **Table 3.48**).

Present Tense Yes/No Questions

The following yes/no questions have a rising intonation (▶ Table 3.49).

Present Tense Wh- Questions

The following information questions have a falling intonation (▶ Table 3.50).

Continuous Tense Yes/No Questions

The following yes/no questions have a rising intonation.

Grammar Note: Was - he/she/it; Were - you/we/they (▶ Table 3.51).

Table 3.46 Question intonation practice

1. Are you in pain?	_____
2. When did the pain first start?	_____
3. Is there pain anywhere else?	_____
4. Where does it hurt?	_____
5. What were you doing when it started?	_____
6. Could you tell me more about your pain?	_____
7. Does anything make it better?	_____
8. When is your physical therapy?	_____
9. Where is his rash located?	_____
10. Is it tender here?	_____

Table 3.47 Past tense yes/no questions

Past tense yes/no questions			Other verb questions			
BE	S	O/C	AUX	S	BV	O/C
Was	your temperature	high?	Did	you	check	your temperature at home?
Was	the pain	sudden?	Did	the pain	come on	suddenly?
Was	your child	healthy at birth?	Did	your child	have	any health problems at birth?

Table 3.48 Past tense Wh- questions

BE verb questions			Other verb questions			
Wh-	BE	S	Wh-	AUX	S	BV
Where	was	the pain?	When	did	the pain	start?
What	was	your temperature?	How high	did	your fever	get?
What	were	your test results?	What	did	your test results	indicate?

Table 3.49 Present tense yes/no questions

BE verb questions			Other verb questions			
BE	S	O/C	AUX	S	BV	O/C
Is	there	pain anywhere else?	Do	you	feel	pain anywhere else?
Is	it	tender?	Does	it	feel	tender?
Are	you	on any medications?	Do	you	take	any medications?
Are	Your	shots up to date?	Do	you	need	vaccinations updated?

Table 3.50 Present tense Wh- questions

BE verb questions			Other verb questions			
Wh-	BE	S	Wh-	AUX	S	BV
Where	is	your pain?	Where	does	it	hurt?
How	is	your appetite?	How often	do	you	eat?
When	are	you most tired?	When	do	you	feel the most tired?

Continuous Tenses Wh- Questions
The following information questions have a falling intonation (▶Table 3.52).

Present Perfect Tense Yes/No Questions
The following yes/no questions have a rising intonation.

Grammar Note: Has - he/she/it; Have - you/we/they (▶Table 3.53).

Present Perfect Tense Wh- Questions
The following information questions have a falling intonation (▶Table 3.54).

Present Perfect Continuous Tense Yes/No Questions
The following yes/no questions have a rising intonation (▶Table 3.55).

Present Perfect Continuous Tense Wh- Questions
The following information questions have a falling intonation (▶Table 3.56).

Modal Verb Tense Questions with "May"
The following yes/no questions have a rising intonation (▶Table 3.57).

Table 3.51 Continuous tense yes/no questions

Past continuous			Present continuous		
was/were	S	V+ing (+C)	is/are	S	V+ing (+C)
Was	your child	doing fine?	Is	your child	doing fine now?
Was	she	behaving normally?	Is	she	behaving normally?
Were	you	hearing ringing in your ears?	Are	you	hearing ringing in your ears?

Table 3.52 Continuous tense Wh- questions

Past continuous				Present continuous			
Wh-	was/were	S	V+ing	Wh-	is/are	S	V+ing
What	were	you	doing?	When	are	you	noticing it most?
When	was	it	most painful?	Where	is	it	hurting the most?
Where	was	the pain	radiating?	Where	is	the pain	radiating?

Table 3.53 Present perfect tense yes/no questions

Present perfect		
have/has	S	PP (+C)
Have	you	had any surgeries performed?
Has	this	ever happened before?
Has	he	been around anyone sick recently?

Table 3.54 Present perfect tense Wh- questions

Present perfect			
Wh-	have/has	S	PP (+C)
How long	have	you	had the fever?
For how long	has	he	been in pain?
What immunizations	has	he	had?

Table 3.55 Present perfect continuous tense yes/no questions

Present perfect continuous			
have/has	S	PP	V+ing (+C)
Has	he	been	coughing lately?
Have	you	been	noticing any recent changes?
Has	your baby	started	eating solids?

Table 3.56 Present perfect continuous tense Wh- questions

Present perfect continuous				
Wh-	have/has	S	PP	V+ing (+C)
When	have	you	been	noticing the pain?
How long	have	you	been	feeling this way?
Where	has	he	been	getting treatment?

Modal Verb Tense Questions with "Could"
The following yes/no questions have a rising intonation (▸Table 3.58).

3.4.5 Grammar Review

Verb Tense Identification
What are the tenses in the following questions?

Example: *Have you ever passed out?* __present perfect__ (▸Table 3.59).

Answers: 1. present continuous; 2. present perfect; 3. simple past; 4. past continuous; 5. simple present; 6. modal.

Verb Tense and Meaning
What is the meaning of the following questions? Underline the implied time frame.

Example: *Have you ever passed out?* yesterday/**sometime before now** (▸Table 3.60).

Answers: 1. right now; 2. sometime before now; 3. specific time-past; 4. ongoing-past; 5. regularly; 6. Possibility.

Speaking Exercises: Past Tense Yes/No Question Patterns (▸Table 3.61).

Practice Checklist
The following is an example checklist for Spoken English Proficiency (SEP) on the CS exam. It is for the purpose of training and it has no relation to the actual checklist on the CS exam. While role-playing, let your study partner evaluate you with this scale. For optimal training, use this checklist with your partner for each practice case.

Table 3.57 Modal verb tense questions with "may"

MAY (implies permission)

May	S	BV	O/C
May	I	untie	your gown?
May	I	help	you sit up?
May	I	take	notes while we speak?

Table 3.58 Modal verb tense questions with "could"

COULD (*implies request*)

May	S	BV	O/C
Could	you	tell	me more about your pain?
Could	you	lower	your gown?
Could	you	estimate	the amount of blood you lost?

Table 3.59 Verb tense identification: review

1. Are you feeling nauseous?	_____
2. Have you had a stroke?	_____
3. When did it start?	_____
4. Were you doing anything unusual?	_____
5. Do you smoke?	_____
6. Would you like to quit smoking?	_____

Table 3.60 Verb tense meaning: review

1. Are you feeling nauseous?	right now/regularly
2. Have you had a stroke?	ongoing-past/sometime before now
3. When did it start?	specific time-past/ongoing-past
4. Were you doing anything unusual?	one time-past/ongoing-past
5. Do you smoke?	right now/regularly
6. Would you like to quit smoking?	possibility/right now

Table 3.61 Speaking exercises: past tense yes/no question patterns

Past tense: BE verb	**Past tense: other verbs**
Remember: (Was/Were) + subject	Remember: Did + subject + base verb
Example: You want to know if: there was any pain Ask: *Was there any pain?*	Example: You want to know if: the pain came on suddenly Ask: *Did the pain come on suddenly?*
You want to know if: the SP had continuous previous medical care the baby was full term it was a natural birth there were any complications the SP's temperature was high	You want to know if: the SP felt thirsty the SP had chest pain the SP checked his or her temperature at home the child had any problems at birth the child ate anything unusual
Ask: *Was your previous medical care continuous?* *Was the baby full term?* *Was it a natural birth?* *Were there any complications?* *Was your temperature high?*	Ask: *Did you feel thirsty?* *Did you have chest pain?* *Did you check your temperature at home?* *Did your child have any problems at birth?* *Did your child eat anything unusual?*

3.4.6 Overall Communication Rating

(▶Table 3.62)

Table 3.62 Overall communication rating

		How well did you understand the physician's speech?	How well did the physician understand you?
Completely understood	(15)		
Mostly understood	(10)		
Somewhat understood	(5)		
Did not understand	(0)		

3.4.7 Physician's Spoken English Proficiency

(▶Table 3.63)

Total Score_____ (60 possible).

Table 3.63 Physician's spoken English proficiency

		Clarity of speech	Necessity to repeat words	Word choice
No errors	(10)			
A few errors	(7)			
Some errors	(5)			
Too many errors	(3)			

4 Chest (Cardiology and Respiratory)

Keywords: cardiology, respiratory, dyspnea, chest pain, palpitation, cough, hemoptysis

4.1 Introduction

For the purpose of the Clinical Skills (CS) exam, both the respiratory and cardiac cases have been combined into one chapter. This is because, most of the time, the history questions for the two types of cases are related. Moreover, cardiac and respiratory exams usually need to be done together.

The following is the foundation that serves all chest cases expected on the exam.

4.2 Medical History

4.2.1 Cardiac Cases

Cardiac symptoms: When asking a patient about cardiac symptoms, remember the mnemonic device **CARD**IAC or picture the four of hearts playing card to help you recall the four symptoms you should ask about (▶ **Table 4.1**).

Laboratory investigations for cardiac cases are explained in ▶ **Table 4.2**.

4.2.2 Respiratory Cases

Respiratory symptoms: When asking a patient about respiratory symptoms, remember that there are six symptoms for the upper respiratory system (three in the nose + three inflammatory states) and three for the lower respiratory system: **CCD** (Chest, Cough, Dyspnea; ▶ **Table 4.3**).

Laboratory investigations for respiratory cases **are explained in** ▶ **Table 4.4**.

4.3 Chest Exam

For the purpose of the CS exam, the best practices for heart and lung examinations are the following (▶ **Video. 4.1**):

- A detailed heart exam with focused lung exam is needed in the cases in which the differential diagnoses (DDs) mostly include cardiac problems such as palpitation and syncope.
- A detailed lung exam with focused heart exam is needed in the cases in which the DDs mostly include pulmonary problems such as sore throat, cough, chest infections, pulmonary tuberculosis (TB), etc.
- Both heart and lung exams are needed in the cases in which the DDs include cardiac and pulmonary diseases such as chest pain, dyspnea, and shortness of breath or if you are in doubt.

Start by informing the standardized patients (SPs) that you will examine their chest from behind. Since you cannot examine through the gown, you will need to untie it, but always ask or tell the SP first. In fact, you should always tell the SP what you are going to do and why, especially if you ask the SP to change position or if you touch them. Once the gown is open, you are ready to begin.

Table 4.2 Laboratory investigations for cardiac cases

Prohibited physical exam	No
Laboratory	Cardiac enzymes (CPK-MB, troponin) Lipid profile Blood gases TSH, BMP (basic metabolic panel)
Imaging	CXR CT scan of the chest Echocardiography
Others	ECG

Abbreviations: CPK-MB, creatine phosphokinase myocardial band; CT, computed tomography; CXR, chest X-ray; ECG, electrocardiogram; TSH, thyroid-stimulating hormone.

Table 4.1 Questions for heart symptoms

	Symptom	Question bank
C	Chest pain	*Do you have chest pain?* *If yes, analyze.*
A	Angina	*Do you get tired while walking upstairs?* *While walking outside, do you get any chest pain? Do you have to stop to catch your breath? If yes, ask: After how many blocks?*
R	Racing heart (palpitation)	*Does your heartbeat race like a horse?/Do you feel irregular beats in your chest?*
D	Dyspnea	*Have you ever had difficulty breathing?* *For paroxysmal nocturnal dyspnea (PND), ask:* *Have you had episodes of difficulty breathing at night?* *For orthopnea, ask:* *Do you have trouble breathing while lying back?/Do you use extra pillows to be more comfortable while sleeping?*
	+ Peripheral edema	*Have you had any swelling in your legs? (There is no need to repeat this if already asked in the general exam.)*

Table 4.3 Questions for respiratory symptoms

Respiratory system	Symptoms	Question bank
Upper 3 in nose	Secretions (outside) Postnasal drip (inside) Nasal allergies	*Have you had a runny nose?* *Do you have postnasal drip?* *Have you been sneezing?*
3 inflammations	Sinusitis	*Do your sinuses feel tender?/Do you have headaches?*
	Pharyngitis Laryngitis	*Do you have a sore throat? Difficulty swallowing?* *Has your voice changed recently?*
Lower	Chest pain Cough + mucus Dyspnea + wheeze	*Do you have any chest pain?* *Have you been coughing lately? If yes, ask:* *Do you cough up any mucus? If yes, ask* ABC questions (see Chapter 1, The Basics, Component 1, Integrated Clinical Encounter) *Have you had any difficulty breathing?* or *Have you felt short of breath? Any chest wheezing?*

Table 4.4 Laboratory investigations for respiratory cases

Prohibited physical exam	No
Laboratory	Sputum studies: (culture and sensitivity, gram stain, and AFB) Blood gases D-dimer (for pulmonary embolism)
Imaging	CXR CT scan of the chest, and CT angiogram
Others	Pulmonary function test A purified protein derivative (PPD) skin test

Abbreviations: AFB, acid-fast bacillus; CT, computed tomography; CXR, chest X-ray.

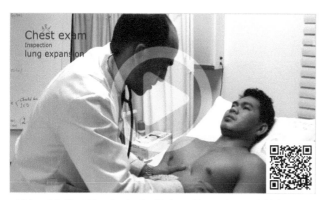

Video. 4.1 Chest Examination for CS. https://www.thieme.de/de/q.htm?p=opn/cs/20/3/11450545-128e49a0

4.3.1 Lung Exam

Inspection:
Inform the SP that you will check their back for any deformities (▶ **Fig. 4.1**).

Palpation:
Start with a test for lung expansion. Put both thumbs on the spine and ask the patient to take a deep breath (▶ **Fig. 4.2**). Then, press gently on each side, one side at a time, to check for pain or tenderness (▶ **Fig. 4.3**). Move to a higher or lower position and repeat. Check the tactile vocal fremitus (TVF) by asking the SP to say "ninety-nine" while touching the chest wall with the ulnar border of your hand (▶ **Fig. 4.4**). Any dulling is indicative of possible consolidation.

Percussion:
Tap the chest looking for any air or excess fluid. Do the percussion test on at least one spot on each side (▶ **Fig. 4.5**).

Auscultation:
Warm the stethoscope as you inform the SP that you will listen to the chest and that they should inhale and exhale deeply while you have the stethoscope pressed to their chest (▶ **Fig. 4.6**).

Then ask the SP to lie back (45 degrees) and to lower the gown, and do another auscultation on the front of the chest. If this is a pulmonary case (e.g., pneumonia, cough), inspect, palpate, and do another percussion test on the front side. Then, do a quick heart examination.

Don't:
Remove the stethoscope until the patient has completely finished exhaling or inhaling (complete cycle).

Palpate, tap, or auscultate on the scapula while examining the lungs.

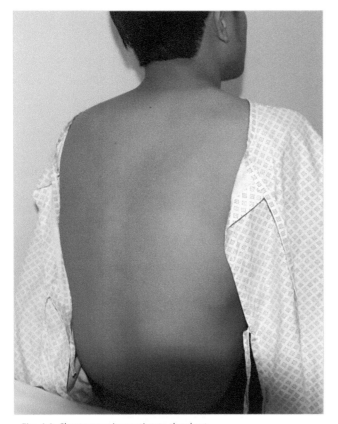

Fig. 4.1 Chest exam: inspection to the chest.

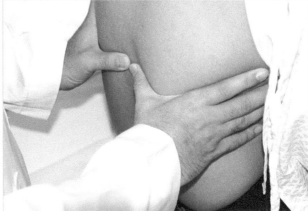

Fig. 4.2 Chest exam: test for lung expansion.

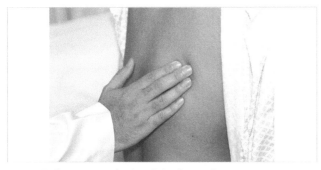

Fig. 4.3 Chest exam: palpation of the chest wall.

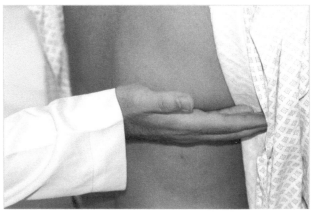

Fig. 4.4 Chest exam: tactile vocal fremitus.

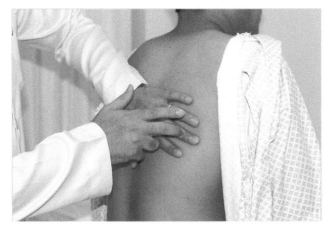

Fig. 4.5 Chest exam: percussion to the lung.

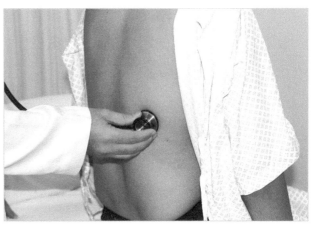

Fig. 4.6 Chest exam: auscultation to the lung.

Practice

Here is a sample script you can use to practice giving lung exam:

"Now, I am going to examine your chest from the back. May I untie your gown? I am starting by looking at your back, just to see if there are any deformities that might affect the chest. Okay, your back looks perfect. Take a deep breath in please. This is a test for chest expansion.

Now I will press on the back of your chest. Does it hurt here? What about here?

Can you say 99 for me, please? Great! Now please say it once more. Thank you!

I will tap on your chest to check for any air or excess fluid around the lungs.

I'm going to listen to your lungs. Please take a deep breath. Sounds fine!

Now, I will listen to your lungs from the front. Could you please lie down for me? Let me first fix the bed and pull out the leg extension so you can be comfortable. Could you lower your gown for me? Thank you!"

If the complaint is mainly respiratory, repeat the steps on the front of the chest and do auscultation of the heart.

4.3.2 Heart Exam

As always, inform the SP of what you are going to do: *"I'm going to examine your heart."*

While the patient is sitting, start by checking the point of the maximal impulse (PMI). Put your hand on the apex of the heart. That is at the fifth intercostal space at the mid-clavicular line.

Listen to the heart at each of the four cardiac areas:
- *Aortic:* at the right second intercostal space, near the sternum (▶**Fig. 4.7**).
- *Pulmonary:* at the left second intercostal space, near the sternum.
- *Tricuspid:* at the left lower sternal border.
- *Mitral:* at the apex (▶**Fig. 4.8**).

With female SPs, and when it is hard to listen to the heart due to the breast, ask them to lift the breast: *"Could you please lift your breast?"*

If it is a respiratory case, this is sufficient for a heart exam. For a detailed cardiac exam, there are three additional steps to complete:
- *Two at the heart:* auscultation at left lateral and leaning forward.
- Two signs at the neck.
- Two peripheral signs.

At the Heart:
Auscultate the heart from the **left lateral decubitus position** for any mitral murmurs (▶**Fig. 4.9**). While you are still wearing the stethoscope, use the bell and ask the SP to roll onto their left side. Do not forget to tell them to roll back when you have finished. Then ask them to **lean forward**, take a deep breath, and then let it out. Next, ask them to hold their breath. Listen at the third left intercostal spaces for aortic regurgitation (▶**Fig. 4.10**).

At the Neck:
Put your stethoscope over the carotid and ask the SP to take a deep breath and to hold it while you listen for a few seconds **for a bruit**. Remember to listen for carotid bruits before

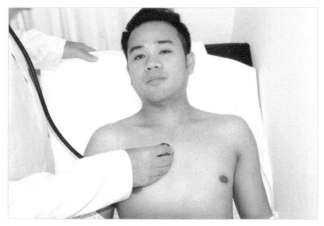
Fig. 4.7 Auscultation at the aortic area.

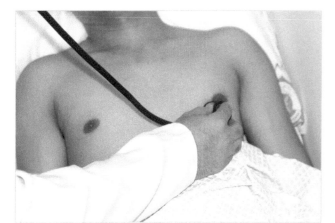
Fig. 4.8 Auscultation at the apex.

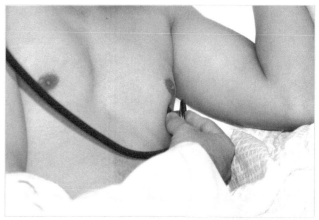
Fig. 4.9 Auscultation of the heart from the left lateral decubitus position.

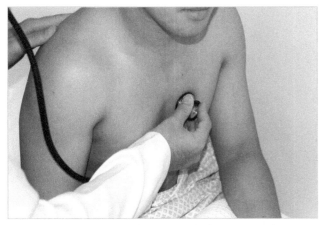

Fig. 4.10 Auscultation of the heart at the third left intercostal space.

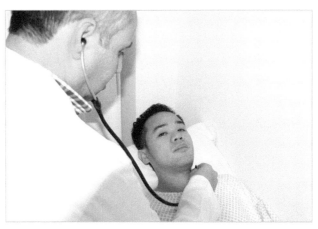

Fig. 4.11 Auscultation for carotid bruits.

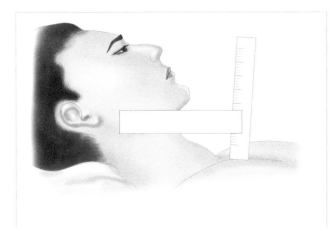

Fig. 4.12 Jugular venous distension (JVD).

palpating the neck in cardiac patients. Repeat on the other side (▶**Fig. 4.11**). The second neck sign is to check for jugular venous distension (**JVD**). It should be done while the SP is lying down with their head at 45-degree angle. Just look briefly and move to the next step (▶**Fig. 4.12**).

Two peripheral signs:
First, check for **peripheral pulsation** (radial, brachial in the upper limb and posterior tibial in the lower leg). Second, check for **peripheral edema** in the lower limbs. Skip steps that were done in the general exam.

Practice

Here is a sample script you can use to practice giving a heart exam:

"Now, allow me to examine your heart. I am feeling the apex of your heart. I am going to listen to your heart. Please breathe normally.

Now could you roll over on your left side? Could you roll back?

Could you lean forward for me? Could you lean a little more forward? Please take a deep breath in, out, could you hold your breath? Thanks, you can breathe normally now. I will re-tie your gown. Thanks

Now I'm going to listen to the veins in your neck, so please take a deep breath and hold it.

Now, I will examine your neck veins. Please look over to your left.

Thanks and you can breathe normally now.

Okay, we have almost finished. I just need to take your pulse. Please hold out your arm.

I am going to examine your leg for any swelling."

Role-Play 1: Sore Throat

Doorway Information

Mr. Donald Mavic, 35 year-old male, has a **sore throat**.

Vital signs:

- Temperature (Temp): 101°F (38.3° C).
- Heart rate (HR): 84/min, regular.
- Blood pressure (BP): 120/80 mm Hg.
- Respiration rate (RR): 16/min.

Examinee tasks:

- Obtain a focused history.
- Perform a relevant physical examination. Do not perform rectal, pelvic, genitourinary, inguinal hernia, female breast, or corneal reflex exam.
- Discuss your initial diagnosis and your workup plan with the patient.
- After leaving the room, complete the patient note (PN) on the given form.

Standardized Patient's Role

You have a sore throat and have had difficulty swallowing for 2 weeks. You feel feverish; you took your temperature at home and it was 101°F. The fever abates when you take Tylenol. You have a mild 3 out of 10 abdominal pain on the left side that is a constant ache.

You are taking over-the-counter (OTC) medication for the pain and fever. Your appetite is decreased and you feel tired. You haven't lost any weight recently.

Your roommate has been sick recently. You had an appendectomy 20 years ago and are allergic to penicillin. You had urethral discharge 6 months ago that was treated. You smoke one pack of cigarettes per day, and you have smoked for 10 years. You consume one alcoholic beverage a day and more on the weekends. You have multiple sexual partners (both male and female) and only occasionally use a condom. You are a full-time tennis teacher.

When the doctor examines you, pretend that the upper left side of your torso is tender.

As the doctor finishes the exam, ask these questions:

Q1: Are the symptoms that I am experiencing indicative of someone having HIV?

Q2: There is a big tennis tournament this weekend, and I am scheduled to play. I would like to participate. What do you think?

Please refer to Chapter 13 (Appendix), to review the general instructions for the SP as well as the Doctor roles.

Role-Play 1: Answer Key

Review the pain and fever questions in previous chapters before starting the history. After you read the doorway information, come up with a preliminary DD. Though findings are rare in most cases on the CS exam, you will need to use a tongue depressor in the exam.

History

Analysis of Chief Complaint

Sore throat:
- *When did it start? Since it started, has it gotten worse or stayed the same?*
- *How bad does it hurt?*
- *Do you have difficulty swallowing?*
- *Does anything relieve your discomfort, such as hot drinks?*
- *Does anything make your sore throat worse, such as smoking?*

Fever: As routine.

Analysis of Differential Diagnosis

Common cold:
Ask about upper respiratory tract symptoms.

Infectious mononucleosis:
- *Do you feel tired?*
- *Are any of your glands swollen?*
- *Does your stomach hurt?*

Infectious diseases:
- *Have you been around anybody sick?*
- *Have you traveled outside the country recently?*
- *What about your shots? Are you up-to-date with them?*

Review of the Local System

Ask about other symptoms of the respiratory tract, such as cough.

Review of Systems

SAW (sleep, appetite, and weight), 2 systems in male (GI and urinary) (see Chapter 1, The Basics, Component 1, Integrated Clinical Encounter).

Past History and Others

PDS for **PDA** for Fast Surgery ± Scar: (see Chapter 1, The Basics, Component 1, Integrated Clinical Encounter), Sex Life: Ask in detail.

Physical Exam

Vital Signs (VS) may change hormones (ADH, NE, LH) that are given by Local Shots.

VS: Obtain VS from doorway information. Document the SP's appearance and decubitus (position).

Head: Check head for tenderness of the sinuses, and look for swollen lymph nodes (LNs). Do eye and full ear, nose, and throat (ENT) exam, especially throat. Use a tongue depressor (▶ **Fig. 4.13**).

Neck: Check for swollen LNs.

LH: Do a focused heart and lung exam unless the SP has other problems that may need a detailed exam (as cough).

Local exam: Palpate abdomen to check for tenderness at left upper quadrant (LUQ; splenomegaly).

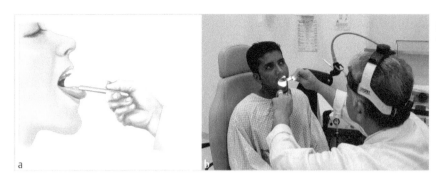

Fig. 4.13 (a, b) Tongue depressor and throat exam.

Communication and Interpersonal Skills Component

Suggested Closure

"Mr. Maci, just to be sure I have understood it right, I am going to repeat what you told me and correct me if I'm wrong. You have a sore throat and have had difficulty swallowing for 2 weeks now. You have a fever and are feeling tired, and your roommate has been sick.

Well, based on your history and my physical examination (PE), your problem may just be a simple viral infection in your throat. However, I cannot eliminate other possible causes at this point in time, without having some tests done. When the results come back, I will sit with you again to tell you the final diagnosis and treatment options."

Counseling

Advise to quit smoking, use safe sex practices, and avoid heavy exercise.

"As you know, smoking is the leading cause of heart attack, stroke, and lung cancers. I usually advise my patients to quit smoking (see more in Chapter 2, The Basics, Component 2, Communication and Interpersonal Skills). You have multiple sexual partners but only occasionally use condoms. As you know, that puts you at risk for STDs, including HIV. How would you feel about taking an HIV test? I need to stress that condom use is recommended to keep you and others safe.

I strongly recommend avoiding any intense physical activity for a couple of weeks, to avoid any serious bleeding in your stomach. Now, do you have any questions for me?"

Suggested Answers to the SP's Questions

Q1: *There is no way that we can definitively know if you have HIV unless you take a test. To answer your question in any other way would be premature.*

Q2: *I understand your desire to participate; however, I must caution you against strenuous exercise in your condition. You could be at risk of serious bleeding in your stomach. Accordingly, I advise you to skip the tennis tournament at this time until we know more about what is causing the trouble?*

Patient Note

History

A 35-year-old male has sore throat for 2 weeks associated with dysphagia, fever that responds to Tylenol, mild LUQ pain, 3/10 dull aching pain, nonradiating. Denies rhinorrhea, cough, chest pain, and dyspnea; has not noticed any swollen glands. His roommate has been sick. **Review of system (ROS):** tired, ↓ appetite, no loss of weight, urinary or bowel problems. **Past medical history (PMH):** appendectomy 20 years ago. **Med:** OTC. **Allergy (All):** penicillin. **SH:** tennis player, smokes 1 pack per day (ppd)/10 y, and drinks heavily on weekends. **Sexual history:** multiple sexual partners (male and female) with occasional condom use. No HIV test done. Past history of urethral discharge that was treated 6 months ago.

Physical Exam

VS: within normal limit (WNL) except for fever = 101°F. No acute distress, alert, oriented ×3.
Head and neck (H&N): PERRLA (pupils equal, round, reactive to light and accommodation), normal tympanic membranes (TMs) exam, nose w/o rhinorrhea, mouth w/o erythema, no tenderness of the sinuses, and no palpable LNs.
Extremities (Ext): Regular pulse, no peripheral edema.
Chest: No deformities, TVF normal, no focal tenderness, CTA/BL (clear to auscultation bilaterally) no rhonchi.
Heart: Normal S1 and S2.
Abdomen: lax, tenderness over LUQ, no rebound, bowel sounds (BS) +.

Differential Diagnosis

History finding(s)	Physical exam finding(s)
1. Viral pharyngitis	
Sore throat	
Feels feverish	Fever = 101°F
Difficulty swallowing	
2. Infectious mononucleosis	
Sore throat	
Feels feverish	Fever = 101°F
Mild LUQ pain	Tenderness over LUQ
Tired, ↓ appetite	
Contact with sick person	
3. HIV infection	
Feels feverish	Fever = 101°F
Multiple sexual partners (male, female), occasional use of condom	
Past history urethral discharge	
Tired, ↓ appetite	

Abbreviations: HIV, human immunodeficiency virus; LUQ, left upper quadrant.

Diagnostic Studies

Pelvic exam

Rapid strep test, monospot test

HIV virus load, CD4 count

Abdominal ultrasound (US)

Role-Play 2: A Telephone Encounter

A telephone encounter with Miss Baldwin, whose father has shortness of breath.

Standardized Patient's Role

Your father is 60 years old. He became short of breath (SOB) 15 minutes ago, and you are calling the hospital, as you are very worried about his breathing difficulty.

Ask the physician as he starts the conversation, **Comment 1**: *"Doc I'm so worried about my father. He cannot breathe. He needs help!"*

The SOB was of acute onset and progressive with no alleviating factors. Your father also has severe 8 out of 10 chest pain on the right side of his chest. The pain is nonradiating. He also complains of an extremely fast heartbeat.

He is bedridden. He had a total hip replacement surgery 2 weeks ago and was discharged from the hospital 2 days ago.

He has peptic ulcer and is taking omeprazole. You remember a similar episode last year when your father had colon surgery. The doctors told you that he had a clot in his lung.

Q1: *"Doctor, could it be another blood clot in this lung?"*
   He is an ex-smoker. He quit 10 years ago (smoked 2 ppd/25 y), and he drinks socially.
   Your mother died 2 years ago. You and your father live together.
   If the physician asks you to bring your father to the ER, say the following.
Q2: *"Doc, I don't have a car, and I've got children at home. Could you just prescribe some medication for now?"*

Please refer to Chapter 13 (Appendix), to review the general instructions for the SP as well as the Doctor roles.

Role-Play 2: Answer Key

SOB is usually an acute case on the CS exam. The SPs complaining of dyspnea and chest pain may hold their hands on their chest, pretending to be in severe pain. They often appear agitated and ask for painkillers.

This role-play is a telephone encounter, but if the SP attends and is an emergency case, it has special concerns. When you enter the room, impress upon the SP that you are motivated to help them, that you are concerned about their condition, that you are sympathetic. Communicate this by your facial expression, your tone of voice, and your body language. It may even be appropriate to soothe a patient by putting your hand on their shoulder. Please refer to Chapter 2, The Basics, Component 2, Communication and Interpersonal Skills for more details.

History

Analysis of Chief Complaint

Shortness of breath
- *When did it start? Since it started, has it gotten worse?*
- *Is it continuous or does it come and go?*

If it comes and goes, ask: *How often does he have shortness of breath?*
- *When was the last time? How long does it last? What makes it better?*
- *What makes it worse?*

Associations: *Does it come with chest pain? Has he ever passed out?*

Analysis of Differential Diagnosis

Cardiac Causes:
Ask CARD questions.

SOB, severe acute chest pain on the left side that radiates to the left arm and is accompanied by other heart attack symptoms, and diaphoresis may indicate **acute coronary syndrome.**

Long history of dyspnea, paroxysmal nocturnal dyspnea (PND), orthopnea, and lower limb edema may point to **congestive heart failure** (CHF).

Respiratory Causes:
Ask questions for upper and lower respiratory symptoms.

Acute onset, recent history of surgery, bone fracture, and prolonged bed rest are symptoms suggestive of **pulmonary embolism.**

Ask: *Has he had any recent surgeries done?/Were the previous few weeks complicated by prolonged bed rest?*

Heavy smokers with chronic cough and thick mucus may indicate chronic obstructive pulmonary disease (**COPD**) exacerbation.

Pneumonia is a possible DD when there is a fever combined with a productive cough.

Bronchial asthma: *Does he have any chest wheezing?*

Others:
Panic attack is a good choice for young, female SPs who are under a lot of stress. *Do you have any kind of stress at work? At home?/Is anything causing you worry?/How is your sleep?*

Review of the Local System

Already asked.

Review of Systems

I SAW two systems.

Past History and Others

D (heart, hypertension [HTN], diabetes mellitus [DM]), S (recent surgery), P (similar episodes), F (heart attack), S (work), ±S (don't ask).

Physical Exam

No physical exam for telephone encounter cases; consider the following for a live SP. **VS** may change hormones (**ADH + NE + LH**) that are given by local shots.

VSs: Usually, there are tachycardia and tachypnea.

Appearance: SP appears acutely distressed.

Head exam: Check for pallor, cyanosis, and do fundus exam.

Neck: Check for carotid bruit and JVD.

Ext: Check for peripheral pulse.

Lung and Heart: Conduct a detailed heart and lung exams.

Communication and Interpersonal Skills Component

Suggested Closure

As with any telephone encounter, once you have finished, ask the patient to come to the hospital for a PE. If the SP expresses reluctance to, or says they cannot, maintain that they need to come immediately:

> *"Ma'am, let me review with you what I know so far. According to you, your father has … and, he is … and …. You told me also he was discharged from the hospital 2 days ago. Based on the history, it could be another blood clot in his lung as he is at risk for that, since he has been bedridden for a long time, and he has just had major surgery, and he had a blood clot last year.*

> *As you might guess, I cannot rely on his medical history alone. I need to see him to do a PE. I'll examine his chest and heart and also run some tests. Really, you need to bring him to the hospital right away. I will inform the ER to call me as you arrive. Do you have any questions?"*

Counseling

Hypertension, DM, and smoking.

Suggested Answers to the SP's Questions, Comments

Comment 1: *"Well, I understand your concern. I will do everything possible to make your father feel better."*

Q1: *"Well, I understand your concern. Please just give me a few minutes to ask you a few questions regarding your father's health. I will take some notes and then answer your question as soon as we have finished with the medical history."*

Q2: *"Your father's condition is a true emergency. Please call 911 now for an ambulance. Bring your children with you if you cannot find a baby sitter. I will contact one of our social workers to assist you. I will have the ER call me when you arrive and I will meet you there. Any other questions? Thanks and see you soon!"*

Patient Note

History

The source of information is the daughter of a 60-year-old man. He became SOB 15 minutes ago. The onset was acute, and the course was progressive with no alleviating factors. It is associated with dyspnea and chest pain in the right side, which is nonradiating, rated at 8/10, sharp and constant, combined with palpitation. He has been bedridden for the last 2 weeks. No orthopnea, PND, cough, or chest wheezing. ROS: Normal appetite and sleep, no fever or edema of the leg, normal urinary and bowel. PMH: peptic ulcer, total right hip replacement surgery 2 weeks ago. Past history of similar episode last year after a colonic surgery. Med: omeprazole. No heparin use. Family history (FH): lives with daughter at home. His wife died 2 years ago. Social history (SH): ex-smoker for 10 years (smoked 2 ppd/25 y), drinks socially, doesn't use street drugs.

Physical Exam

N/D (not done).

Differential Diagnosis

History finding(s)	Physical exam finding(s)
1. Pulmonary embolism	
Acute SOB, dyspnea	
Chest pain, palpitation	
Bed ridden and recent surgery	
2. Acute MI	
Acute SOB	
Chest pain, palpitation	
60-year-old	

Abbreviations: MI, myocardial infarction; SOB, short of breath.

Diagnostic Studies

Arterial blood gas (ABG), D-dimer, cardiac enzymes

Serum electrolytes

ECHO, chest X-ray (CXR), CT angiogram, Doppler US lower limbs

Electrocardiogram (ECG)

Role-Play 3

Mr. Richard Davis, 35-year-old male patient, complains of cough.
Vital signs:
- Temp: 100.4°F (38°C).
- HR: 94/min, regular.
- BP: 120/80 mm Hg.
- RR: 16/min.

Standardized Patient's Role

You have been coughing for 3 days now. It was mild, but is now much worse. When it started, it was a dry cough, but now you cough up whitish-yellow mucus. You haven't seen any blood.

You have had a common cold with a runny nose for the last week, but you are much better. You still have a mild sore throat, post-nasal drip, and a mild headache. You took an OTC medicine and that has helped, but cough is still worse at night. You feel pressure in your sinuses. You have mild chest pain (4/10) all over your chest that ↑ when you take a deep breath. Your 8-year-old child had the flu last week.

You and your father have bronchial asthma (BA). You usually have two episodes of sinusitis per year as you have nasal allergies. You are sensitive to pollen and pets. You are taking albuterol MDI (metered-dose inhaler) and Claritin. You smoke 1/2 ppd/10 y and drink socially.

When the doctor examines you, pretend that your sinuses are tender.

Ask the doctor:
Q1: *"Doc, could you prescribe me some antibiotics?"*
Q2: *"Could I have caught this flu from my son?"*

Role-Play 3: Answer Key

On the CS exam, coughing is usually due to **respiratory tract infections,** exactly like those you would encounter in a family doctor's office. If the patient has a long history of heavy smoking, or they have thick sputum, consider **COPD** as a DD. Patients with **CHF** may have also cardiac dyspnea, PND, and orthopnea. Consider **pulmonary TB** if there is fever with chills, night sweating, and recent history of travel outside the United States. Rarely on the CS is g**astroesophageal reflux disease** (GERD) a cause for chronic cough. Do not forget to ask about medication history. Remember use of **angiotensin-converting enzyme (ACE) inhibitors** is a common DD for cough on the CS exam.

History

Analysis of Chief Complaint

Cough and Fever.

Analysis of Differential Diagnosis

Respiratory:
Respiratory tract infections: Ask the respiratory symptoms questions (upper and lower).

For **pulmonary TB**: *Do you have night sweats? Chills? Any unintentional loss of weight?*

For infectious diseases: *Have you been around any sick people recently? Have you traveled outside the United States recently? Are your immunization shots up-to-date?*

Cardiac:
Ask CARD questions.

Others:
Medication side effect of "**ACE inhibitor**": *Have you started to take a new medicine when this problem came on? Do you think this issue is a side effect of any new medicine?*

Gastrointestinal system causes such as **GERD**: *Do you have any heartburn?*

Review of the Local System

Respiratory symptoms questions were already asked.

Review of Systems

Past History and Others

As routine, stress on medications (ACE inhibitor), allergies (allergic rhinitis and BA), and smoking.

Physical Exam

VS: Obtain VS from doorway information. Document them in your PN; fever refers to respiratory tract infection.
ADH, NE: Do full ENT exam and tenderness of the sinuses, and check for LNs. For cardiac causes and hypertensive cases, do fundus exam and listen to the carotid bruit.
LH: A detailed lung exam with a focused heart exam is needed. If you suspect cardiac causes, also do a detailed heart exam.

Communication and Interpersonal Skills Component

Suggested Closure

As routine.

Counseling

Smoking.

Suggested Answers to the SP's Questions

Q1: *"I understand your concern, but I need to run some blood work first to see what's going on. If it's a bacterial infection, antibiotics will be effective. However, if it's viral or anything else, antibiotics will be useless or even harmful, because as you may know, antibiotics are only for bacterial infections."*

Q2: *"Well, you have flu symptoms, so it's possible that you have contracted the flu from your child, but I can't say for sure at this time. I will need to run some tests to be sure."*

History

A 35-year-old male complains of cough for 3 days, gradual in onset, present all the time, worse at night, and better with OTC meds. Started as dry cough, then associated with little whitish-yellow thin mucus with no blood, mild sore throat, postnasal drip, mild headache, and tender sinuses. Has mild chest pain (4/10) all over his chest, getting worse in taking a deep breath. Denies any voice change, difficulty breathing, heartburn, orthopnea, recent travel, exposure to TB patient, or use of new medication. He has been around his 8-year-old son who had flu last week. ROS: Normal sleep and appetite, no change in weight and no urinary or bowel habit problems. PH: bronchial asthma, sinusitis. Meds: albuterol MDI, loratadine. ALL: pets and pollen. FH: father with asthma. SH: tobacco use 1/2 ppd/10 y, drinks socially. Irrelevant sexual history.

Physical Exam

VS: WNL apart from fever (100.4°F). Alert and conscious with no acute distress.
HEENT (head, eye, ear, nose, throat): tender sinus, no enlargement of LNs, ears have normal TM, nose is w/o rhinorrhea, noncongested nasal turbinates, throat w/o erythema.
Ext: No pallor or cyanosis. **Chest:** no chest deformities, normal TVFs, no air or fluid per percussion, CTA, B/L no wheezes or crepitation, normal S1 and S2, no murmurs.

Differential Diagnosis

History finding(s)	Physical exam finding(s)
1. Acute bronchitis	
Cough with mucus	
Feels feverish	Fever (100.4°F)
History of common cold	
Mild chest pain 4/10 all over the chest	
2. Acute sinusitis	
Cough with mucus	
Feel feverish	Fever (100.4°F)
History of common cold and sinusitis	Sinus tenderness
Post nasal drip	
3. Pleurisy	
Diffuse chest pain	
Pain increases with deep inspiration	

Diagnostic Studies

Sputum culture

CXR

Return to clinic if acutely worsening after 1 week (suggestive of bacterial infection)

Role-Play 4: Rapidly Beating Heart

Doorway Information

Mrs. Anna Rodriguez, 20-year-old, complains of a **rapidly beating heart**.
Vital signs:
- Temp: 98.6°F (37°C).
- HR: 84/min, regular.
- BP: 110/70 mm Hg.
- RR: 20/min.

Standardized Patient's Role

For the past 3 weeks, your heart has been felt like it is going to explode at times. It does not happen often, but yesterday it happened three times. It persists for a few minutes, and the last time it happened was 3 hours ago. When the feeling comes on, it is accompanied by mild chest pain, on the left side of your chest. It is nonradiating and you rate the intensity of the pain at 4 out of 10.

You also have had difficulty sleeping recently. It takes around 1 to 2 hours to fall asleep. You remember having a similar episode last year, just before final exam week, and you are worried about passing the exam. Your last menstrual period (LMP) was 2 weeks ago and regular. You had a pap smear done 2 years ago and it was normal.

You are a college student, drink four cups of coffee a day, smoke 2 ppd/5 y, and drink socially. You are sexually active, monogamous with your boyfriend, and always use condoms.

Ask the doctor
Q1: *Do you think I will pass my exams?*
Q2: *Why does my heart beat so fast when I'm nervous? Is that normal?*

Role-Play 4: Answer Key

Palpitation is a common complaint on the CS exam. Why? Stress is so common in life and is often the cause of what patients perceive as palpitations. Think about high-pressure jobs, everyday worries, broken hearts, caffeine consumption, smoking, and sleepless nights. Causes of palpitation are organic (cardiac causes, hyperthyroidism, pheochromocytoma) and stress/psychiatric/others (anxiety disorder and caffeine overconsumption).

This is reflected on the CS exam. Many of the SPs will complain of a rapid heartbeat. The cause of the SPs' palpitation is often something simple. The test makers don't want to confuse you—they want to see how you apply your knowledge in a basic medical situation.

History

Analysis of Chief Complaint

Ask questions for complaints that come in episodes (see Chapter 1, The Basics, Component 1, Integrated Clinical Encounter).
- *When did it start? Since it started, has it gotten worse or stayed the same?*

Association:
- *When it comes on, do you get lightheaded?*
- *What about dizziness?*
- *Do your hands shake?*
- *Have you ever passed out?*

Analysis of Differential Diagnosis

Cardiac (valvular, HTN, IHD, and cardiomyopathy): ▶Fig. 4.14 shows ECG with supraventricular tachycardia (SVT). Ask CARD questions.
Hyperthyroidism: Ask the questions for hyperthyroidism.
Pheochromocytoma: *Is it accompanied by a headache?*
When it comes on, do you start sweating?
Anxiety disorder: *Do you have any kind of stress at home? At work?*
Are you worried about anything? Have you been sleeping well?
Caffeine overconsumption: *Do you drink coffee? How many cups do you drink per day?*
Others: Anemia and drug abuse.

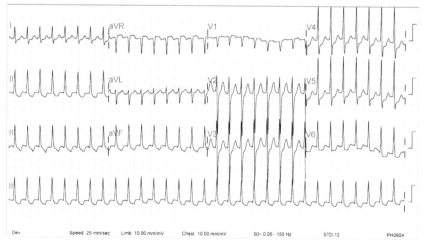

Fig. 4.14 ECG with supraventricular tachycardia.

Review of the Local System

As a standard.

Review of Systems

As a standard.

Past History and Others

D (heart diseases, thyroid problems), **P** (similar episodes), **D** (any sympathomimetic), **F** (heart disease in the family), **S** (stress, caffeine, smoking, alcohol).

Physical Exam

VS: Obtain VS from doorway information, look for tachycardia in the VS, document that in your PN.
ADH, NE: As routine, pay particular attention to the **thyroid** and check for *hand tremors*.
LH: A detailed heart exam with a focused lung exam is needed.
Local: Do a quick abdominal exam; feel for any organomegaly to eliminate the possibility of pheochromocytoma.

Communication and Interpersonal Skills Component

Suggested Closure

"Miss Rodriguez, let me review what we know so far. You are worried about your heart and you feel that it has been beating abnormally fast. You told me also that you are quite nervous and worried about an upcoming final exam. In addition, you admit to being a heavy smoker and drinking a lot of coffee. One or more of these things could be causing your condition. The problem may simply be related to your anxiety. However, I cannot eliminate anything without first running some tests. So, we can be sure to find out what is causing your rapid heartbeat. Also, we need to take some pictures of your heart just to be sure that everything is doing fine. When the results come back, then we can sit and I will give you my final diagnosis at that time. Do you have any other questions or concerns?"

Counseling

Coffee, smoking, sleep.

Suggested Answers to the SP's Questions

Q1: *"I sure hope you get an A+. I'm going to do what I can to maximize your health so you don't have to worry about that on exam day."*

Q2: *"Good question. A temporarily rapidly beating heart is not so abnormal. Simply speaking, nervousness stimulates the sympathetic nervous system. This system is a part of the greater nervous system. It prepares different parts of our body to handle large amounts of stress. One way in which it does this is by stimulating the heart to beat faster and stronger to satisfy the body's needs. I can give you a pamphlet if you would like to know more about his phenomenon."*

Patient Note

History

A 20-year-old woman complains of palpitation. The problem started few weeks ago. Initially, it was infrequent, but now it occurs one to three times a day. The last one was 3 hours ago and lasted for few minutes. It worsens when the patient experiences stress, consumes caffeine, or lacks sleep. It is accompanied by mild chest pain (4/10) on the left side and is nonradiating. Patient has never passed out, experienced light headedness, orthopnea, or PND. Denies heat intolerance. ROS: insomnia, good appetite, no urinary or bowel problems, LMP was 2 weeks ago, last Pap smear 2 years ago and it was normal. PMH: previous episode last year, which also occurred just prior to final exam week. Med: sleep meds. NKDA. FH: irrelevant. SH: college student, smokes 2 ppd/5 y, drinks 4 cups of coffee/d, drinks socially. Sexual history: active with one boyfriend.

Physical Exam

VS: WNL apart from tachycardia (pulse: 100), appears anxious.
H&N: PERRLA, normal thyroid gland, no JVD, pallor, or cyanosis.
Ext: normal peripheral pulsation, no tremors.
Chest: CTA/BL.
Heart: PMI not displaced. Normal S1 and S2, no gallop or rub.
Abdomen: soft, no organomegaly.

Differential Diagnosis

History finding(s)	Physical exam finding(s)
1. Anxiety disorder	
Palpitation and Insomnia	Tachycardia (pulse: 100/min)
Nervous, worried about passing exams	Appears anxious
No heat intolerance	Normal thyroid exam
Heavy smoker	No recent weight loss or organomegaly
2. Cardiac arrhythmia	
Palpitation	Tachycardia (pulse: 100/min)
Chest pain	No recent weight loss
No heat intolerance	Normal thyroid exam
3. Caffeine induced	
Palpitation	Tachycardia (pulse: 100/min)
Drinks 4 cups/d	No recent weight loss
No heat intolerance	Normal thyroid exam

Diagnostic Studies

Complete blood count (CBC), vanillylmandelic acid (VMA) in urine and thyroid-stimulating hormone (TSH)

Echo, CXR

ECG

Introduction to Chest Pain Cases on the CS Exam

Before starting the encounter and while reading the doorway information for a chest pain case, look at the age and VS. On CS exam, chest pain at a young age with normal VS has a DD that is different than an SP at an older age with abnormal VS (tachycardia and/or tachypnea).

Chest pain is a common case on the CS exam and sometimes there is more than one case with chest pain with different diagnoses. It may come as an acute or nonacute case on the exam.

History

Analysis of Chief Complain

Chest pain → analyze pain as usual.

Analysis of Differential Diagnosis

Think of the chest from the outside-in: chest wall, pleura, lung, heart, and others; please look at the diagram (▶ Fig. 4.15). Mark the following causes on the fig. 4.15 that will help you to remember them on the exam (if you draw this picture on the exam too).

Chest wall: Costochondritis.
- *Was it preceded by any chest trauma?*
- *Did you hurt your chest?*
- *Does the pain change when you change position?*
- *Do you feel the pain anywhere else?* (Pain usually changes with position and is nonradiating.)

Pleura
Pleurisy:
- *Does the pain get worse when you take a deep breath? Have you had any recent respiratory tract infection?*

Pneumothorax:
- *Have you had a chest injury?*

Lung:
Pneumonia and pulmonary embolism; ask about lower respiratory tract symptoms.

Pericardium: Pericarditis and pericardial effusion.
- *Have you had any recent respiratory tract infection?*

Heart: Acute coronary syndrome (angina and MI [myocardial infarction]), cardiac, arrhythmia, and aortic dissection. Ask CARDiac questions.

Others: Panic attack and GERD.

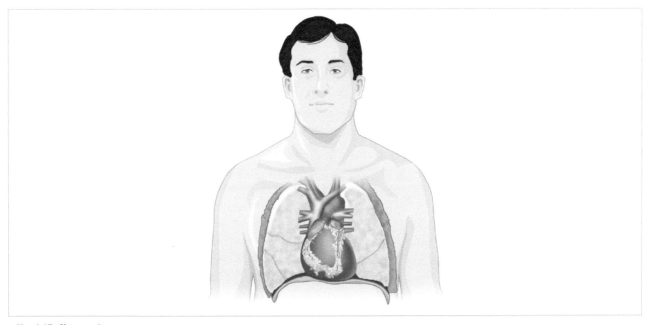

Fig. 4.15 Chest cavity contents.

Although the DD of chest pain is wide, there are clues to help you narrow the focus.

Age: In young patients, consider panic attack, costochondritis, pericarditis, and pleurisy, mitral valve prolapse.
- In young and athletic people, consider costochondritis and hypertrophic cardiomyopathy (syncope). With fever and productive cough, bronchopneumonia or pneumonia may be considered.
- *Old age with many risk factors (smoking, HTN, hypercholesterolemia, DM):* Consider acute coronary syndrome.

Recent history of **surgery,** prolonged bed rest, or recent leg pain or swelling may be indicative of **pulmonary embolism.**

Recent history of URT infection increases suspicion of **pericarditis** (pain that increases when lying back and decreases when leaning forward) and **pleurisy** (pain that increases with deep inhalation or cough).

Do not forget **GERD.** It may also produce chest pain.

Though rarely encountered on the CS exam, consider the uncommon cases of **aortic dissection** and **ruptured aortic aneurysm.**

Note: In noncardiac causes of chest pain, pain is usually chronic, localized, and tender.

Review of the Local System

Ask respiratory or cardiac questions that are relevant to the case.

Review of System

As a routine.

Physical Exam

As a routine with special stress on:
VS: Look for any tachycardia, tachypnea.
Appearance: SP may be in acute distress (in pain).
Do a general exam, documenting the following:
- Fundus exam (if HTN and/or DM exist).
- Pallor and cyanosis.
- Carotid auscultation and JVD.

Local (LH): Do a lung and heart exam; do a detailed exam of the affected system.

Role-Play 5: Chest Pain (I)

Doorway Information

Mrs. Jessica Andrews, 30 years old, complains of **chest pain.**
Vital signs:
- Temp: 98.6°F (37°C).
- HR: 84/min, regular.
- BP: 110/70 mm Hg.
- RR: 16/min.

Standardized Patient's Role

As the doctor enters, appear worried and nervous.

For the last 2 months, you have had many social conflicts at home with your husband. That has upset you and made you nervous lately. You and your husband have been arguing a lot regarding your children's futures.

You have pain in your chest that comes in waves, two to three times a week and lasts for 20 to 30 minutes. When it hurts, you also have difficulty breathing, an abnormally rapid heartbeat, and you sweat a lot. During the last episode, you were choking, and you felt as if you were going to die.

These episodes sometimes occur when you are in a crowded place. Relaxing improves the condition. You are also having trouble falling asleep. It often takes you more than an hour to fall asleep. Your bladder is overactive, and you have irritable bowel disease.

You take oral contraceptive pills and oxybutynin. You have visited many doctors; unfortunately, they haven't reached a final diagnosis.

You are working as a physician assistant. It is a stressful job. You drink at least four cups of coffee a day and you smoke cigarettes—one pack a day for the last 10 years.

Your mother has a thyroid problem, but your father is healthy. You and your husband are sexually active.

Your LMP was 2 weeks ago. You had a Pap smear 2 years ago; the results were normal.

At the end of the PE, ask the doctor:
Q1: *Are these symptoms related to my nervousness?*
Q2: *Is it a heart attack?*

Role-Play 5: Answer Key

Communication and Interpersonal Skills Component

Suggested Closure

"I have finished the PE and let's talk about what is on my mind. You told me that your chest pain comes in episodes and is accompanied by difficulty in breathing and a rapid heartbeat. Also you mentioned that your work causes you stress and that you are under pressure and feeling nervous. Based on your history and present circumstances, and my physical exam, it seems like you are having panic attacks. However, I cannot rule out other possible causes. For example, your problem may be related to the quantity of coffee that you drink, or it could be something with your thyroid like your mother has. To be sure, we need to run an ECG, which is …, and we need to take a CXR. When the results come back, we'll sit down together and I'll give you my final diagnosis and treatment options. Now, about your question about nervousness—have I already answered it, or do you still have concerns? Thank you very much for coming to see me." (Shake hands.)

Counseling

Difficulty sleeping (see Chapter 10, Neurology).

Suggested Answers to the SP's Questions

Q1: *"As I just explained, it is most probably due to stress. Any other concerns?"*

Q2: *"You are too young to be at risk for heart disease, yet your smoking may be a contributing factor. To be sure, we need to run an ECG, which is …, and we need to take a CXR."*

Patient Note

History

A 30-year-old female patient complains of chest pain. It comes in episodes two to three times/week for the last 2 months, lasts about 30 minutes, and is accompanied by dyspnea, palpitation, and sweating. When it comes on, she feels a choking sensation and feels like she will die. It is exacerbated by being in small, crowded places, is relieved when she relaxes. She has had difficulty falling asleep. Also, she and her husband have had arguments about their children's future. She is not depressed, does not have intolerance to heat, and does not have blurry vision. Appetite is normal, no recent weight loss, no bowel or urinary problems. LMP: 2 weeks ago; last pap smear was 2 years ago and it was normal. She has seen many doctors with no diagnosis reached. PMH: inflammatory bowel disease and over-active bladder. Med: OCPs (oral contraceptive pills) and oxybutynin. FH: mother with thyroid problem. SH: physician assistant, caffeine 4 to 5 cups/d. Smokes 1 ppd/10 y, social drinker, sexually active, monogamous with her husband.

Physical Exam

VS: WNL. The patient is alert and oriented ×3. Head: PERRLA, mouth without erythema, no pallor. Neck: normal thyroid. Ext.: no peripheral edema, palpable peripheral pulse, no tremors. Lung: CTA/BL. Heart: normal S1 and S2 with no murmurs. Neuro: intact sensation and muscle 5/5.

Differential Diagnosis

History finding(s)	Physical exam finding(s)
1. Panic attack	
Episodes of chest pain, dyspnea	Normal chest exam
Choking, impending death	Normal thyroid
Social stress with her husband	
2. Hypochondriasis	
Many doctor visits	Normal physical exam
No diagnosis reached	

Diagnostic Studies

CBC

TSH

Role-Play 6: Chest Pain (II)

Doorway Information

Mr. Carlini, 60-year-old male, who has **chest pain.**

Vital signs:
- Temp: 98.6°F (37°C).
- Pulse: 104/min, regular.
- BP: 160/110 mm Hg.
- RR: 24/min.

Standardized Patient's Role

When the doctor enters, put your hand on your chest, and pretend that you have severe pain in your chest. Take your breath deeply and rapidly. Then tell him:

Q1: *Doc, please help me quickly. My chest feels like there is a knife in it.*

You have had acute chest pain for an hour. It was so bad that it woke you up. It has been getting worse and goes along the left side of your neck. The pain is a squeezing and crushing sensation, and you rate it at 9 out of 10. It is constant and nothing seems to make it better. You are SOB, have a rapid heartbeat, and are sweating profusely. For many years, you have had mild chest pain, and you become SOB after walking more than four to five blocks. You had a similar episode 1 month ago. Oxygen and some medication relieved it that time. You have had high blood pressure for 20 years. You take nitrates and hydrochlorothiazide (HCTZ) but not always regularly. Your cholesterol is high, and you have been taking simvastatin for 10 years. Your father died from a heart attack when he was 65 years old. You have smoked one pack of cigarettes per day for 30 years.

Ask the doctor:

Q2: *Am I having a heart attack?*

Q3: *Can you give me a painkiller?*

Role-Play 6: Answer Key

As you start the encounter, show that you are very concerned about the chest pain; tell him that you are going find out what the problem is as quickly as you can. Remain standing throughout the exam.

Communication and Interpersonal Skills Component

Suggested Closure

"Mr. Carlini, let's sit down and review your case. You said that your chest pain came on suddenly, 1 hour ago, so severe that it woke you up, is that right? You had a similar episode 1 month ago that was treated with oxygen and meds. Based on your history and my physical exam, I think it may be angina or heart attack, which are caused by a decrease in blood and oxygen to the muscles of the heart. I am really concerned about your condition, and I consider it possibly life-threatening. Since this is an emergency, I'm going call the nurse-in-charge right now to get started on your blood tests. So, the first thing we will do is to take an ECG, which is ..., and take some CXR. As soon as we have the results, I'll be back to give you my final diagnosis and the treatment options.

Also, I recommend that you be admitted to the hospital to be kept under observation so that if anything develops we can deal with it immediately. How does that sound?"

Counseling

Smoking and HTN.

Suggested Answers to the SP's Questions

Q1: *"I understand your concern; I will do everything possible to make you feel better."*

Q2: *"Well, based on your medical history and my physical exam, and as I explained, it could be a heart attack because ..., but it may be something else. To be sure, however, I need to run a couple of tests: ... and ...."*

Q3: *"I understand that you are in pain, but unfortunately I can't do that until I have a final diagnosis. If I gave you a painkiller right now, it could interfere with my ability to diagnose what is causing the pain. So, I am asking you to be patient and hold on until we know more."*

History

A 60-year-old male patient complains of chest pain that had a sudden onset 1 hour ago. It has gotten worse since then. It is on the left side of the chest and radiates to the left arm. The pain is crushing (9/10), constant, associated with diaphoresis, palpitation, and dyspnea. It is not affected by change of position or movement, no alleviating factors. When walking, he typically has to stop after four to five blocks to catch his breath. No chest trauma, swelling of the legs, PND, orthopnea, cough, or heartburn. ROS: no recent change in weight, others irrelevant. PMH: HTN 20 y, hypercholesterolemia for 10 years. Previous episode 1 month ago. Med: nitrates, HCTZ, and statin. NKDA. FH: father died of MI. SH: smokes 1 ppd/30 y and no alcohol.

Physical Exam

VS: BP is 160/110 mm Hg, pulse rate 104/min, RR 24/min, and Temp is 98.6°F. The patient is in acute distress and in pain. **H&N:** PERRLA, normal fundus exam, no pallor, cyanosis, JVD, or carotid bruit. **Ext.:** no swelling of the lower limbs, normal peripheral pulse. **Cardiac:** PMI; not displaced, no visible thrill, normal S1and S2, no gallop or additional sounds, no JVD. **Chest:** no deformities, no tenderness, normal TVFs and percussion, CTA/BL without rhonchi or crepitation.

Differential Diagnosis

History finding(s)	Physical exam finding(s)
1. Acute MI	
Acute chest pain (crushing, severe 9/10, radiates to the left side)	Appears distressed
Dyspnea and distressed	Tachypnea and tachycardia
Smoker 20 y, HTN, hypercholesterolemia	ECG with ST elevation (if ECG provided; ▶ **Fig. 4.16**)
Previous angina relieved by nitrates	
2. Unstable angina	
Acute chest pain (crushing, severe 9/10, radiates to the left side)	Appears distressed
Dyspnea and distressed	Tachycardia and tachypnea
Smoker 20 y, HTN, hypercholesterolemia	
Previous angina relieved by nitrates	ECG changes (if ECG provided, ▶ **Fig. 4.17**)

Abbreviations: ECG, electrocardiogram; HTN, hypertension; MI, myocardial infarction.

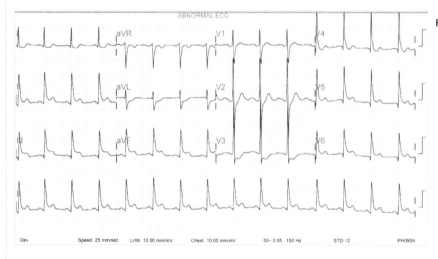

Fig. 4.16 ECG with ST elevation.

(Continued)

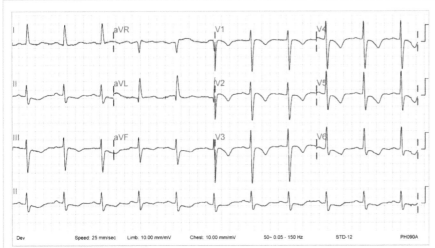

Fig. 4.17 ECG changes in myocardial ischemia.

Diagnostic Studies

Cardiac enzymes, ABG and serum electrolytes

CXR

Echo
Cardiac angiography—if highly suspicious for MI

ECG (with and without stress)

Role-Play 7: Chest Pain (III)

Mr. Adams, 28-year-old male, has chest pain.

Vital signs:
- Temp: 98.6°F (37°C).
- HR: 84/min, regular.
- BP: 110/70 mm Hg.
- RR: 16/min.

Standardized Patient's Role

Your chest pain started 2 weeks ago. It came on suddenly, during a wrestling match. Since then, the pain has lessened but not disappeared. The pain is in the right part of the chest, nonradiating, and mild (4/10). You describe the pain as a dull ache. The pain increases when you move your right arm and when you take a deep breath; it lessens when you rest and massage the affected area.

You had the flu last week. It improved with OTC medications.

You have no dyspnea, fever, or other symptoms. You have smoked a pack a day for 10 years, and you drink socially. You are sexually active with one girlfriend and use condoms. Your father died of lung cancer.

When the doctor examines you, express tenderness over the right side of your chest.

Ask the doctor:
Q1: *There is a wrestling match this weekend with my team. Do you think it's okay if I wrestle?*
Q2: *I have an ointment. Should I use it?*

Role-Play 7: Answer key

Communication and Interpersonal Skills Component

Suggested Answers to the SP's Questions

Q1: *"I understand your desire, but until I run some tests on you and get the results back, my best medical advice is to tell you to refrain from such physical activity."*

Q2: *"There are many OTC ointments and they are usually quite effective, so I don't see any harm in it. By the way, what is the name of the ointment you have?"*

If the SP knows: reply accordingly.

If not: *"Why don't you call me when you get home and let me know what it is. Then I will look it up."*

Patient Note

History

Please type the history notes as learned in the previous cases.

Physical Exam

Please type the PE notes as learned in the previous cases.

Differential Diagnosis

History finding(s)	Physical exam finding(s)
1. Costochondritis (musculoskeletal pain)	
Chest pain started while wrestling	Right side of the chest is tender
Increases when right arm is moved	CTA, B/L no wheezes
Relieved by massage	Heart is RRR with no murmurs
2. Pleurisy	
Chest pain	
Increases with deep inspiration	CTA, B/L no wheezes
Has had flu last week	Heart is RRR with no murmurs

Abbreviations: CTA, B/L, clear to auscultation bilaterally; RRR, regular rate and rhythm.

Diagnostic Studies

Cardiac enzymes (CPK-MB [**creatine phosphokinase myocardial band**], troponin)

ECG

CXR

Role-Play 8

Mr. Kenneth King, a 65-year-old male patient, came to the clinic and has been **coughing up blood**.

Vital signs:
- Temp: 98.6°F (37°C).
- HR: 90/min, regular.
- BP: 120/80 mm Hg.
- RR: 16/min.

Standardized Patient's Role

You are a 60-year-old male. You have had rust-colored sputum for the last 3 months. Yesterday, you coughed up about a half cup of blood that was bright red in color with no blood clots.

You have had difficulty breathing for many years that is controlled with medications (steroids and albuterol inhaler). Also, you have a cough with yellowish-green sputum. Sometimes you have chest wheezes if you run or are exposed to heavy dust or pollen in the spring.

You have chest pain in the right side of your chest, 4/10, which you describe as a dull ache. The pain is constant. It gets worse when you take a deep breath. Nothing makes it better.

You need two pillows to sleep comfortably with breathing problems. You lost 10 lb in the last 6 months.

Your father died from lung cancer. At this time, ask, **Q1**: *Doc, do I have lung cancer like my father had?*

You are retired; you worked for 30 years in the steel industry, and there was a lot of air pollution. You quit smoking 5 years ago. You smoked 2 packs daily for 25 years; you drink socially, and are sexually active with your wife.

As the doctor examines you, express tenderness on the right side of your chest.

Role-Play 8: Answer Key

In consideration of the CS exam, look at the doorway info. In addition to the main complaint, "coughing of blood," if you find fever, consider TB, pneumonia/bronchopneumonia among the differentials. You can consider COPD and lung cancer with no fever.

History

Analysis of Chief Complaint

Hemoptysis (ABCDE) + chest pain.

Analysis of Differential Diagnosis

With no fever—PE, COPD, lung cancer. With fever—TB, pneumonia.

COPD: Smoker for a long time, chronic cough and sputum. (The SP could show you CXR showing finding suggestive of COPD as in ▶Fig. 4.18.)

Lung cancer: Smoker for a long time, loss of weight, and may have positive family history.

TB: Fever, sweating, chills, traveling outside the United States, contact with sick person, night sweating, loss of weight, and chronic cough.

Pneumonia and bronchopneumonia: Fever, cough, sputum, Upper respiratory tract (URT) infection, and contact with sick person.

Review of the Local System

Respiratory system.

Review of System

As standard.

Past History and Others

A usual stress on **D** (blood thinner meds) **F** (of lung cancer) **S** (smoking, occupational hazards).

Physical Exam

VS, ADH, NE, LH: **H** (Full ENT exam), **N** (LNs), **E** (finger clubbing). Do chest with a detailed respiratory exam.

Communication and Interpersonal Skills Component

Give standard answers.

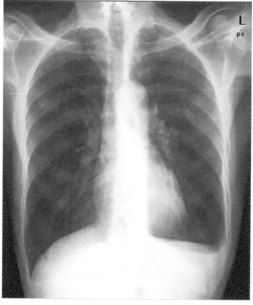

Fig. 4.18 X-ray showing finding suggestive of chronic obstructive pulmonary disease.

Patient Note

History

A 65-year-old male patient who came with complain of hemoptysis. It started 3 months ago with sputum streaked with blood. He coughed up fresh blood yesterday, about half cup; has no blood thinner use; the blood was bright red in color with no clots; he is not dizzy and has no bleeding anywhere else. He has cough with yellowish-green sputum, chest pain, on the right side, nonradiating, dull aching, 4/10, and constant. He complains of dyspnea, chest wheezes on exertion and orthopnea, uses two pillows to sleep comfortably. No rhinorrhea, sinus tenderness, or sore throat, no fever, chills, or night sweating. He has no PND. **ROS:** lost 10 lb/6 months. **PMH:** COPD. **Med:** steroid and albuterol inhaler, allergic to pollen and dust. **FH:** father died from lung cancer. **SH:** retired, worked in the steel industry, smokes 2 ppd/25 y, quitted 5 y ago, socially drinks, and is sexually active, monogamous with his wife.

Physical Exam

VS: WNL. **H&N:** no pallor, no cyanosis, TMs clear, nose without rhinorrhea, throat without erythema, no palpable LNs. **Ext:** no clubbing, cyanosis, no peripheral edema. **Chest:** no deformities, tenderness over the right side of the chest, normal TVFs and percussion, CTA/BL. No wheezes, rales or crepitations. **Heart:** Normal S1 and S2, no murmurs or gallop.

Differential Diagnosis

History finding(s)	Physical exam finding(s)
1. Chronic obstructive pulmonary disease	
Hemoptysis	
Smoker for 25 y	
Dyspnea, orthopnea	
2. Lung cancer	
Hemoptysis and weight loss	
Smoker for 25 y	
Family history of lung cancer	Tenderness over the right side of the chest

Diagnostic Studies

CBC, sputum culture

Sputum for AFB, PPD test

CXR and CT chest

5 Abdomen (Gastroenterology and Urology)

Keywords: abdominal pain, hemoptysis, vomiting, diarrhea, constipation

5.1 Introduction

In this chapter, the doorway info may include the following:
- *Abdominal pain:* upper abdominal, right upper quadrant (RUQ), right lower quadrant (RLQ), left-sided, and flank pain.
- *Changes in the bowel habits:* diarrhea and constipation.
- *Urology cases:* weak urinary stream, incontinence, and weak penile erection.
- *Bleeding disorders:* vomiting of blood, dark stool, dark urine, and bleeding per rectum.
- *Others:* heartburn, yellowish discoloration of the skin and eyes, and difficulty swallowing.

5.2 Questions for Medical History

5.2.1 For Gastrointestinal Symptoms

Abdominal pain: *Do you have any pain in your belly?*

Upper gastrointestinal (GI) symptoms:
- *Do you feel nauseous? Have you vomited? Have you vomited any blood?*
- *Do you have difficulty swallowing? Do you have heartburn?*

Lower GI symptoms:
- *Have you had any recent changes in your bowel movements?*
- *Have you noticed if your stool was dark?*

For rectal and anal problems:
- *Do you have rectal pain?*
- *Have you noticed any masses coming out of your rectum?*
- *Have you ever been diagnosed with hemorrhoids?*
- *Have you noticed any blood on the toilet paper?*

5.2.2 Urology Symptoms

Nonurologic cases on the Clinical Skills (CS) exam usually need only one question to figure out any urologic complaints: *Do you have any problems in passing urine?*

In urology cases of *benign prostatic hyperplasia (BPH), hematuria, urinary incontinence, etc.,* the matters should be discussed in detail.

Hematuria: *Have you ever noticed any blood in your urine?*

Irritative urinary symptoms: (daytime, night + IUD), IUD is intrauterine device as a mnemonic.

Daytime frequency: *Do you go to the bathroom more often than usual?/How many times do you go to the bathroom to urinate per day?*

Nocturia: *Do you have to wake up at night to urinate?* If yes; *how many times?*

Incontinence: *Are you incontinent for urine? /If yes: Do you have any urine leakage while sneezing or coughing?*

Urgency: *Do you have to rush to the bathroom to urinate?*

Dysuria: *Does it burn while you are urinating?*

Obstructive urinary symptoms (difficult to start and to end, straining that results in weak stream):

Hesitancy: *Do you have difficulty starting your urine stream?*

Straining: *Do you have to push down to urinate?*

Weak stream: *Do you have a weak stream?*

Incomplete emptying: *Do you feel as if your bladder still contains urine after urination?*

5.3 Abdominal Examination

Please pay attention of proper draping technique. Before exposing the abdomen by moving the gown up, use a sheet to cover the legs and the lower part of the abdomen first.

5.3.1 Inspection

Inform the Standardized Patient (SP) that you are going to examine his or her belly and ask him or her to lie back. Fake scars (appendectomy or cholecystectomy) are commonly seen while doing an inspection.

Say to the SP: *"I need to examine your belly right now. Could you lie back please? Let me first fix the bed and pull out the leg extension so you can lie back and be comfortable. I'm looking at your belly for any swelling, discoloration, or any scars."*

5.3.2 Palpation

Do superficial palpation starting from the RLQ, moving toward the left side. Alternatively, start opposite of where the patient says it hurts, and ending on the most tender area. Remember to be gentle and on the CS exam, there is no need for deep palpation to check for organomegaly/masses, but you can pretend you are doing this and say so—the patient will understand. You can ask the SP to bend his or her knees (to relax the abdominal muscles). Warm your hands before starting (▶ Fig. 5.1).

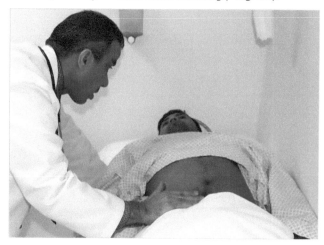

Fig. 5.1 Examination of the abdomen, palpation.

Say to the SP: *"Now, I'll press on your belly. Could you bring your knees up? It helps in relaxation of the abdominal muscles. Does it hurt here? What about here? I am so sorry; I didn't mean to hurt you."*

5.3.3 Percussion

Do gentle percussion in the four quadrants, but percussion to check for liver span usually isn't mandatory (▶ Fig. 5.2).

Say to the SP: *"I'm going to tap on your belly."*

5.3.4 Auscultation

Warm your stethoscope and listen at least to two areas: over the cecum (at the RLQ) and around the umbilicus (▶ Fig. 5.3).

Say to the SP: *"I am going to listen to your belly."*

5.3.5 Rebound Tenderness

Tell the SP that you will press little bit more, then release your hand quickly. If it hurts when you let your hands go, it is a sign of positive rebound tenderness (a sign of peritoneal irritation; ▶ Fig. 5.4a, b).

Say to the SP: *"I am going to press a little bit more on your belly and then I am going to release my hands."*

Special maneuvers for appendicitis: see individual cases.

When a local exam is necessary: *"Sir/Ma'am, I need to do a pelvic exam. Would you mind if I call nurse-in-charge to get you ready?"* Don't forget to write it down in the workup.

Notice: Sometimes auscultation of the abdomen is better to be done before deep palpation as the latter may change the bowel movements.

5.4 Diagnostics Studies

5.4.1 For Gastrointestinal Cases

Prohibited physical exam (PE): rectal exam.

Lab: complete blood count (CBC), stool analysis for occult blood, pancreatic enzymes, liver function test.

Imaging: X-ray (abdomen), ultrasonography (US; abdomen and pelvis), and CT scan.

Others: upper GI endoscopy, lower GI (colonoscopy and anoscopy).

5.4.2 For Urology Cases

Prohibited PE: pelvic and rectal exams.

Lab: urine analysis, urine culture, CBC, serum creatinine, prostate-specific antigen (PSA).

Imaging: X-ray KUB, US KUB, and CT KUB. KUB is kidney, ureter and bladder.

Others: cystoscopy, urodynamic studies.

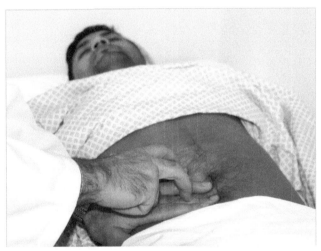

Fig. 5.2 Examination of the abdomen, percussion.

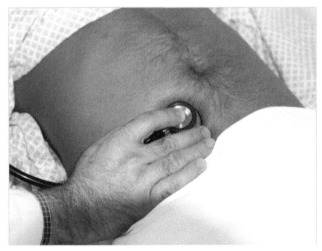

Fig. 5.3 Examination of the abdomen, auscultation.

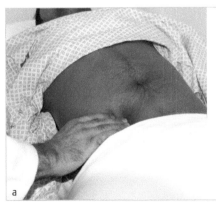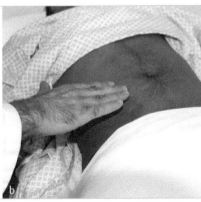

Fig. 5.4 (a, b) Rebound tenderness.

Role-Play 9

Doorway Information

Mrs. Donna Martin, 32-year-old female patient, has **upper abdominal pain**.

Vital signs:
- Temperature (Temp): 98.6°F (37°C).
- Blood pressure (BP): 100/70 mm Hg.
- Pulse rate (PR): 84/min, regular.
- Respiratory rate (RR): 100/min.

Examinee tasks:
- Obtain a focused history.
- Perform a relevant PE. Do not perform rectal, pelvic, genitourinary, inguinal hernia, female breast, or corneal reflex exam.
- Discuss your initial diagnosis and your workup plan with the patient.
- After leaving the room, complete the patient note (PN) on the given form.

Standardized Patient's Role

You came to the clinic because of upper abdominal pain. You have had it for 1 year, but it has gotten worse in the last 3 months. The pain travels up and sometimes you have a sour taste in your throat. You have heartburn under your breast bones. The pain is not constant and comes three to five times a week. It gets worse when you eat big meals or lie back. Antacids (Tums) and ome-prazole help.

Your appetite is good, and you haven't lost any weight.

You had the same symptoms during your last pregnancy. You take antacids and ibuprofen for chronic knee pain. You take also ome-prazole that was prescribed by your family doctor; you took it for 1 year and it alleviated your symptoms but you stopped taking it 3 months ago. If the doctor asks why, tell him or her you have no health insurance (**Comment 1**).

Your mother was treated for peptic ulcers. You live with your husband and two children. You are a teacher. You smoke 1 pack per day for 10 years (1 ppd/10 y) and drink 1 to 2 cups daily; you thought many times to stop drinking and you feel guilty about that.

When the physician does the physical exam on you, act as if the upper part of your abdomen is tender.

As the doctor finishes the exam, ask:
Q1: *Do I have stomach ulcers like my mother had?*
Q2: *What is an endoscopy? I remembered that my mother had one done.*

Please refer to Chapter 13 (Appendix), to review the general instructions for the SP as well as the Doctor roles.

Role-Play 9: Answer Key

Upper abdominal pain (younger patient)

History

Analysis of Chief Complaint

Abdominal pain.

Analysis of Differential Diagnosis

Gastroesophageal reflux disease (GERD): Young age, heartburn with a sour taste that travels up the throat, not referred to the neck or arms. It gets better with antacids and proton pump inhibitors (PPI) and worse with heavy meals and lying back.

- *"Do you have heartburn? Do you notice a sour taste in your throat?"*
- *"Does anything make it worse?" "Does anything make it better?"*
- *"Do you have a cough? Have you ever choked?"*

Peptic ulcer: Pain that relates to diet, usually worse when meals are delayed, alleviated by antacids or food and past history of similar episodes.

Gastritis: Long use of nonsteroidal anti-inflammatory disease (NSAID), vomiting of blood, and dark stool.

Pancreatitis: Dyspepsia with malabsorption, chronic alcohol use/gallstones, and pain radiates to the back.

Review of the Local System

GI system questions.

Review of Systems

SAW (Sleep, appetite, and weight), 3 systems in female (GI, Urology, Gyne).

Past History and Others

As routine questions + **D** (Tums and PPI and NSAID), **S** (smoking and alcohol).

Physical Exam

H (jaundice, pallor, use a tongue depressor to examine the throat and teeth). Do auscultation for Lung and Heart (LH) only. Do a detailed abdominal exam. **Special maneuvers:** Rebound tenderness and Murphy's sign.

Communication and Interpersonal Skills Component

Suggested Closure

As routine questions.

Counseling

Diet, smoking, and alcohol (CAGE questionnaire).

Suggested Answers to the Standardized Patient's Questions

Comment 1: Doc: *"Why did you stop taking your medicine?"*
SP: *I don't have health insurance and I couldn't afford it.*
Doc: *"I see. Well, you should know that we have social workers here who have more experience in dealing with such issues. Would you mind if I contact one of them?"*

Q1 and Q2: Give your answer as explained before.

History

A 32-year-old female patient complains of having epigastric pain with heartburn and sour sensation in the throat for the last year, which has gotten worse in the last 3 months, 3 to 5 times/wk. Worsens after big meals and lying down. Tums relieve pain. No vomiting, difficulty swallowing, hematemesis, or dark stool. No chest pain, dyspepsia, palpitation, or cough. Review of systems (ROS): normal appetite, no recent changes in weight, no urinary/bowel movement problems. Past medical history (PMH): previous symptoms during last pregnancy. Medication (Med): Tums, NSAID, omeprazole that stopped 3 months ago. No known drug allergy (NKDA). Family history (FH): mother had peptic ulcer. Social history (SH): smokes 1 ppd/10 y, drinks 1 to 2 cups of coffee daily. CAGE = 2/4. Lives with husband and two children.

Physical Exam

Vital signs (VS): within normal limits (WNL). Patient is alert, conscious, and oriented ×3. **Head and neck (H&N):** moist mucous membranes, throat without erythema, no pallor, or jaundice. No palpable lymph nodes (LNs). Normal thyroid. **Extremities (Ext):** No peripheral edema. **Chest:** CTA/BL (clear to auscultation bilaterally). **Heart:** normal S1 and S2. **Abdomen:** nondistended (ND), mild tenderness of epigastric area. No rebound or organomegaly, BS +, Murphy's sign –ve.

Differential Diagnosis

History finding(s)	Physical exam finding(s)
1. Gastroesophageal reflux disease	
Epigastric pain, sour throat sensation	Epigastric tenderness
Increased by heavy meal and lying back	
Relieved by antacids and proton pump	
2. Peptic ulcer disease	
Epigastric pain	Epigastric tenderness
Relieved by antacids	
Family history and proton pump use	
3. Gastritis	
Epigastric pain	Epigastric tenderness
Prolonged nonsteroidal anti-inflammatory drugs use	

Diagnostic Studies

Complete blood count, amylase, antibodies to *Helicobacter pylori*

Upper gastrointestinal endoscopy

Role-Play 10

Mr. Bill Brown, a 60-year-old male patient, has **upper abdominal pain.**

Vital signs:
- Temp: 98.6°F (37°C).
- HR: 84/min, regular.
- RR: 16/min.
- BP: 120/80 mm Hg.

Standardized Patient's Role

You have had upper abdomen pain for many years. Spicy food worsens the pain. Tums (antacids) and Zantac relieve the pain. For the last 3 months, the pain has been getting worse (5/10). It is localized and constant and is accompanied by heartburn. You have vomited twice in the last 3 weeks; the vomit was streaked with blood. You have also had dark-colored stool and abdominal bloating. You have been feeling tired and dizzy and have lost over 10 lb in the last 3 months. You have rheumatoid arthritis (RA) and take 200 mg of ibuprofen daily.

Your parents passed away; your mother has RA and peptic ulcer and your father died of stomach cancer. You are a heavy smoker—two packs of cigarettes a day for the last 25 years, and you drink three cups of alcohol daily. People's comments about your drinking make you very annoyed and you have tried many times to stop alcohol drinking, but you couldn't. You are sexually active with your wife.

When the physician does the physical exam upon you, act as if the upper part of your abdomen is tender.

As the doctor finishes the exam, ask:

Q1: *Doc, a friend of mine had an endoscopy for the same problem that I'm having. Do you recommend that I have one done?*

Q2: *This friend also told me that they took a biopsy. What exactly is a biopsy?*

Role-Play 10: Answer Key

Upper abdominal pain (older age)

History

Analysis of Chief Complaint

Abdominal pain, vomiting, and dark stool.

Analysis of Differential Diagnosis

GERD, peptic ulcer, gastritis and pancreatitis: ...see the previous case.

Stomach cancer: old age, anorexia, early satiety, loss of weight, and dark stool.

Rarely on CS exam:
- **Diabetic gastropathy:** In a patient with uncontrolled diabetes mellitus (DM), there also may be symptoms suggestive of peripheral neuropathy and retinopathy.
- **Referred pain from MI** (myocardial infarction).

Review of the Local System

GI system questions.

Review of Systems

I SAW 2/3 systems.

Past History and Others

As routine + P (any hematemesis and black stool), D (Tums and PPI and NSAID), F (FH of cancer), S (smoking and alcohol).

Physical Exam

H (jaundice, pallor), N (enlarged LNs). Do auscultation for LH only. Do a detailed abdominal exam and schedule for pelvic and rectal exams. **Special maneuvers:** rebound tenderness and Murphy's sign.

Communication and Interpersonal Skills Component

Suggested Closure

As routine.

Counseling

Diet, smoking, and alcohol (CAGE questionnaire).

Suggested Answers to the Standardized Patient's Questions

As routine.

Patient Note

History

A 60-year-old male patient complains of epigastric pain with heartburn, gradual onset and progressive course, nonradiating, 5/10, and constant, worsened by spicy food and relieved by antacids. Twice vomited streaked with blood with melena, no dysphagia or change in bowel habits apart from abdominal bloating.

ROS: lost 10 lb/3 mo, diet has many spicy foods.
PMH: RA for many years.
Med: Tums, ibuprofen, and Zantac. NKDA.
FH: mother with peptic ulcer and RA; father died of stomach cancer.
SH: smokes 2 ppd/25 y, drinks 3 cups daily, CAGE = 2/4, monogamous with his wife.

Physical Exam

VS: WNL, no acute distress. **HEENT (head, eyes, ears, nose, throat):** no pallor or jaundice. Throat without erythema, nonpalpable supraclavicular LN. **Ext:** No peripheral edema, normal joint exam. **Chest:** CTA/BL. **Heart:** Normal S1 and S2. **Abdomen:** No visible scars, masses or pulsation. Soft, tender epigastric area, no rebound, no organomegaly, BS +.

Differential Diagnosis

History finding(s)	Physical exam finding(s)
1. Peptic ulcer disease	
Epigastric pain	Epigastric tenderness
Worsened by spicy food and relieved by antacid	Normal chest and heart exam
Drinks 3 cups daily	
Hematemesis and melena	
Mother has peptic ulcer	
2. Cancer stomach	
Epigastric pain	Epigastric tenderness
Loss of weight	Lost 10 lb/3 mo
Drinks 3 cups daily	
Hematemesis and melena	
Father has stomach cancer	
3. Gastritis	
Epigastric pain	Epigastric tenderness
Taking Ibuprofen	
Hematemesis and melena	

Diagnostic Studies

Rectal exam

Stool for OB (occult blood), CBC (complete blood count), amylase, serology for *Helicobacter pylori*

Upper gastrointestinal endoscopy

Role-Play 11

Mrs. Linda Thomas, a 50-year-old female, has **right upper abdominal pain.**
Vital signs:
- Temp: 100.4°F (38°C).
- PR: 100/min, regular.
- RR: 16/min.
- BP: 130/90 mm Hg.

Standardized Patient's Role

Other than your abdominal pain, your health has been excellent, and nothing has been troubling you.

You have had abdominal pain and dyspepsia for a long time. You notice that it increases when you consume fatty food. You have come to the ER with abdominal pain, which you would rate 6/10. A few hours ago, the pain increased to 8/10. It is a sharp, spasmlike pain in the right side of the upper part of your abdomen and radiates to your right shoulder. You feel nauseous and have vomited clear fluid.

You had a similar episode 3 months ago, but with no fever; they scanned your abdomen and informed you that there were multiple stones in your gallbladder. Your mother has gallstones, too.

You have been menopausal for 1 year. You have had high BP for 20 years and DM for 10 years. You take 50 mg of atenolol and 500-mg metformin, both once daily. You have no allergies, smoke (1 ppd/25 y), drink socially, and live with your husband.

During the physical examination: Express tenderness on the right side of the upper part of your abdomen. Express pain when the doctor pushes down and when releases the pressure. If the doctor puts his or her hand under your ribs and asks you to take a deep breath, act like it hurts so much while inhaling that you cannot continue.

Role-Play 11: Answer Key

History

Analysis of Chief Complaint

Abdominal pain + fever.

Analysis of Differential Diagnosis

Acute cholecystitis: Usually female, constant pain that radiates to the right scapula. Pain is brought on by fatty food and is not relieved by antacids. Usually with fever and associated with gallstones (▶ **Fig. 5.5**).

Biliary colic: Recurrent episodes of RUQ pain with no fever. Usually with similar episodes.

Pancreatitis: Pain radiates to the back, alleviated by leaning forward. History of heavy drinking.

Rarely seen on the CS exam:
- **Acute hepatitis:** Fever, vomiting, travel outside the United States (Hepatitis A), and jaundice.
- **Perforated peptic ulcer:** Severe RUQ pain, tenderness, rebound tenderness, long history of heartburn.
- **Right basal pneumonia:** Cough with mucous and fever.

Review of the Local System

GI system questions.

Review of Systems

I SAW three systems.

Past History and Others

As routine questions + **D** (NSAID, antacids, PPI), **F** (possible history of gallstones), **S** (alcohol for pancreatitis).

Physical Exam

VS: (possible fever), **A, D:** (lying back in pain), **H** (jaundice). Do auscultation for **LH** only. Do full abdominal exam and schedule for pelvic and rectal exams. **Special maneuvers:** rebound tenderness and Murphy's sign.

Murphy's sign: Place your hand under the right costal margin (▶ **Fig. 5.6**). Ask the SP to take a deep breath. If the SP stops breathing temporarily, it's positive (a sign for cholecystitis in RUQ pain cases). Explain to the SP:

"I am going to press little bit more. Could you take a deep breath?"

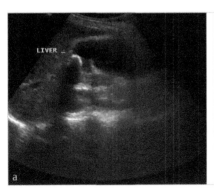
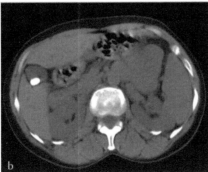

Fig. 5.5 Scan showing gallstones, **(a)** Ultrasonography, and **(b)** nonenhanced CT.

Communication and Interpersonal Skills Component

Suggested Closure

"Ms. Thomas, let's go over your case. You told me that you have abdominal pain that … and …. You had a similar episode 3 months ago, is that right? Well, based on your history and my physical exam, my preliminary diagnoses are inflammation of the gallbladder, or biliary colic from a moving stone. However, I cannot eliminate other possibilities at this point, so I need to order the following tests: …. Now, your case is an emergency, so I strongly recommend that you be admitted to the hospital till we can see what is causing this. As soon as we get the lab results from the tests, we'll sit down together to discuss the final diagnosis and the treatment options."

Counseling

Diet and smoking.

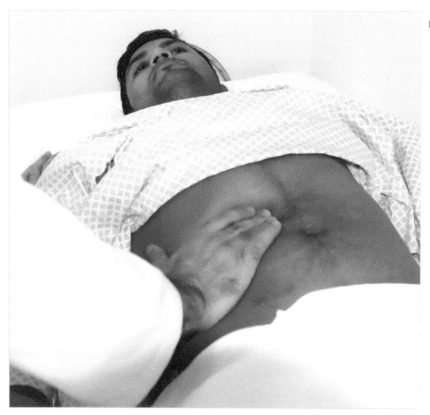

Fig. 5.6 Murphy's sign.

Patient Note

History

A 50-year-old female patient complains of abdominal pain started a few hours ago with a gradual onset and progressive course. Pain is in the RUQ, radiating to the right shoulder, constant, spasmlike, 6 to 8/10, and is accompanied by nausea and one episode of vomiting clear fluid. Consumption of fatty food exacerbates pain. No heartburn, dysphagia, or change in bowel movement. No hematemesis, melena, jaundice, chest pain, or cough. **ROS:** normal appetite, postmenopausal for 1 year. **PMH:** hypertension (HTN) 20 years, DM 10 years, previous episode 3 months ago relieved by pain med. **Med:** Atenolol 50 mg and metformin 500 mg. NKDA. **FH:** mother has gallbladder stones. **SH:** smokes 1 ppd/25 y, drinks socially, and lives with her husband.

Physical Exam

VS: Temp: 100.4°F, pulse 100, RR 16, and ABP 130/90. The patient is lying back and is in pain. **H&N:** no jaundice, throat without erythema, normal thyroid. **Ext:** no peripheral edema, normal skin. **Chest:** CTA/BL. **Heart:** normal S1 and S2. **Abdomen:** no visible scars, masses, or pulsation. + BS. RUQ is tender with + rebound. No organomegaly and + Murphy's sign.

Differential Diagnosis

History finding(s)	Physical exam finding(s)
1. Acute cholecystitis	
Pain in right upper quadrant (RUQ) and radiates to the right shoulder	Tenderness of RUQ area with + rebound
Pain increases with fatty food	+ Murphy's sign
Has fever	Temp = 100.4°F
2. Biliary colic	
RUQ pain	Tenderness of RUQ
Similar episode three months ago	
Mother has gallbladder stones	

Diagnostic Studies

CBC, LFTs, lipase and amylase

Abdominal US

CT abdomen

Role-Play 12 (▶Video. 5.1)

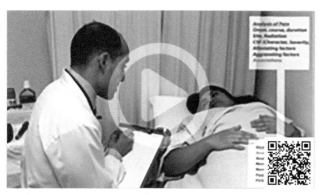

Video 5.1 This is a live demo of a 30-year-old female who has right-sided abdominal pain https://www.thieme.de/de/q.htm?p=opn/cs/20/3/11450546-08cbf8b7

Doorway Information

Mrs. Sharon Thompson, a 30-year-old female, has **right-sided abdominal pain.**
Vital signs:
- Temp: 101°F (38.3°C).
- Pulse: 100/min, regular.
- RR: 20/min.
- BP: 120/80 mm Hg.

Standardized Patient's Role

You have abdominal pain that was ill defined when it started 5 hours ago. Now it is centered in the lower right side of the abdomen. It feels a spasm, sharp, 6/10, nonradiating, and constant. You feel nauseated and have vomited twice—both times a clear fluid. You are feverish, but you haven't taken your temperature.

Last week, you had vaginal discharge that was greenish and foul smelling. You took an over-the-counter (OTC) vaginal suppository, but you don't remember the brand. The discharge is less now. Last year, you had one episode of pelvic inflammatory disease (PID). You don't have any medical problems and you've never had an operation. Your last menstrual period (LMP) was 2 weeks ago and never got pregnant.

You smoke one pack daily and drink socially. You are sexually active with multiple sexual partners and only occasionally use condoms. You contracted gonorrhea 6 months ago.

During the exam: Lie back in the bed and act like you are in pain as the physician enters the room. Tell him or her your right lower abdomen hurts when the physician presses on it and when he or she releases the pressure. If he or she moves your legs, say that the maneuvers cause some pain on the right lower abdomen.

At the end of the exam, ask:
Q1: *Do I have appendicitis?*
Q2: *Can you give me pain meds?*
Q3: *Do I need to have surgery?*

Role-Play 12: Answer Key

Right lower abdominal pain (female + fever)

History

Analysis of Chief Complaint

Abdominal pain + fever.

Analysis of Differential Diagnosis

Acute appendicitis, gynecological causes (PID), and urinary tract infection (UTI). In acute appendicitis, pain usually starts around the umbilicus, and then pain moves to the RLQ area, also with nausea, vomiting, and low-grade fever.

Review of the Local System

As a standard.

Review of Systems

As a standard.

Past History and Others

As a standard.

Physical Exam

VS: tachycardia and fever, **A** (in pain), **D** (lying back supine). Do auscultation for **LH** only. Do full abdominal exam and ask for pelvic and rectal exams. Do special maneuvers for appendicitis (see below) and costovertebral angle (CVA) tenderness.

Rovsing's sign: Press on the left lower quadrant (LLQ) and ask the SP where it hurts. If it hurts in the RLQ, it's positive. Tell the SP, *"I'll press here. Does it hurt?"*

Obturator sign: Flex the hip nearly at 90 degrees together with a flexed knee and then internally rotate the hip joint. It's positive if the SP expresses pain at the RLQ (▶ **Fig. 5.7a**).

Explain to the SP: *"Please relax. I'm going to lift and rotate your leg little bit; any pain or discomfort in your abdomen?"*

Psoas sign: Ask the SP to lie on his or her left side and extend his or her right hip and knee (▶ **Fig. 5.7b**). Pain means a positive test.

Explain to the SP: *"Can you roll over on your left side? I'm going to move your leg again. Tell me if it hurts."*
Alternatively, tell the supine patient to flex the right hip; provide resistance to flexion by pressing down on the knee with your palm.

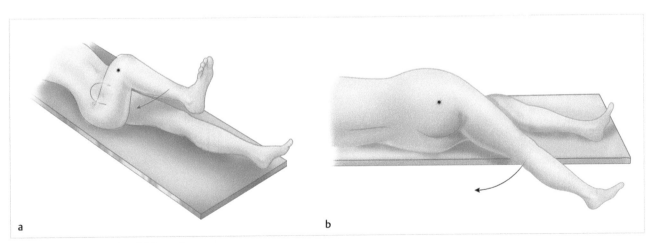

Fig. 5.7 (a) Obturator sign. (b) Psoas sign.

Communication and Interpersonal Skills Component

Suggested Closure

As emergency case with possible admission.

Counseling

Safe sex precautions.

Suggested Answers to the Standardized Patient's Questions

Please answer following guidelines.

Patient Note

History

A 30-year-old woman complains of abdominal pain that started 5 hours ago; it was initially ill defined and came on gradually. Now, located in the RLQ, the pain is nonradiating, sharp, colicky (6/10), and constant. Patient is feverish and nauseous and has twice vomited clear fluid. LMP was 2 weeks ago. She was treated for vaginal discharge last week. **ROS:** no urinary problems or recent changes in bowel movements; LMP was 2 weeks ago. **PMH:** PID last year. NKDA and gonorrhea 6 m ago. **FH:** parents are healthy. **SH:** smokes 1 ppd/5 y and drinks socially. Is active with multiple sexual partners; only occasionally uses condoms.

Physical Exam

VS: Temp = 101°F, 100, 20, 120/80. Patient was in pain, lying supine. **H&N:** no pallor or jaundice. **Ext:** No peripheral edema, normal pulsation. **Chest:** CTA/BL. **Heart:** normal S1 and S2. **Abdomen:** no visible scars, BS+. **Percussion:** normal in Bowel sounds in all 4 quadrants (sometimes abbreviated as +BS x4Q). McBurney's point is tender with rebound tenderness noted; Rovsing's signs and psoas are +, obturator sign and CVA tenderness are (–).

Differential Diagnosis

History finding(s)	Physical exam finding(s)
1. Acute appendicitis	
Ill-defined abdominal pain that moved to right lower quadrant (RLQ)	Tenderness over the RLQ area
Feels feverish	Fever (101°F)
Nausea and vomiting	+ Rebound tenderness, psoas, and Rovsing's signs
2. Pelvic inflammatory disease (PID)	
Pain in RLQ	Tenderness over the RLQ area
Feels feverish	Fever (101°F)
Multiple sex partners, occasional condom use	+ Rebound tenderness
Vaginal discharge and past history of PID and gonorrhea	

Diagnostic Studies

Pelvic and vaginal exam

CBC, UA, HVS (high vaginal swab)

Abdominal US and CT scan

Role-Play 13

Doorway Information

Mrs. Dana Miller, a 35-year-old female patient, came to the ER for **left-sided abdominal pain.**
Vital signs:
- Temp: 101°F (38.3°C).
- PR: 100/min, regular.
- RR: 20/min.
- BP: 120/80 mm Hg.

Standardized Patient's Role

Before the doctor enters, lie down and groan with pain as the he or she enters the exam room.

You have left flank pain that radiates to the lower part of your abdomen. It started gradually yesterday as mild pain, but today it's sharp, 8/10, and constant. The pain increases as you move around. You feel nauseous and have vomited once with no blood. Also, you have severe dysuria and go to the bathroom more often than usual. You took your temperature yesterday and it was 100°F, but now it feels higher. The pain increases as you move around and decreases a little bit with Tylenol.

You were hospitalized 3 months ago with left renal colic, and CT was done that showed stone in the left ureter and you don't have health insurance for stone endoscopy. Please show the doctor the CT shown in ▸ Fig. 5.8. You are sexually active with multiple male partners, and you do not usually use condoms. You have a little vaginal discharge with a bad fishy odor. Your LMP was a week ago.

You were treated 6 months ago for gonorrhea. You have allergic rhinitis. You take Claritin and are allergic to penicillin. You don't smoke.

During the PE: When the doctor touches your abdomen or back, say that it hurts on the left side of your abdomen, and again complain of pain when he or she lets up on the pressure with his or her hands.

Tell the doctor as he or she finishes: *"Please give some pain meds now. My kids are home alone, and I need to go."*

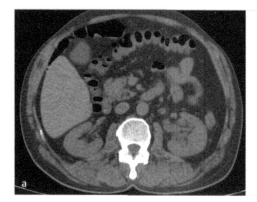
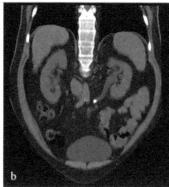

Fig. 5.8 Nonenhanced CT. **(a)** Axial section showing mild left hydronephrosis. **(b)** Coronal section showing mild left hydroureteronephrosis down to stone on the left ureter.

Role-Play 13: Answer Key

LLQ pain (female + fever)

History

Analysis of Chief Complaint

Abdominal pain, fever, malodorous vaginal discharge.

Analysis of Differential Diagnosis

Acute pyelonephritis and pelvic inflammatory disease.

Review of the Local System

GI system questions.

Review of Systems

As routine questions.

Past History and Others

As routine questions.

Physical Exam

VS: tachycardia and fever, **A** (pain), **D** (lying back supine). Do auscultation for **LH** only. Do a detailed abdominal exam and ask for pelvic and rectal exams.

Special maneuvers: CVA tenderness.

Ask the SP to get up, and at the renal angle, which is the angel between the back muscles and the last rib (CVA), place the palm of your left on it and strike by your right hand (▶ **Fig. 5.9**). Do it if you suspect a renal pathology (renal and ureteric colic or pyelonephritis).

Before doing CVA, inform the SP: *"Could you get up please? We are almost done. I'm going to tap on your back. Does it hurt?"*

Suggested Answers to the Standardized Patient's Questions

Q1: *"Ms. Miller, I understand your desire for pain medication. However, giving any painkiller may change the quality of your pain, and it may make it hard for us to make a diagnosis. Please be patient and I appreciate your cooperation. Now, about your kids—we have a social worker here. Do you mind if I contact him to see if we can arrange for a babysitter until your tests have been completed?"*

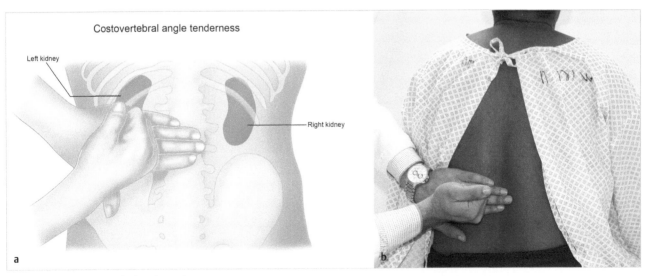

Fig. 5.9 (a, b) Costovertebral angle tenderness exam.

Patient Note

History

Please type the history notes as learned in the previous cases.

Physical Exam

Please type the PE notes as learned in the previous cases

Differential Diagnosis

History finding(s)	Physical exam finding(s)
1. Acute pyelonephritis	
Left-sided abdominal pain	Abdominal tenderness, + costovertebral angle
Fever, dysuria, and urinary frequency	Temperature is 101°F
Was diagnosed with ureteral stone 3 mo ago	
2. Pelvic inflammatory disease	
Left-sided abdominal pain	Abdominal tenderness
Fever, vaginal discharge	Temperature is 101°F
Multiple sexual partners with occasional use of condom	
History of gonorrhea 6 mo ago	

Diagnostic Studies

Pelvic and vaginal exam

UA including culture and sensitivity (C/S) and serum creatinine

Pregnancy test and cervical secretion culture

Abdominal computed tomography

Role-Play 14

Doorway Information

Mr. Kenneth Smith, a 35-year-old man, has **left-sided abdominal pain.**
Vital signs:
- **Temp:** 100.5°F (38°C).
- **PR:** 90/min, regular.
- **RR:** 16/min.
- **BP:** 110/70 mm Hg.

Standardized Patient's Role

You have abdominal pain in the left lower part of your abdomen. The pain came on gradually this morning and has not changed over time. It's a constant, nonradiating, dull ache, and 6/10. You feel bloated and have had bloody, mucous diarrhea. For the last few years, you have had rectal pain and a sensation of incomplete evacuation. You have also been suffering from mild fevers, skin rashes, and mild joint pain. You have lost 8 lb in the last 6 months.

You feel feverish; you took your temperature at home and it was 100.5°F.

You also urinate frequently and have a burning maturation. You passed a kidney stone spontaneously last year and had a similar episode of pain few months ago. You had a colonoscopy 2 years ago; the doctor told you that your colon was inflamed. You take steroids. Your father had colon cancer at 60. You don't smoke or drink alcohol. You are sexually active and monogamous with your wife.

During the exam: pretend that your left lower abdomen hurts when the physician presses on it and when he or she releases the pressure.

If the doctor asks about anything other than your abdominal pain, say that nothing else is wrong.

At the end of the exam, ask:
Q1: *Do I have colon cancer?*
Q2: *Should I have another colonoscopy?*

Role-Play 14: Answer Key

Left lower abdominal pain (male + fever + bloody stool).

History

Analysis of Chief Complaint

Abdominal pain + fever.

Analysis of Differential Diagnosis

Inflammatory bowel disease, acute diverticulitis (usually >40 years), and UTI.

Inflammatory bowel disease: Young age, bloody diarrhea, loss of weight, and systemic symptoms (fever, joint pain, skin rash).

Acute diverticulitis: older than 40 years, LLQ pain, fever, long history of constipation, ± rectal bleeding.

Colon cancer: older age (on the CS exam, usually older than 50 years), abdominal pain/constipation, FH of colon cancer, loss of weight, blood in stool, and anemia.

Review of the Local System

As previously explained.

Review of Systems

As previously explained.

Past History and Others

As a routine.

Physical Exam

VS: fever, A (pain), E (skin rash, joint tenderness). Do auscultation for LH only. Do full abdominal exam. **Special maneuvers:** Do CVA tenderness and schedule pelvic and rectal exams.

Communication and Interpersonal Skills Component

Suggested Closure

As emergency case with possible admission.

Counseling

Safe sex precautions.

Suggested Answers to the Standardized Patient's Questions

Q1: Give standard answer.
Q2: *"I understand your concern; could you fax me the report of your last colonoscopy?"*

SP: *Sure.*

Physician: *"Okay, let me take a look at the report and I'll give you a call after that."*

Patient Note

History

A 35-year-old man complains of abdominal pain that started this morning. Onset was gradual and pain has not worsened. Located in the LLQ, pain is nonradiating, constant, and dull (6/10); associated with bloating, hematochezia, and tenesmus. Patient is not constipated, urinates frequently, has dysuria, feels feverish, has a mild skin rash and joint pain, and has lost 8 lb over the last 6 months. **PMH:** kidney stones a year ago and colonoscopy 2 years ago. Previous episodes with the last one being few months ago. **Med:** steroids. NKDA. **FH:** father died of colon cancer at 60 years. **SH:** denies smoking and drinking, monogamous with his wife.

Physical Exam

VS: WNL apart from fever (100.5°F), alert, oriented ×3. **H&N:** no pallor or jaundice, throat without erythema. **Ext:** no peripheral edema. **Chest:** CTA/BL. **Heart:** normal S1 and S2. **Abdomen:** ND, LLQ tender, + rebound, BS +, no organomegaly.

Differential Diagnosis

History finding(s)	Physical exam finding(s)
1. Inflammatory bowel disease	
Pain in left lower quadrant (LLQ)	Tenderness in LLQ
Feels feverish	Fever (100.5°F)
Bloody diarrhea	+ Rebound tenderness
Weight loss	
2. Urinary tract infection	
Pain in the LLQ	Tenderness of LUQ area
Feels feverish	Fever (100.5°F)
Dysuria and frequent urination	

Diagnostic Studies

Pelvic and rectal exam

UA, urine culture, CBC

US (abdomen, pelvis)

Colonoscopy

Role-Play 15

Doorway Information

Mr. Kevin Brown, a 65-year-old male, came to the clinic because he has **bleeding per rectum/dark stool**.
Vital signs:
- **Temp:** 98.6°F (37°C).
- **PR:** 90/min, regular.
- **RR:** 16/min.
- **BP:** 120/80 mm Hg.

Standardized Patient's Role

You are a 65-year-old man, and for the last 3 months, your stool has had streaks of blood. You have had pain on the left side of your abdomen, and you couldn't ask for medical advice.

Yesterday, you were very frightened when you saw bright red blood came from your rectum although there were no blood clots.

Say at this time: *"Doc, the blood frightened me so much, and I'm so worried!"* (**Comment 1**)

Your appetite is normal. You are not on any special diet, but your diet doesn't have enough vegetables or fruits.

You have also constipation (2 times/wk) with straining. When the nurse took your weight, you discovered that you have lost 10 lb over the last 6 months.

You have were diagnosed with DM 25 years ago and take insulin.

Your father died of colon cancer when he was 70 years old.

You worked as a driver but are now retired. You quit smoking 10 years ago (smoked 1 ppd/20 y) and are not sexually active.

As the doctor examines you, express tenderness on the left side of the abdomen.

At the end of the encounter, ask:
Q1: *Do I have colon cancer?*

Role-Play 15: Answer Key

Dark stool/bleeding per rectum is a common case on the CS exam. Dark or black stool means bleeding from the upper GI tract (esophagus, stomach, or duodenum), while fresh red bleeding is colorectal or anal in origin.

While looking at the doorway information, pay attention to the age, because anal fissure and piles are common in young patients—blood in the toilet paper usually is the complaint. Colon cancer is common in older age. Moreover, look for fever that may refer to inflammatory bowel disease or infectious/gonococcal proctitis.

History

Analysis of Chief Complaint

Dark stool/bleeding per rectum, ask **ABCDE** questions (See chapter 1, The Basics, Component 1, Integrated Clinical Encounter).

Analysis of Differential Diagnosis

Anal fissure/hemorrhoids:
Do you have to push down in the restroom?/Do you have constipation?
Do you feel any mass coming from the rectum?/Have you been diagnosed with hemorrhoids?/Have you noticed any blood on the toilet paper?

Diverticulosis: *Do you have constipation?* With acute diverticulitis; there is fever and severe abdominal pain

Colon cancer: *Has any one in your family had a colon cancer?*
Have you had a colonoscopy done? If yes: *When?*

Inflammatory bowel disease: *Do you have a fever? Joint pain? Skin rash?*

Infectious colitis: Ask questions for infectious diseases (see Chapter 1, The Basics, Component 1, Integrated Clinical Encounter).

Gonococcal proctitis: Take a detailed sexual history.

Review of the Local System

GI symptoms.

Review of Systems

As standard.

Past History and Others

As standard.

Physical Exam

As standard.

Suggested Answers to the Standardized Patient's Questions and Comments

Answers as explained in previous cases.

Patient Note

History

A 65-year-old man complains of bleeding per rectum. For the last 3 months he has stool streaks with blood, but he had fresh bleeding yesterday, bright red in color, with no blood clots, he does not feel dizzy, no bleeding anywhere else, doesn't take any blood thinner meds. He has also constipation (twice a week) with abdominal distension, no cold intolerance. He didn't feel any anal masses, has mild left-sided abdominal pain, and no vomiting.

ROS: normal appetite, food has low-fiber, no urinary problems; lost 10 lb/6 mo.
PMH: DM 25 years, no previous history of similar episode.
Med: insulin. NKDA.
FH: father died from colon cancer.
SH: retired, ex-smoker 10 years ago (1 ppd/20 y), and not sexually active.

Physical Exam

VS: WNL, alert and oriented ×3.
H&N: no pallor, jaundice, throat without erythema, normal thyroid. No palpable LNs.
Ext: no peripheral edema.
Chest: CTA/BL.
Heart: normal S1 and S2.
Abdomen: soft, ND, tenderness over the left iliac area, no rebound, BS +, no organomegaly.

Differential Diagnosis

History finding(s)	Physical exam finding(s)
1. Colon cancer	
Dark stool	
Abdominal pain, distension	Tenderness over the left iliac fossa
Loss of weight	Weight loss (10 lb/6 mo)
Family history	
2. Diverticulosis	
Dark stool	Tenderness over the left iliac fossa
Constipation	
Low fiber diet	

Diagnostic Studies

Rectal exam

Stool analysis for OB and CBC

CT scan abdomen

Anoscopy and colonoscopy

Role-Play 16

Mr. Kevin Brown, a 65-year-old male patient, has **vomiting of blood**.

Vital signs:
- Temp: 98.6°F (37°C).
- PR: 100/min, regular.
- RR: 18/min.
- BP: 100/60 mm Hg.

Standardized Patient's Role

You are a 65-year-old man. Early this morning you vomited a little blood (2–3 tablespoons) and 3 hours later you vomited about half cup of blood. This made you very scared, and you immediately came to the ER. The blood was bright red with no blood clots. You haven't had such a problem before. Also, you noticed that you had darker stool than normal last week.

You also have abdominal pain that comes and goes. It's in the upper part of your abdomen, radiating to the back, 5/10, and burning. It gets worse when you eat spicy food and smoke. It is alleviated with antacids (Tums).

For the last 5 years, you have had peptic ulcers, and you take Tums and Pantoprazole.

You discovered that you have lost 6 lb over the last 3 months. You have migraine headaches, and you usually take ibuprofen.

Your father died of stomach cancer.

You work as a manager in the headquarters of a big food company, and you have a lot of stress at work. You smoke (1 ppd/25 y), drink one alcoholic beverage daily, and are sexually active with your wife.

As the doctor examines you, express tenderness on the upper part of the abdomen.

At the end of the encounter, ask:

Q1: *Do I have stomach cancer?*

Q2: *I remember my father had an endoscopy for his stomach. What is that?*

Role-Play 16: Answer Key

In this case, don't forget to ask about the color of the stool; in most of the cases, it may be associated with dark stool (melena).

History

Analysis of Chief Complaint

Vomiting of blood, ask **ABCDE** questions.

Analysis of Differential Diagnosis

Mark the following causes on the ▶ **Fig. 5.10** that will help you to remember them on the exam (if you draw this picture on the exam too).

Esophageal varices:
- *Have you noticed any yellowish discoloration of your eyes or skin?* (Jaundice)
- *Do you have any tendency to bleed? Do you bruise easily?* (Hepatocellular failure)
- *Have you noticed any swelling in your legs?*

Mallory–Weiss tear:
- *Was it preceded by heavy drinking?/Was it preceded by retching?*

Acute gastritis:
- *Was the bleeding preceded by taking any medicine such as NSAID or aspirin use?*

Stomach cancer:
- *Do you feel full quickly when you eat?/Do you have vomiting?*
- *Have you had any recent changes in your body weight?*

Peptic ulcer disease:
- *Do you have heartburn?/Are you currently using Tums or antacids?*

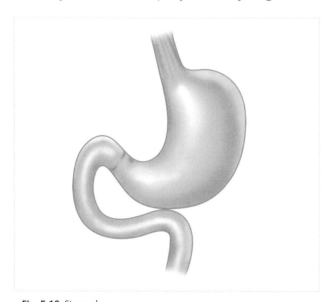

Fig. 5.10 Stomach.

Review of the Local System

As routine.

Review of Systems

As routine.

Past History and Others

As routine.

Physical Exam

As explained in the previous cases

Communication and Interpersonal Skills Component

Suggested Closure

As emergency case.

Counseling

Smoking, alcohol, and diet.

Suggested Answers to the Standardized Patient's Questions

Please answer as explained.

Patient Note

History

A 65-year-old male patient who came to the ER with hematemesis twice, the last about half of a cup a few hours earlier; he has no blood thinner use. The blood is bright red in color with no blood clots. He does not feel dizzy and has no bleeding anywhere else. He also has epigastric pain that radiates to his back, 5/10, is burning and not constant, increased with spicy food and smoking, and relieved by Tums. The bleeding was not preceded by retching, coughing, or heavy drinking. No dysphagia, abdominal pain anywhere else, jaundice, or lower limb edema. **ROS:** melena for 1 week, lost 6 lb/3 mo. **PMH:** peptic ulcer for 5 years. **Med:** ibuprofen, Tums, and pantoprazole. NKDA. **FH:** father died from stomach cancer. **SH:** manager in food industry with a lot of stress, smoker (1 ppd/25 y), drinks one alcoholic beverage daily, sexually active, monogamous with his wife.

Physical Exam

VS: 98°F, 100, 18, 100/60, and the patient is alert, oriented ×3. **H&N:** No pallor or jaundice and normal thyroid. No palpable LNs. **Ext:** no peripheral edema. **Chest:** CTA/BL. **Heart:** normal S1 and S2. **Abdomen:** no visible scars, soft, ND, tenderness over the epigastric area. BS +, no organomegaly.

Differential Diagnosis

History finding(s)	Physical exam finding(s)
1. Peptic ulcer bleeding	
Vomiting of blood	
Epigastric pain	Epigastric tenderness
Pain ↑ by spicy food and ↓ by tums	
2. Stomach cancer	
Vomiting of blood	
Epigastric pain	Epigastric tenderness
Loss of weight	6-lb loss
Father with stomach cancer	
3. Acute gastritis	
Vomiting of blood	
Epigastric pain	Epigastric tenderness
Takes ibuprofen	

Diagnostic Studies

Rectal exam

Stool analysis for OB, CBC, LFTs, *Helicobacter pylori* serology

Abdominal US

Upper GI endoscopy

5.5 Vomiting

On CS exam, vomiting is usually a secondary complaint (to the chief complaint) in many cases such as the following:

Abdominal cases: epigastric, RUQ, RLQ, flank... pain.

OB/Gyn (obstetrics and gynecology): pregnancy, ectopic pregnancy, PID...

Neurology: headache, dizziness and vertigo.

Psychiatry: anorexia nervosa and malingering

Endocrine (DKA [diabetic ketoacidosis]): Ask, *"Do you feel excessive thirst? Do you urinate frequently?"*

It is rare for vomiting to be on the CS exam as a chief complaint—commonly in gastroenteritis. In such cases, analyze it as routine, and then ask: *"Do you have other symptoms besides vomiting?"*

Proceed and ask more according to the SP further complaints and symptoms. Presence of fever in the doorway information can really help in narrowing the differential diagnosis. Consider gastroenteritis, PID, UTI, and other inflammatory diseases.

For no fever, think about questions for the conditions below:

Pregnancy: *"Are you sexually active? Are you using any contraception? When was your LMP? Is there any chance you could be pregnant?"*

Anorexia nervosa: *"Have you lost weight recently? Are your menstrual cycles regular? Are you preoccupied with gaining weight?"*

Medication-induced vomiting: *"Has it coincided with taking a new prescription or any OTC medicines?"*

Vertigo: *"Do you feel dizzy? Have you felt the room spinning around you?"*

5.6 Diarrhea

5.6.1 Analysis of Chief Complaint

As the routine questions (see Chapter 1, The Basics, Component 1, Integrated Clinical Encounter). To assess the degree of diarrhea/dehydration, you can also ask: *"Do you feel dizzy or light-headed?"*

5.6.2 Analysis of Differential Diagnosis

You can use this mnemonic: When HIV guy traveled, he got gastroenteritis. When he took antibiotics, he got inflammatory bowel disease and malabsorption.

HIV: Take sexual history in detail.

Traveler's diarrhea/infectious disease: *"Have you traveled outside the country recently? Have you been around any sick person?"*

Gastroenteritis: *"Have you been vomiting? Do you have any pain in your belly? Did you eat something unusual recently? Was diarrhea preceded by eating out? Does anyone in your family have the same complaint?"*

Antibiotic use: *"Are you currently taking any medicine? Are you currently taking any antibiotics?"*

Inflammatory bowel disease: *"Do you have a fever? Have you had any recent changes in weight? Do you have joint pain? Do you have a skin rash? Have you noticed any blood in your stool?"*

Malabsorption: Not common on the CS exam.

Role-Play 17

Mr. Hal Smith, 25 years old, has been **vomiting and has diarrhea** (▶**Fig. 5.11**).
Vital signs:
- Temp: 98°F (36.7°C).
- PR: 90/min, regular.
- RR: 16/min.
- BP: 110/70 mm Hg.

Standardized Patient's Role

You have vomited three times in the last 6 hours. The vomit had bits of food in it, but no blood. You have cramps in your abdomen, and the pain is partially relieved by diarrhea (two times). There is no mucous or blood. The pain is ill defined in your abdomen and is 4/10 in severity. You took your temperature at home. It was normal. You don't feel thirsty or dizzy.

All these symptoms started 6 hours ago after eating at a local restaurant. Your mother and father, who also ate there, have the same symptoms, but theirs are milder than yours. You are healthy with no medical diseases and have never had surgery. You just finished a course of amoxicillin for 7 days for acute sinusitis.

You are a college student. You don't smoke, but you do drink socially. You do not use drugs. You are sexually active with your girl-friend and you always use a condom.

Your parents are healthy and have no major health problems.

If the doctor asks you about anything other than vomiting, just say that your health has been fine.

When the doctor examines you, pretend that your upper abdomen (epigastric area) is tender.

When the physician starts the exam, ask:
Q1: *Do you think these symptoms are related to the food that I ate in the restaurant?*

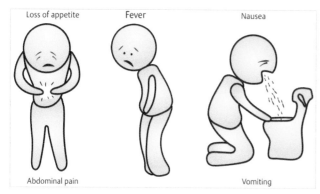

Fig. 5.11 Vomiting.

Role-Play 17: Answer Key

History

Analysis of Chief Complaint

Vomiting ± diarrhea, fever, abdominal pain (▶ **Fig. 5.11**).

Analysis of Differential Diagnosis

Gastroenteritis, food poisoning, etc.

Review of the Local System

As routine.

Review of Systems

As routine.

Past History and Others

As routine.

Physical Exam

Quick general exam, auscultate the lung and heart and do a full abdominal exam.

Communication and Interpersonal Skills Component

Suggested Closure

"Okay, now I have finished my exam; so let's review your case. You have vomiting, diarrhea, and abdominal pain. These symptoms started after eating with your parents at a restaurant. Also, you mentioned …. Based on your medical history and my physical exam, the problem could be inflammation of the stomach. This was probably caused by the restaurant food and it should be resolved soon. However, I can't totally eliminate other possible causes. So, we need to do … and …. When I get the results of these tests back, I'll give you my final diagnosis and the treatment options."

Suggested Answers to the Standardized Patient's Questions

"This is a good question, but please give me a few minutes to finish the PE first. I'm writing your questions down on my paper and I'll answer you as soon as I'm done, okay?"

As you finished: *"Have I answered your question?"*

History

A 25-year-old man complains of vomiting that started 6 hours ago after a meal at restaurant. He has vomited three times with no blood; does not feel thirsty or dizzy. He has cramping abdominal pain, 4/10, relieved partially by diarrhea (no blood). He feels nauseous. No difficulty swallowing or bloody stool. No blurry vision or headache. **ROS:** normal appetite, no recent changes in body weight or urinary problems. **PMH:** irrelevant. **Med:** N/D. **FH:** his parents who ate with him have the same condition but milder. **SH:** college student, denies smoking and drinks socially. He is sexually active with his girlfriend.

Physical Exam

VS: WNL. Alert and oriented ×3. **H&N:** no signs of dehydration, mucous membranes moist, throat without erythema, no palpable LNs. Normal thyroid. **Ext:** normal skin turgor, regular peripheral pulse. **Chest:** CTA/BL. **Heart:** normal S1 and S2. **Abdomen:** no visible scars, soft, ND, mildly tender epigastric area, no rebound or organomegaly, BS +, CVA not tender.

Differential Diagnosis

History finding(s)	Physical exam finding(s)
1. Viral gastroenteritis	
Nausea, vomiting and diarrhea	Epigastric tenderness
Cramping abdominal pain	No rebound
Ate outside home	
Family members share the same complaint	
2. Bacterial gastroenteritis	
Nausea, vomiting, and diarrhea	Epigastric tenderness
Cramping abdominal pain	No rebound
Ate outside home	
Family members share the same complaint	
Pseudomembranous colitis	
Diarrhea	
Just finished a course of amoxicillin	

Diagnostic Studies

Complete blood count, serum electrolytes

Role-Play 18

Doorway Information

Mrs. Nancy King, a 35-year-old woman, has **constipation.**

Vital signs:

- **Temp:** 98.6°F (37°C).
- **PR:** 84/min, regular.
- **RR:** 16/min.
- **BP:** 120/80 mm Hg.

Standardized Patient's Role

Put a transverse scar on your neck, as if you've had surgery for your thyroid.

You have been constipated for 6 months. You used to have bowel movements every day, but recently only twice a week, and you have to strain down with mild abdominal pain.

Your job as a sales representative doesn't allow you much time to cook and so you mostly eat fast food, with few vegetables and fruits.

You have been feeling tired and have been sleeping more than usual. Moreover, you feel cold when others don't feel that.

You have gained 8 lb in the last 6 months. Your menstruation has been irregular; your LMP was 2 weeks ago. Your bladder is overactive, and you take oxybutynin. You had a thyroidectomy for a benign disease 5 years ago and you take thyroid replacement therapy. You had two previous C-sections. You don't smoke or drink, and you live with your husband. Your father died of colon cancer at 60 years, and your mother suffers from depression.

When the doctor examines you, act normally, display no tenderness or soreness.

At the end of the encounter, ask:

Q1: *My father died of colon cancer. Do you recommend that I have a colonoscopy?*

Role-Play 18: Answer Key

History

Analysis of Chief Complaint

Constipation:

"When did it start? Since it started, has it gotten worse? How often do you defecate in a week? Tell me about your stool. Is it hard? Have you noticed any blood in your stool? Do you have rectal pain?"

Analysis of Differential Diagnosis (D+3M)

1. Diet-related
2. Mechanical: Intestinal obstruction and Colon cancer
3. Metabolic (hypothyroidism)
4. Medication: Anticholinergic, Opiates, and Iron

1. Diet:
- *Could you tell me a little bit more about your diet?*
- *What do you usually eat? Are you currently on any special diet?*
- *Does your diet have enough fiber?*
- *How often do you eat vegetables and fruit?*

2. Mechanical:
- *Have you been vomiting?*
- *Do you feel any swelling or distension in your belly?*
- *Have you noticed any blood in your stool?*
- *Have you lost weight recently?*

3. Metabolic: Ask hypothyroidism questions.

4. Medication: *Are you currently taking any medicine?*

Review of the Local System

As routine.

Review of Systems

As routine.

Past History and Others

As routine questions + D (hypothyroidism), S (any recent surgery), P (any previous episodes), D (anticholinergics).

Physical Exam

General exam is as a routine, plus palpate the thyroid. Do auscultation for **LH** only. Do a full abdominal exam and schedule for pelvic and rectal exams.

Communication and Interpersonal Skills Component

Suggested Closure

As routine questions.

Counseling

Food, for fiber-rich diet.

Suggested Answers to the Standardized Patient's Questions

"Well, I can certainly understand your concern. How old was your father when he got colon cancer?" Wait for the SP response. "I ask because the guideline for colonoscopy is to be offered to males at age 50, or who are 10 years younger than the age at which the youngest first-degree relative was affected. So, colonoscopy is recommended for you at the age of 45 years because and as you told me that your father got colon cancer when he was 55 years old."

Please refer to the Chapter 13, Appendix to review preventive medicine review.

Patient Note

History

A 35-year-old female patient complains of constipation for 6 months. She has bowel movement twice a week. The stool is hard with no blood. Defecation requires her to strain with mild abdominal pain. Her diet consists mainly of fast food with little fiber, is intolerant to the cold, feels tired and sleepy. No nausea, vomiting, dysphagia, or heartburn. No hematemesis or melena.

ROS: normal appetite, no fever, gained 8 lb/6 mo, LMP was 2 weeks ago, irregular menstrual cycles.

PMH: overactive bladder, thyroidectomy, two C-sections.

Med: thyroid replacement and oxybutynin. NKDA.

FH: father died of colon cancer, mother with depression.

SH: does not smoke or drink. Sexually active and monogamous with her husband.

Physical Exam

VS: WNL. Patient is alert, oriented ×3.

H&N: no pallor, throat without erythema, scar of possible thyroidectomy. No palpable LN.

Ext: normal skin no peripheral edema.

Chest: CTA/BL.

Heart: normal S1 and S2.

Abdomen: soft, NT, ND, BS +, no organomegaly.

Differential Diagnosis

History finding(s)	Physical exam finding(s)
1. Hypothyroidism	
Constipation	Scar from thyroid surgery
Cold intolerance	
Menstrual irregularities	
Past history of thyroidectomy, on thyroid replacement	
2. Medication-induced constipation	
Constipation	
Oxybutynin (anticholinergic)	
3. Diet-related constipation	
Constipation	
Low-fiber diet	

Diagnostic Studies

Rectal examination

TSH, free T3, and T4, CBC

Screening colonoscopy

Urology Cases

As the following cases are not so common on the CS exam, we see that the following information is quite enough.

Role-Play 19

Mrs. Gloria Peter, a 55-year-old woman, has **urinary leakage.**

Vital signs:

- Temp: 98.6°F (37°C).
- PR: 96/min, regular.
- RR: 16/min.
- BP: 110/70 mm Hg.

Standardized Patient's Role

You are a 55-year-old woman who came to the clinic as you have leakage of urine. It was mild for the last couple of years; however, it has been bothering you lately. You use three pads daily. The problem makes you to feel self-conscious.

You can't hold your urine and usually you release a few drops of urine before finding a toilet. Moreover, coughing, sneezing, and lifting heavy objects aggravate the problem.

Your LMP was 4 years ago. You've had five pregnancies, and all ended with normal deliveries. You and your mother have bronchial asthma (BA) and you use an albuterol inhaler. You have also peptic ulcer and take omeprazole.

You have smoked a pack of cigarettes daily for 20 years, are sexually active with your husband, and use local estrogen cream that helps in your sexual life.

Role-Play 19: Answer Key

History

Analysis of Chief Complaint

DD:
- Urge incontinence.
- Stress incontinence.
- Mixed incontinence.
- Total incontinence.
- Retention with overflow incontinence.

Ask about onset, course, alleviating and precipitating factors.
- *How often does it occur?*
- *How does this problem impact your life?*
- *Do you use sanitary napkins?"* If yes: *How many pads do you use a day?*

Analysis of Differential Diagnosis (▶Fig. 5.12)

- *Do you have to rush to the bathroom to urinate? (Urgency)*
- *Are you able to hold urine till you find a toilet?*
- *Have you had any leakage of urine while going to the bathroom?* (Urge incontinence).
- *Does it occur while sneezing or coughing?* (Stress incontinence)
- *Do you have difficulty starting to urinate?*
- *Does the urine come out continuously?* (Total incontinence)

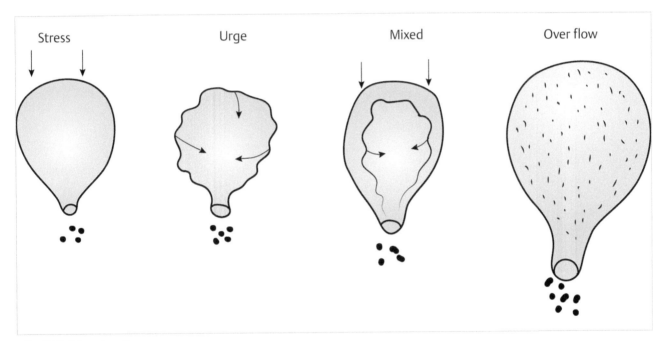

Fig. 5.12 Urinary incontinence.

Review of the Local System

Urology questions.

Review of Systems

Stress also on the following:
- *OB/Gyn history:* number and type of deliveries.
- History of neurological diseases.
- History of pelvic trauma/surgeries.

Past History and Others

As routine.

Physical Exam

As routine.

Communication and Interpersonal Skills Component

Counseling

"I am going to give you some recommendations that may help lessen your problem.

*I strongly advise you to follow a **timed voiding** pattern. It is a technique used to empty the bladder on a regular basis—not only when the urge to void is felt. The normal interval between voiding during the day is usually 3 to 4 hours. Simply, you train the bladder into a new voiding pattern.*

This way, you try to calm the urge in order to wait to go to the bathroom until the next scheduled voiding interval."

*"Could you keep for me a **voiding diary**? It is a simple record for various things about bladder function such as the frequency of urination, the volume of urine, and the volume of fluid intake, in addition to urge/incontinence episodes and pad usage."*

*"Also, I want to stress on **pelvic floor exercise**. As you may know, it is a series of exercises that strengthens your pelvic floor and helps reduce the risk of incontinence. I am going to give you a leaflet that explains how to do it."*

*"Finally, I want to remind you that **weight control and reduction** is an effective nonpharmaceutical therapy for urinary incontinence."*

Patient Note

History

A 55-year-old female patient complains of urinary leakage for 2 years. Initially mild but now requires 3 pads/d.

The leakage increases when coughing, sneezing, and lifting heavy objects. She is usually dry at night. The problem bothers her and makes her very self-conscious. Sometimes she needs to rush to the bathroom to urinate. No abdominal pain, dysuria, or difficulty urinating. No hematuria; bowel movements are normal; postmenopausal for 4 years, G5P5. Normal deliveries, no tingling nor numbness elsewhere. **PMH:** BA, peptic ulcer. **Med:** albuterol inhaler, PPI. NKDA. **FH:** mother with BA. **SH:** smokes 1 ppd/20 y, sexually active, monogamous, uses estrogen vaginal cream.

Physical Exam

VS: WNL and alert, oriented ×3. **H&N:** no pallor, jaundice, mouth without erythema, normal thyroid. No palpable LNs. **Ext:** no peripheral edema. **Chest:** CTA/BL. **Heart:** normal S1 and S2. **Abdomen:** lax, ND, NT. BS (+)ve, no organomegaly.

Differential Diagnosis

History finding(s)	Physical exam finding(s)
1. Stress urinary incontinence	
Leakage of urine	
Increases when sneezing, coughing	
2. Urge urinary incontinence	
Leakage of urine	
Rush to the bathroom to urinate	
3. Mixed urinary incontinence	
Leakage of urine	
Has stress and urge incontinence	

Diagnostic Studies

Pelvic exam, stress test

Urinalysis, urine culture

Cystogram and urodynamics

Role-Play 20

Mr. Richard, a 62-year-old man, has **weak penile erection**.
Vital signs:
  Temp: 98.6°F (37°C).
  PR: 96/min, regular.
  RR: 16/min.
  BP: 170/110 mm Hg.

Standardized Patient's Role

You are a 62-year-old male patient and have had a sexual problem for the last 6 months. It is so embarrassing, the reason that makes you reluctant to ask for medical advice. When you explain your complaint, tell your doctor, *"My problem is so embarrassing!"* (**Comment 1**)

You have sexual desire; however, your erection is too weak to commence sex with your wife. Ejaculation is also delayed with infrequent nocturnal erection.

This problem started gradually but worsened with time. You have had high BP and diabetes for 20 years. You take propranolol and insulin. For the last couple of years, your BP and diabetes haven't been under control, probably because you are not complaint with your meds. If the doctor asks you about the reason, tell him or her that you no longer have health insurance since you have retired from your work (**Comment 2**). You also have to stop after four to five blocks to catch your breath and rest because of leg cramps.

You also have had depression for 1 year and your psychiatrist has added daily buspirone.

Your father died from a heart attack, and your mother has Alzheimer's disease. You stopped smoking 10 years ago, but you smoked 1 pack of cigarettes a day for 20 years. You drink socially.

During the physical exam: Pretend that the sensation in your legs is a little impaired compared to your arms.

Role-Play 20: Answer Key

This is relatively uncommon on the CS exam.

DD:
- Psychogenic ED.
- Organic ED (vascular, neurologic, venous).
- Medication side effects.

History

Analysis of Chief Complaint

After asking about onset, course, alleviating and precipitating factors, ask:
- *What degree of impotence do you have?*
- *Are you able to have sexual intercourse or not?*
- *Do you have sexual desire?* (libido)
- *Do you have morning/nocturnal erection?* (persists in psychogenic ED)

Analysis of Differential Diagnosis

For psychogenic erectile dysfunction (ED):
- *"Do you have any kind of interpersonal conflicts or problems with your spouse? Is your home life or work stressful in any way?/ Do you feel depressed?/Do you feel sad?"*

For organic ED:
- *"Do you have high BP? Do you have diabetes?"* If yes, ask:
- *"Do you have any chest pain? Do you have any problems with your vision?"*
- *"While walking, do you have to stop to catch your breath? While walking, have you had any cramps in your legs?"*
- *"Have you noticed any changes in the sensations in your legs?"*
- *"Have you had any major accidents?"* (Venous leak)

Review of the Local System

Ask questions regarding urinary system.

Other components of history, physical exam, and CIS: Follow the standard as explained in the previous cases.

History

A 62-year-old male patient who has had erectile dysfunction for 6 months. It came on gradually and has been progressive. Ejaculation is delayed and nocturnal erection is infrequent, but libido is normal. Has no social or personal problems with his spouse. He has leg claudicating for five to six blocks, no vision problems, chest pain, headache, dizziness, no history of TIA (transient ischemic attack), and has never passed out. **ROS:** no urinary nor bowel problems. **PMH:** HTN and DM 20 years and depression 1 year ago. **Med:** propranolol, insulin, buspirone. NKDA. **FH:** father died of heart attack; mother has Alzheimer's. **SH:** ex-smoker for 10 years (smoked 1 ppd/20 y), drinks socially.

Physical Exam

VS: BP: 170/110, others WNL, alert, conscious. **H&N:** PERRLA (pupils equal, reactive to light and accommodation), intact red reflex. No carotid bruit or jugular venous distention. **Ext:** no hair no skin changes, pulse +2 bilateral. **Chest:** CTA/BL. **Heart:** normal S1 and S2. **Neuro:** intact sensation to pinprick and light touch in both upper limbs and impaired in the lower limbs.

Differential Diagnosis

History finding(s)	Physical exam finding(s)
1. Organic erectile dysfunction (vascular/neurogenic)	
Gradual onset, progressive course	
HTN, DM for 20 y, leg claudicating	Impaired sensation on the lower limbs
No loss of libido	
2. Medication-induced ED	
Weak penile erection	
Taking buspirone and propranolol	

Diagnostic Studies

Pelvic and penile exam

FBS and HB A1c and hormonal profile

Nocturnal penile tumescence

Penile Doppler US

Role-Play 21

Doorway Information

Mr. Adam Smith, a 60-year-old male patient, has **dark urine**.

Vital signs:
   Temp: 98.6° (37°C).
   PR: 90/min, regular.
   RR: 18/min.
   BP: 110/70 mm Hg.

Standardized Patient's Role

You came to the ER as you noticed that you have had blood in your urine for the last few days but had half of a cup of bright red blood with no clotting 2 hours ago.

You have had difficulty in urinating and when you do, the stream is weak. You notice that you are going to the bathroom more often than you used to in the daytime and at night (three times). You take medication for a prostate condition. The prescription is tamsulosin: you have been taking 0.4 mg at bedtime for the past 10 years.

You remember passing a kidney stone (about 7 mm) 10 years ago. You have lost nearly 6 lb during the last 3 months.

Your father died from urinary bladder cancer when he was 65 years old.

You work as a painter, smoke (1 pack daily for 25 years), and drink socially. You live with your wife and have no other sexual partners.

As the doctor examines you, express tenderness in the lower abdomen.

Ask your doctor:
Q1: *Do I have cancer?*
Q2: If the doctor informs that you may need a cystoscopy, ask him or her what a cystoscopy is.

Role-Play 21: Answer Key

History

Analysis of Chief Complaint

Dark urine (ABCDE).

Analysis of Differential Diagnosis

Urologic: trauma, infections, stone disease, BPH, and cancer (▶ **Fig. 5.13**). Mark the following causes on the fig. 5.13 that will help you to remember them on the exam (if you draw this picture on the exam too).
- *Did you injure your back or your belly?*
- *Do you have a fever?*
- *Does it burn while you are urinating?*
- *Have you ever passed a kidney stone?*
- Ask the questions for obstructive and irritative lower urinary tract symptoms (LUTS; see the questions for BPH in the Chapter 5, Abdomen (Gastroenterology and Urology), Urology section):
- *What do you do for work?* (Chemical/textile workers are at risk for bladder cancer.)

Nephrologic: glomerulonephritis.
- *Have you noticed any puffiness in your face?*
- *Do you have any swelling in your legs or in your hands?*
- *Have you had any recent respiratory tract infection?*

Others: Food, medication, and exercise-related hematuria.
- *Does it occur with any specific kind of food? With heavy exercise?*
- *Has it come with a new prescription?*

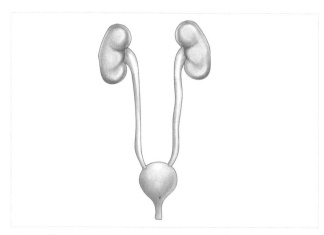

Fig. 5.13 Urinary tract.

Review of the Local System

Do you have flank pain? Any back pain? Do you have any problem passing urine?

Review of Systems

As routine.

Past History and Others

D (BPH, stone disease...), P (? previous episodes), D (alpha blockers), F (of cancer), S (occupational hazards, smoking...). Sexual history with little detail.

Physical Exam

Document for pallor, do full abdominal exam and CVA tenderness, and finally ask for the necessity of a pelvic exam.

Patient Note

History

A 60-year-old man who complains of hematuria for days, no blood thinner use, about half of a cup, bright red in color with no clots, doesn't feel dizzy. It was not preceded by specific food, trauma, or exercise. No fever, renal colic, or dysuria. He has had obstructive LUTS (difficulty in urinating, weak stream) and irritative symptoms (frequency and nocturia) that improved with meds. No puffiness of eyes, no peripheral edema. **ROS:** lost 6 lb/6 mo, normal bowel movements. **PMH:** BPH for 10 years; passed a renal stone 10 years ago. **Meds:** tamsulosin. NKDA. **FH:** father died from bladder cancer. **SH:** painter, smoker 1 ppd/25 y, social drinker, sexually active, monogamous with wife.

Physical Exam

VS: WNL and alert, oriented ×3. **H&N:** no pallor, throat without erythema, normal thyroid. No palpable LNs. **Ext:** no peripheral edema. **Chest:** CTA/BL. **Heart:** normal S1 and S2. **Abdomen:** Soft, tenderness over the suprapubic area, ND, BS +, CVA nontender.

Differential Diagnosis

History finding(s)	Physical exam finding(s)
1. Benign prostatic hyperplasia	
Hematuria	
Obstructive and irritative LUTS	
Takes tamsulosin	
2. Prostate cancer	
Hematuria	
Obstructive and irritative LUTS	
Lost weight	Lost 6 lb/6 mo
3. Bladder cancer	
Hematuria	Tenderness over the suprapubic area
Irritative LUTS	
Smoker for 20 y, family history of bladder cancer and works as a painter	
Lost weight	Lost 6 lb/6 mo

Diagnostic Studies

Rectal and genital exams

UA, CBC, serum creatinine and PSA

Renal and pelvic US

CT abdomen with contrast

Cystoscopy

6 Obstetrics and Gynecology

Keywords: vaginal bleeding, vaginal discharge, pregnancy, hot flashes, menopause

6.1 Introduction

In this specialty, the following are common on doorway information: abdominal pain, vaginal bleeding/discharge, missing last menstrual period (LMP)/pregnancy, and hot flashes/menopause.

The complaints you are most likely to encounter on the Clinical Skills (CS) exam are abdominal pain and vaginal bleeding and the least common case is vaginal discharge. No matter what type the case is, you should always take a detailed gynecological and obstetric (OB/Gyn) history. Sample questions are listed in the following section.

We used **PPC** mnemonics for all females (see Chapter 1, The Basics, Component 1, Integrated Clinical Encounter); however, this part of the history should be asked in detail in OB/Gyn cases.

6.2 Gynecological History: The routine (PPC) + Bleeding (3M + C)

- *When was your last menstrual Period?*
- *Is your cycle regular?*
- *How often do you have your menstrual period?*
- *How many days does it last?*
- *Have you had a **P**ap smear done? When? Was it normal?*
- *Do you use any kind of **C**ontraception?*
- *How old were you when you had your **F**irst menstrual period? (**M**enarche)*
- *How many pads do you use on a heavy day? (**M**enorrhagia)*
- *Have you ever bled between cycles? (**M**etrorrhagia)*
- *Have you ever noticed any bleeding or spotting after intercourse? (Post–**C**oital bleeding)*

6.3 Obstetric History (Gravida, Para, Abortion)

- *Have you ever been **pregnant**? If no: Don't ask more questions.*

If yes:
- *How many times have you been **pregnant**?*
- *How many times have you given **birth**?*
- *Did you have a natural birth or a C-section?*
- *Have you ever had a miscarriage or an **abortion**? If yes:*
- *How many times? Was it first, second, or third trimester? Do you have any idea what caused it?*

Role-Play 22

Doorway Information

Mrs. Sharon Evans, a 25-year-old woman, complains of **lower abdominal pain.**

Vital signs:

- **Temperature (Temp):** 98°F (36.7°C).
- **Pulse Rate (PR):** 108/min, regular.
- **Respirator Rate (RR):** 20/min.
- **Blood Pressure (BP):** 90/60 mm Hg.

Examinee tasks:

Obtain a focused history.

Perform a relevant physical examination (PE). Do not perform rectal, pelvic, genitourinary, inguinal hernia, female breast, or corneal reflex examinations.

Discuss your initial diagnostic impression and your workup plan with the patient.

After leaving the room, complete your patient note (PN) on the given form.

Standardized Patient's Role

When the doctor enters, lie back in the bed and complain of severe pain in your abdomen.

When the doctor starts asking about your medical history, say (**comment 1**): *"Doc, I'm so worried. I've been bleeding from my vagina."*

You came to the ER with severe sharp abdominal pain that started 1 hour ago. It was sudden and severe; you rate your pain as 9/10. The pain is in the lower left side of the abdomen. It is constant and gets worse when you cough. Nothing makes your pain better. Occasionally, you find blood in your underwear. It is not a lot but is bright red in color. For the last 2 weeks, you have had morning sickness and your breasts are tender.

You had the first menstrual period in your life at the age of 13 years. Your menses are usually regular, occurring every 28 days and lasting for 5 days. However, the last one should have come 3 weeks ago, but it didn't. You had a Pap smear 2 years ago; the result was normal. You have been pregnant once, 2 years ago. However, you miscarried at 2 months.

You are sexually active with multiple male partners who only occasionally use condom. You work in a restaurant, smoke 1 pack per day for 5 years (1 ppd/5 y), drink one beer daily and more on weekends.

When the doctor begins examining you, complain of sever tenderness on the lower left side of the abdomen. Complain when the doctor presses the hand down and when he lets it go. Then, ask **Q1:** *"Do I have a miscarriage"?*

Please refer to Chapter 13 (Appendix), to review the general instructions for the SP as well as the Doctor roles.

Lower Abdominal Pain in a Female SP (►Fig. 6.1)

When any female SP presents with acute abdominal pain, first figure out the possibility of pregnancy. Look at the patient's age on the doorway information to see if she is in the child-bearing range. Ask *"When was your LMP? Have you missed a period? Is there any chance you could be pregnant?"*

If you found out that there is a possibility of pregnancy, ask about for vaginal bleeding. *"Do you have any vaginal bleeding or spotting?"* If yes, analyze as usual (ABCDE).

Possible causes include ectopic pregnancy and miscarriage.

In the cases of abdominal pain without significant vaginal bleeding and no possibility of pregnancy (another common scenario of abdominal pain in a female on the CS exam), the following are included:

- Ovarian torsion.
- Ruptured ovarian cyst.
- Pelvic inflammatory disease (for cases with fever).

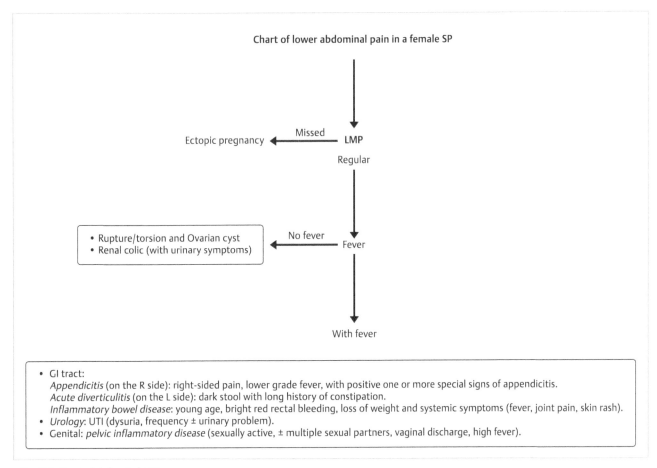

Fig. 6.1 Chart of abdominal pain.

Role-Play 22: Answer Key

Abdominal pain (female + missed LMP).

History

Analysis of Chief Complaint

Abdominal pain + vaginal spotting.

Analysis of Differential Diagnosis

Ectopic pregnancy and miscarriage.

Review of the Local System

OB/Gyn system questions.

Review of Systems

As routine questions.

Past History and Others

As routine questions + **S** (previous gynecological surgery), **D** (contraceptive use), ± **S** (full sexual history).

Physical Exam

As a standard + full abdominal exam. **Special maneuvers:** Rebound tenderness, ask for SP's permission to do a local/pelvic examination, and document it in the PN.

Communication and Interpersonal Skills Component

Suggested Closure

> *"Mrs...., let us review your case. I need to be sure that understand it right. You have severe abdominal pain and vaginal spotting, both started 1 hour ago. Also, you have had morning sickness for the last few weeks and your breasts are tender. You are sexually active and you missed your last period. Based on your history and my physical exam, you could be pregnant, and you should have a pregnancy test done so we can be sure. At this point, I have a preliminary diagnosis. You may have a problem that is related to a possible pregnancy. Also, I would like you to be admitted to the hospital. Your BP is low. This may be due to significant blood loss, so that is the best care for you till we are sure that everything is fine. Now, I'll call the nurse to collect the samples for you and I'll be right back in a minute to inform you of the results."*

Counseling

Safe sex precautions.

Suggested Answers to the Standardized Patient's Questions and Comments

Comment 1: *"I'm sorry to hear that. I know that it must be uncomfortable and scary for you. However, don't worry because I'm going to do everything possible to help you stop bleeding as soon as possible."*

Q1: *"I think I have addressed this concern as best as I can at this point; do you have any other questions for me?"*

Patient Note

History

A 25-year-old woman complains of severe abdominal pain, began suddenly 1 hour ago, worsening with time, in the left lower quadrant (LLQ), nonradiating, sharp, 9/10, constant ↑ with coughing; nothing alleviates the pain. Accompanied with nausea, vaginal spotting of bright red blood, not dizzy. Not preceded by trauma or sexual intercourse. LMP was 7 weeks ago; missed the last one for 3 weeks. No bowel or urinary problems, menarche was at 13 years old, regular cycle 28/5. No menorrhagia or abnormal discharge, last Pap smear was 2 years ago and was normal, G1P0, the pregnancy that ended by spontaneous abortion 2 years ago.

Review of system (ROS): irrelevant.

Past medical history (PMH): healthy, evacuation for spontaneous abortion 2 years ago. No known drug allergy (NKDA).

Family history (FH): parents are healthy.

Social history (SH): works at a local restaurant, smokes 1 ppd/5y, drinks 1 beer/d, more on weekends, no use of street drugs. Sexually active, multiple sexual partners, occasional use of condom, never tested for HIV.

Physical Exam

Vital signs (VS): 98°F, 108, 20, 90/60. Appears anxious, lying back in pain.

Head and Neck (H&N): no pallor or cyanosis.

Lung and heart: normal S1, S2, CLA/BL (clear to auscultation bilaterally).

Extremities (Ext): regular peripheral pulsation, no pallor.

Abdomen: no scars or deformities, bowel sounds is positive (sometimes abbreviated as BS +), and tenderness at LLQ, + rebound, no organomegaly.

Differential Diagnosis

History finding(s)	Physical exam finding(s)
1. Ectopic pregnancy	
Missed the last period	
Acute LLQ pain	Tenderness over the LLQ
Vaginal bleeding	Hypotension, tachycardia
2. Abortion	
Missed the last period	
Vaginal bleeding	Hypotension, tachycardia
Acute LLQ pain	Tenderness over the LLQ

Diagnostic Studies

Pelvic and vaginal exam

Pregnancy test and quantitative beta-hCG (beta-human chorionic gonadotropin)

Pelvic ultrasonography (US; ► **Fig. 6.2a**)

Diagnostic laparoscopy (if pelvic US is not diagnostic or in emergency situation; ► **Fig. 6.2b**)

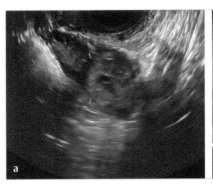 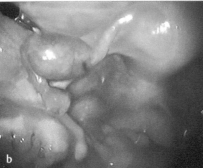

Fig. 6.2 (a) Ultrasonography showing ectopic pregnancy on the tube. (b) Laparoscopic view showing ectopic pregnancy on the left fallopian tube.

Role-Play 23

Doorway Information

Mrs. Linda Brown, a 30-year-old female patient, came to the ER with severe **lower abdominal pain**.
Vital signs:
- **Temp:** 101°F (38.3°C).
- **PR:** 104/min, regular.
- **RR:** 20/min.
- **BP:** 100/60 mm Hg.

Standardized Patient's Role

As the doctor enters, lie back in the bed complaining of severe abdominal pain (on left lower abdomen). You came to the ER because you have severe burning abdominal pain, which started a few hours ago and has been getting worse. This pain rates 7/10, is localized to the lower left abdominal area, radiates to the pelvis, and is constant. The pain worsens when you cough or move around. Nothing seems to make it better. You are nauseous, but you only had a single incidence of vomiting of clear fluid.

When you urinate, there is a burning sensation with increasing frequency. There is also a foul-smelling vaginal discharge, which is white-greenish in color, but there is no blood. You use one to two pads a day.

You are a woman in good health with no diseases, and you have never had an operation. You had your first period at the age of 13 years, and your menses are regular (every 28 days), last around 5 days, and you never have been pregnant. You contracted gonorrhea 6 months ago and a kidney infection 1 year ago. Both of those have been cured, and you are not currently taking any medication.

You are a teacher, you don't smoke but drink socially, and are sexually active with multiple partners, with no condom use, and you take oral contraceptive pills (OCPs). You had a Pap smear 2 years ago; the result was normal.

When the doctor begins examining you, complain of tenderness on the lower part of the left side of the abdomen. Complain when the doctor presses the hand down and when he or she lets it go. Also, express tenderness if the doctor taps on your back.

At the end of the encounter, ask:

Q1: *"Doc, I don't have time to stay in the hospital. I can't miss work. Please just give me a prescription for some pain meds and let me go."*

Role-Play 23: Answer Key

Lower abdominal pain: Young female + fever.

History

Analysis of Chief Complaint

Abdominal pain + vaginal discharge + fever.

Analysis of Differential Diagnosis

Pelvic inflammatory disease, urinary tract infection, and others.

Review of the Local System

OB/Gyn system questions.

Review of Systems

Ask routine questions.

Past History and Others

Ask routine questions.

Physical Exam

As standard + full abdominal exam. **Special maneuvers:** rebound tenderness, costovertebral angle (CVA) tenderness. Ask for SP's permission to do a local and a pelvic examination; document it in the PN.

Communication and Interpersonal Skills Component

Suggested Closure

As emergency case.

Counseling

Safe sex precautions.

Suggested Answers to the Standardized Patient's Questions

Q1: Ask her first, *"Why don't you want to be admitted to the hospital?"* Wait for her response. You can say, *"Well, although … is your concern, your health is my concern, too. You have abdominal tenderness and a fever, and I recommend that you be admitted to the hospital till we find out what's going on. Although I can't force you to stay, it's in your best interest, and besides, the problem may get much worse."*

Patient Note

History

A 30-year-old woman complains of abdominal pain, sudden onset and progressive course, on LLQ, radiates to pelvis, sharp, 7/10, constant, ↑ when coughing and moving, denies any alleviating factors. Associated with dysuria, nausea, one instance of vomiting, clear and not bloody, has foul-smelling white-greenish vaginal discharge. **ROS:** LMP 5 days ago, menarche at 13 years, regular 28/5, never been pregnant, no bowel problems, or recent loss of weight. **PMH:** previous urinary tract infection (UTI) episode (pyelonephritis). **Med:** over-the-counter (OTC). NKDA. **SH:** works as a teacher, denies smoking, drinks socially. Sexually active, multiple male partners, does not use condoms or OCPs, and had gonorrhea last year.

Physical Exam

VS: 101°F, 104, 20, 100/60. Alert, orient ×3, lying back in pain. **H&N:** no pallor, PERRLA, throat without erythema. **Ext:** no peripheral edema. **Lung and Heart:** S1, S2 normal, CTA/BL. **Abdomen:** no scars or deformities, bowel sounds in all 4 quadrants (sometimes abbreviated as +BS ×4Q). Tenderness in the LLQ and left lumber area, + rebound. No organomegaly. CVA tenderness on the left side.

Differential Diagnosis

History finding(s)	Physical exam finding(s)
1. Pelvic inflammatory disease	
Pain in LLQ	Tenderness in LLQ
Feels feverish	Fever (101°F)
Vaginal discharge	
Sexually active, no condom	
Gonorrhea last year	
2. Urinary tract infection	
Pain in LLQ and left lumbar	Tenderness in LLQ
Feels feverish	Fever (101°F)
Dysuria	CVA+

Diagnostic Studies

Pelvic exam

CBC (complete blood count), UA (urinalysis), urine culture, Pap smear, HVS (high vaginal swab)

Pregnancy test

US (abdomen and pelvis)

CT (abdomen and pelvis)

Role-Play 24

Mrs. Sally Smith, a 24 year-old woman, missed her last period and came to the clinic after having **a positive result on a home pregnancy test.**

Vital signs:

- **Temp:** 98°F (36.7°C).
- **PR:** 90/min, regular.
- **RR:** 16/min.
- **BP:** 110/70 mm Hg.

Standardized Patient's Role

You have been married for 6 years and have a 5-year-old boy. Your husband stopped condom use as a contraceptive a few weeks ago, as you wish to have a new baby. As you missed the last period that was supposed to be 1 week ago, you bought a pregnancy test and are very happy, as it came out positive. For the last few days, you have felt nauseated. You have had morning sickness, tender breasts, and frequent urination.

You are fairly healthy, and you don't take any meds apart from multivitamins that you have started since you found out you are pregnant. As you remember, your first menses came when you were 12 years old; it was regular. It now comes every 28 days and lasts usually for 5 days. You had one natural birth 5 years ago. You had a Pap smear 2 years ago; the result was normal.

You work as a technician at a medical lab, have smoked five cigarettes daily for 5 years and drink socially. You never had any sexually transmitted diseases.

At the end of the encounter, ask:

Q1: *Can I work out? Is there anything I should not be doing?*

Q2: *How do I know if there is a problem with my pregnancy? What do I need to be aware of?*

Amenorrhea is a cessation of menstruation; it can be primary or secondary. Secondary amenorrhea is the more common on the CS exam.

Differential Diagnosis for Secondary Amenorrhea

- Pregnancy.
- **Two endocrine causes:** hyperprolactinemia and hypothyroidism.
- **Two ovarian causes:** premature ovarian failure and polycystic ovary disease.

Analysis of Differential Diagnosis

Pregnancy:

- *Is there any chance you could be pregnant?*
- *Are you sexually active?*
- *Do you use any kind of contraception?*

Ask about the following: nausea, morning sickness, heaviness of the breasts, etc.

Hyperprolactinemia:

- *Do you have any milk discharge from breasts?*
- *Do you have headaches, blurry vision, and vomiting?* (signs of increased intracranial pressure)

Hypothyroidism: see questions in Chapter 1, The Basics, Component 1, Integrated Clinical Encounter.

Premature ovarian failure:

- *Do you have any hot flashes?*

Polycystic ovary disease (PCOD):

- *Have you noticed any new hair or abnormal hair growth? Any changes in your voice?*

Role-Play 24: Answer Key

Amenorrhea caused by pregnancy (▶ Fig. 6.3).

Pregnancy on the CS exam may appear on the doorway information in a variety of ways, such as noting that there was a positive pregnancy test result, or that the SP missed her LMP (amenorrhea).

If you see a positive pregnancy test result on the doorway information, take note of the SP's emotional state when you enter the exam room. If she is smiling and appears happy, you may assume that the pregnancy was planned or is welcome. Return her smile. If, on the other hand, the SP seems sad, this could be a sign that the pregnancy was unplanned or unwanted. Be reserved and sympathetic until you know what the situation is. Plan to use the last 3 minutes for counseling and closure.

Note: This case presented with positive pregnancy test, so there's no need to ask all the questions presented for the differential diagnosis of secondary amenorrhea. However, these questions should be asked for cases that present with missed menstrual period.

History

In general, taking the history and doing the physical exams are straightforward.

When you take the history, focus on symptoms of early pregnancy and the symptoms of warning. Also, ask about immunizations, diet and exercise habits, and vices (▶ Table 6.1).

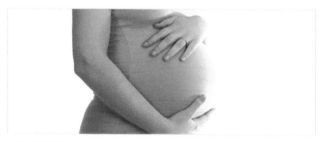

Fig. 6.3 Woman with pregnancy.

Table 6.1 Suggested questions for pregnancy case

Start asking about pregnancy with:
Was this a planned pregnancy, or has it come as a surprise?/Has this pregnancy come at a good time in your life?

Early symptoms of pregnancy	Ask about: missed LMP, nausea, morning sickness, vomiting, breast tenderness, and frequent urination
Pregnancy warning symptoms	*Have you been vomiting frequently?* *Have you fainted?* *Have you had any severe abdominal pain?* *Have you noticed any vaginal bleeding?*
Immunizations	*Have you had shots for measles? Varicella? German measles? Influenza?*
Diet	*Could you tell me a little bit more about your diet?*
Exercise	*How often do you work out?* *How long do you work out each time?*
Vices	*Do you smoke?* *Do you drink?* *Are you using any drugs, like cocaine, marijuana, heroin, or anything else that I should know about?*
Sex life	Sexual history

Finish with a detailed sexual history and figure out if the pregnancy is planned or not, and if she wants to have the child. *Remember, you are not giving advice or suggesting her to have an abortion, you are merely asking to find out about her psychological frame of mind.*

Communication and Interpersonal Skills Component

Suggested Closure

"Mrs...., have a seat. I want to tell you what I've come up with so far. You have told me you got a positive pregnancy test at home, in addition to nausea, morning sickness, and ..., ..., ... for the last few weeks. You are sexually active with no contraceptive use and you missed your last period. Given your medical history and the results of the physical exams, I would say it's highly possible that you are pregnant. To be 100% sure, we need to repeat the test again and I would like to get a urine sample for analysis and culture, and a blood sample for blood grouping and Rh factor, and finally, we'll test your immunization status."

Counseling

Use Triple 2 rule (see Chapter 2, The Basics, Component 2, Communication and Interpersonal Skills, Communication Skills Part).

End your counseling with: *"And if you are pregnant, I'll be happy to see you regularly throughout your pregnancy. After we know if you are pregnant, we can discuss immunizations such as influenza."*

Suggested Answers to the Standardized Patient's Questions

Possible SP's questions	Answers
Q1: *Are there any precautions regarding my physical activity? Can I work out? Is there anything I should not be doing?*	*"Generally, strenuous physical exercise is not permitted, otherwise you can remain active the entire pregnancy."*
Q2: *How do I know if there is a problem with my pregnancy? What do I need to be aware of?*	*"The danger signs of pregnancy problems are severe abdominal pain and any fainting or vaginal bleeding. Don't hesitate to call us at any time. We are available 24/7. Here is my business card."*

History

A 24-year-old woman came to the clinic as she had a positive pregnancy test result. She has nausea, morning sickness, tender breasts, and frequent urination for the last few weeks. Denies headache, blurry vision, and vaginal bleeding.

ROS: normal sleep, appetite, no recent loss of weight, normal bowel movements. Menarche at 12 years, LMP was 5 weeks ago, regular 28/5, last Pap smear was 2 years ago that was normal, G1P1, normal vaginal delivery, no current use of contraception.

PMH: N/D.

Med: vitamins. NKDA.

FH: no familiar diseases. **SH:** technician, smoker 0.5 ppd/5 y, drinks socially, sexually active, monogamous with her husband. No STDs, never tested for HIV.

Physical Exam

VS: WNL. Alert, orient ×3.

H&N: no pallor, PERRLA, throat without erythema.

Ext: no peripheral edema.

Lung and Heart: S1, S2 normal, CTA/BL.

Abdomen: No scars or deformities, soft, + BS in 4 QU. non tender (NT), and non distended (ND).

Differential Diagnosis

History finding(s)	Physical exam finding(s)
1. Pregnancy	
Missed the LMP and + pregnancy test	Normal exam
Nausea, vomiting, morning sickness, and breast tenderness	
Sexually active, no contraception	

Diagnostic Studies

Pelvic exam

Pregnancy test, CBC, Rh factor, UA, urine culture

Serology (measles, varicella, VDRL [Venereal Disease Research Laboratory test])

Role-Play 25

Mrs. Carolina Williams, a 52-year-old woman, came to the clinic complains of **hot flashes**.
Vital signs:
- **Temp:** 98°F (36.7°C).
- **PR:** 90/min, regular.
- **RR:** 16/min.
- **BP:** 120/80 mm Hg.

Standardized Patient's Role

You came to the clinic as you have hot flashes for the last 3 months; they usually come without any warning beforehand, four to five times a day. They last maybe for a few minutes and occasionally came with irregular heartbeats and sweating. They are generally tolerable, but sometimes they make you nauseated and disturb your sleep.

You are not feeling good not only from hot flashes, but also because your sexual life has started to be affected. You have vaginal pain during sex with your husband, but he is very supportive and cooperative.

You have high BP and take propranolol 10 mg daily. You had a laparoscopic cholecystectomy done many years ago. You are allergic to penicillin.

As you remember, your first menstrual period was at 13 years; it was regular. It came every 28 days, lasted for 5 days. However, it was less than usual for the last year and the last time you had it was 3 months ago. You had two full-term pregnancies and all were ended with normal deliveries.

Your mother died from breast cancer. You smoke five cigarettes daily and drink socially. You have only your husband as your sexual partner.

At the end of the encounter, ask:
Q1: What is hormonal replacement therapy (HRT)?

Role-Play 25: Answer Key

In the cases like this one, take a focused history, do a quick PE, and then allow a few minutes for closure and counseling.

History

Analysis of Chief Complaint

- *How long have you been having hot flashes?*
- *How often do you have them?*
- *How long do they last?*
- *Is there any warning beforehand?*
- *How much would you say the hot flashes bother you?*

Problems associated with menopause: osteoporosis, atrophic vaginitis, depression, and others, such as sweating, palpitation, or difficulty in sleeping.

- *Do your bones ache?/Do you have any pain in your back/legs?*
- *Have you been sexually active lately?*
- *Have you been having any problems while/with having sex?*
- *Do you feel sad or depressed?*
- *Do you have any problems besides hot flashes?*

Analysis of Differential Diagnosis

Ask questions inquiring for hyperthyroidism.

Review of the Local System

A detailed OB/Gyn history.

Review of Systems

As routine.

Past History and Others

As routine, but pay particular attention to the heart, previous thromboembolic diseases, calcium or HRT medications, family history of breast cancer.

Physical Exam

No specific exam is needed; just give the SP a quick general exam, with a chest and heart, and an abdominal exam plus a brief neurological exam.

Counseling is mandatory. Schedule the SP for a counseling session and follow-up.

Communication and Interpersonal Skills Component

Counseling

"In general, I have some recommendations for you: You probably already know this, but you should stop smoking and drinking (see Chapter 2, The Basics, Component 2, Communication and Interpersonal Skills). Exercise regularly. My suggestion is 20 minutes a day, five times a week. Eat healthy foods.

Maybe later we will add calcium and vitamin supplements (▶ Fig. 6.4). I can also prescribe estrogen vaginal cream because you experience pain during intercourse.

Have you had a mammogram done?" (If not, recommend one.)

Suggested Answers to the Standardized Patient's Questions

Q1: *"HRT has its advantages and disadvantages. It works for hot flashes as well as helping with sex. However, there may be some side effects. It can increase the risk of breast cancer and heart disease. Your mother died from breast cancer and this should be taken in consideration. We will figure out this issue later. Now, do you have any other questions or concerns for me?"*

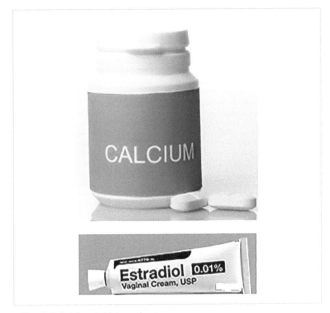

Fig. 6.4 Calcium tablets and estrogen cream.

Patient Note

History

A 52-year-old woman has had hot flashes for 3 months. They occur four to five times per day and appear without warning. They last only for few minutes, but disturb her sleep and have a daytime nausea. She experiences no back pain or pain anywhere else. She has occasional dyspareunia, but her husband is supportive. She doesn't feel good, but is still interested in her daily life; she also has sweats and has heart palpitations. Menarche was at 13 years, LMP was 3 months ago and has been occurring less often than usual in the previous 6 months, it was regular 28/5. G2P2, natural births, Pap smear was normal long time ago. **ROS:** no urinary or bowel problems, good appetite with no recent weight loss. **PMH:** hypertension (HTN) and lap. Cholecystectomy many years ago. **Med:** propranolol l0 mg. **All (allergy):** penicillin. **FH:** mother died from breast cancer. She lives with her husband, smokes 5 cigarettes/d, drinks socially, sexually active, and is monogamous with her husband.

Physical Exam

VS: WNL, alert, oriented ×3, no acute distress.
Head: PERRLA, no pallor, throat without erythema.
Neck: normal thyroid, no palpable LNs.
Ext: no peripheral edema.
Chest and heart: normal S1, S2, no murmurs, CTA/BL.
Abdomen: soft, non tender (NT), and non distended (ND), no rebound, + BS, no organomegaly.

Differential Diagnosis

History finding(s)	Physical exam finding(s)
1. Menopause	
LMP 3 mo ago	Free physical exam
Hot flashes	
Feeling sad	

Diagnostic Studies

Local vaginal exam

TSH (thyroid-stimulating hormone), T3, FSH (follicle-stimulating hormone)

Screening mammogram

Pelvic US

Role-Play 26

Mrs. Donna Mitchell, a 25-year-old woman, has **vaginal bleeding**.

Vital signs:

- **Temp:** 98.6°F (37°C).
- **PR:** 100/min, regular.
- **RR:** 16/min.
- **BP:** 90/50 mm Hg.

Standardized Patient's Role

You are 25-year-old woman. Yesterday, you had vaginal spotting, but it was mild. Since then, it has gotten worse since this morning, and you have used four pads.

As the doctor starts his or her history say (**Comment**): *"Doc, I'm so worried. I've got vaginal bleeding."*

You are not taking any blood thinner meds. The blood in the pads is bright red in color, and you didn't notice any blood clots.

You also have abdominal pain, in the lower part of your abdomen, and it feels like cramps, (4/10), and it comes and goes. Nothing makes it better.

Your menses is regular. It comes every 28 days and lasts for 5 days. You missed your last period that was supposed to be 3 weeks ago. Since then, you have had morning sickness and breast tenderness and a home pregnancy test was positive.

You had a pap smear done 2 years ago that was normal. You got pregnant once 2 years ago that ended in birth, a full-term baby by C-section.

You are sexually active with your husband only with no contraceptive use.

You are working at a local restaurant. You are a smoker 1 ppd/5 y, drink socially, and more on the weekends.

As the doctor examines you, lie back in pain expressing tenderness on the lower abdomen.

Suggested question to ask the doctor:

As the doctor starts his or her exam, ask:

Q1: *Am I having miscarriage?*

Role-Play 26: Answer Key

As we have learned, always keep yourself focused. If you see vaginal bleeding in the doorway information, look at the age first. This complaint in young females of in child-bearing period usually refers to cases of miscarriage or ectopic pregnancy on the CS exam. In this case, vaginal bleeding is the main complaint with mild lower abdominal pain, so miscarriage is the first possible differential diagnosis.

History

Analysis of Chief Complaint

Vaginal spotting **ABCDE** + abdominal pain.

Analysis of Differential Diagnosis

Abortion and ectopic pregnancy.

Review of the Local System

OB/Gyn history in detail.

Review of Systems

As routine.

Past History and Others

Take a full sexual history.

Physical Exam

VS: Do full abdominal exam, test for rebound tenderness, and finally ask for the necessity of pelvic and vaginal exams.

Communication and Interpersonal Skills Component

If the SP who has vaginal bleeding with possible miscarriage appears sad, depressed, answers monosyllabically or remains silent, be sympathetic and try saying, *"I understand this is really hard for you, but please remember that I'm here to help you. Just let me know if there is any way that I can assist you."*

Suggested Closure

As a routine emergency case (see case 22).

Counseling

Smoking and alcohol.

Suggested Answers to the Standardized Patient's Questions

As standard.

Patient Note

History

Please type the history notes as learned in the previous cases.

Physical Exam

Please type the PE notes as learned in the previous cases.

Differential Diagnosis

History finding(s)	Physical exam finding(s)
1. Abortion	
Vaginal bleeding	
Suprapubic cramping abdominal pain	Tenderness over the suprapubic area
Missed her LMP and sexually active with no contraception use	Hypotension, tachycardia
Morning sickness, breast tenderness, and + home pregnancy test	
2. Ectopic pregnancy	
Vaginal bleeding	
Abdominal pain	Abdominal tenderness
Missed her LMP and sexually active with no contraception use	Hypotension, tachycardia
Morning sickness, breast tenderness, and + home pregnancy test	

Diagnostic Studies

Pelvic and vaginal exam

Pregnancy test and quantitative hCG, CBC, UA

Pelvic US

Role-Play 27

Mrs. Marian Brown, a 60-year-old woman, has **vaginal bleeding.**
Vital signs:
- **Temp:** 98.6° F (37°C).
- **PR:** 90/min, regular.
- **RR:** 16/min.
- **BP:** 120/80 mm Hg.

Standardized Patient's Role

You are a 60-year-old woman, and you came to the clinic as you have noticed vaginal bleeding for 1 month, as if your period is returning. The last period was 5 years ago. You feel self-conscious as you must buy pads. At this time, say, *"Doc, It's so hard for me, it's hard...."*

You use five to six pads per day, but you don't use any blood thinner meds. The blood is dark red with a few blood clots. Yesterday, you felt dizzy when you stood up suddenly. You don't have bleeding from anywhere else in your body.

You remember some vaginal spotting after you had sex with your male partner 2 weeks ago. You have lost about 6 lb over the last 3 months.

You remember, you had menarche when you were 11 years old, and it stopped 5 years ago. Your menses used to be regular (coming every 28 days) and last for 5 days. You don't have any abnormal bleeding in between.

You got pregnant twice that were ended in miscarriage. You are not aware neither did pap smear.

Currently you are sexually active with one male partner, but earlier and for 3 years, you had three male partners. You tried to have your partners use condoms, but sometimes they didn't.

You were diagnosed with high BP 15 years ago and is controlled by propranolol.

You are working at a community hospital, are a smoker 1 ppd/20 y, drink two beers a day, and more on the weekends. You never thought to cut down on your alcohol, but you feel guilty as you know it's not good for your body. Sometimes you get annoyed by people's comments regarding your drinking. You don't drink early in the morning.

Your mother died from uterine cancer.

As the doctor examines you, express mild tenderness over the lower part of your abdomen.

Ask your doctor:
Q1: *Is it necessarily to do a pelvic exam for me?*
Q2: *Doc, as I heard that HRT protects against osteoporosis, could you prescribe it to me?*

Role-Play 27: Answer Key

Vaginal bleeding: Vaginal bleeding on the doorway information at older age without the possibility of pregnancy has different differentials than at younger age. Jot down the listed differential diagnosis below on your scratch paper. After analysis of the complaint, ask the SP if she is still menstruating and end your physical exam by asking for pelvic and vaginal exams and type them first in the workup section in the PN.

Causes are listed as follows:
- **Endometrial causes:** Polyp, hyperplasia, fibroid (▶**Fig. 6.5a, b**), endometrial carcinoma.
- **Cervical causes:** cervicitis, cervical cancer.
- **Vaginal causes:** vaginitis.
- **Hormonal causes:** dysfunctional uterine bleeding (DUB).

History

Analysis of Chief Complaint

Vaginal bleeding (ABCDE).

Analysis of Differential Diagnosis

- *Do you have any vaginal discharge? If yes, analyze* **ABCD.**
- *Have you noticed any bleeding after sexual intercourse?*
- *Have you noticed any sores around the vagina?*
- *Have you noticed any recent changes in your weight?*

Review of the Local System

As routine.

Review of Systems

As routine.

Past History and others

As routine.

Physical Exam

As standard and as previously explained.

Communication and Interpersonal Skills

Suggested Answers to the Standardized Patient's Questions and Comments

Comment 1: As standard.

Q1: *"I understand your concern. I prefer to do a pelvic exam to understand more about your disease. I'll be as gentle as I can. Sounds good?"*

Q2: *"I understand your concern. HRT may be helpful in osteoporosis for postmenopausal women, but unfortunately it's contraindicated in the presence of any vaginal bleeding, so we are not able to prescribe HRT for you now until we figure out the cause of the bleeding."*

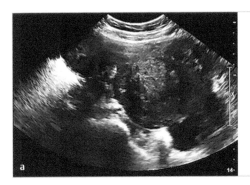 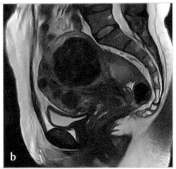

Fig. 6.5 Showing uterine fibroid. **(a)** Ultrasonography and **(b)** MRI.

Patient Note

History

A 60-year-old woman with complain of vaginal bleeding; she uses five to six pads a day, no blood thinner meds use, the blood is dark red with few blood clots. She felt dizziness when she stood up yesterday, no bleeding from anywhere else. No use of contraception, no vaginal discharge or vulval ulcers. Postcoital spotting 2 weeks ago, menopause at 55, menarche was at 11 years, cycles were regular 28/5. G2P0, last pap smear normal. **ROS:** no fever, normal appetite, loss of weight 6 lb/3 mo, no bowel or no urinary complaint. **PMH:** HTN. **Med:** propranolol. NKDA. **FH:** mother died from uterine cancer. **SH:** works at a hospital, smokes 1 ppd/20 years, drinks two beers a day, CAGE = 2/4. Was sexually active with multiple male partners with infrequent condom use; currently with one male partner with usual condom use. Never tested for HIV.

Physical Exam

VS: WNL. Alerted, oriented ×3, no acute distress.
Head: PERRLA, no pallor, throat without erythema.
Neck: normal thyroid, no palpable LNs.
Ext: no peripheral edema.
Chest and heart: normal S1, S2, no murmurs, CTA/BL.
Abdomen: soft, mild tenderness in the suprapubic area, no rebound, ND, BS +, no organomegaly.

Differential Diagnosis

History finding(s)	Physical exam finding(s)
1. Endometrial carcinoma	
Postmenopausal bleeding	Tenderness over the suprapubic area
Family history in mother	
Weight loss (6 lb/3 mo)	Low weight
2. Endometrial hyperplasia	
Postmenopausal bleeding	
Old age	
3. Cervical cancer	
Postcoital bleeding	
Multiple sexual partners	
Did not do pap smear	
4. Senile vaginitis	
Postcoital bleeding	

Diagnostic Studies

Pelvic and vaginal exam
CBC
US and CT (abdomen, pelvis)
Endometrial biopsy

7 Pediatrics

Keywords: pediatrics for USMLE CS, fever, diarrhea, jaundice

7.1 Introduction

On the Clinical Skills (CS) exam, pediatric cases are a bit different from other types of cases. This is because there are no child standardized patients (SPs). So, the patient, that is, the child, will not be present. You only will have the parent or guardian to talk with, sometimes through a telephone conversation. During the interview, remember to find out how the adult is related to the child. He/ She could be a parent, stepparent, caretaker/ nanny, babysitter, or legal guardian (▶ Video 7.1).

Of course, whether you are meeting the guardian in the exam room or speaking with them over the phone, *you will not be able to perform a physical examination (PE)*. You will not be rushed for documentation, as you are during cases involving adult patients. Since there is no physical exam, that part is usually left blank when you write the Patient Note, so you will have more time for the interview. Your time management will be different. Begin with the history, allot more time than usual for taking the history, and go into more detail than you would normally.

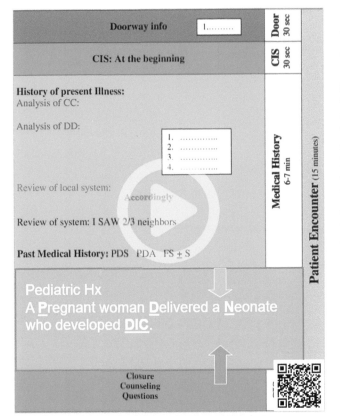

Video. 7.1 This demo gives you a solid road map to study and practice different pediatric cases. The video provides a set of questions that should be asked in almost all pediatric cases. https://www.thieme.de/de/q.htm?p=opn/cs/20/3/11450542-b8ed59e9

Do not forget that you will need time to address the issues unique to pediatric cases (pregnancy, delivery, developmental history, immunization, and others). In closing the interview, take more time than you normally do for counseling: discussing probable causes, treatment options, etc.).

At the end of the encounter, ask the guardian to make an appointment so that you schedule a time to meet with the patient. The severity of the case determines when and how you can examine the child.

If the child's complaint is a true **emergency** (e.g., shortness of breath or foreign body [FB] aspiration) ask the guardian to call 911 and arrange to meet the child in the ER.

If the problem is **not so urgent** but is still significantly worrying (e.g., fever, diarrhea, or cough) ask the guardian to bring the child in as soon as possible.

For **chronic conditions,** for example, weight loss or nocturnal enuresis, schedule an appointment at a mutually agreeable time. No matter what the nature of the medical problem is, the child's safety should be your number one concern.

Note: In **telephone calls,** don't be afraid to ask for clarification. Ask the caller to **speak up** or **speak slower**. Also, you can ask the caller to repeat a question or paraphrase it. You can rephrase it to be sure that you have heard the question correctly.

7.2 Strategy for Taking the History

Start with the history of present illness (HPI). You see that it is the first category in ▶ **Table 7.1**. Then move to the patient's routine information, which is his or her general medical history. The mnemonic device, "**PDS** for **PDA** results in Fast Surgery" should help you remember the questions for the past medical history (see Chapter 1, The Basics, Component 1, Integrated Clinical Encounter).

Finally, ask about the pediatric history. You should follow the questions in the order they are given, in order to avoid forgetting any of the topics. Choose one of the following mnemonic devices to help you remembering the questions in order:

- Pediatricians Do Not Do Investigations Childishly.
- A Pregnant woman Delivered a Neonate who developed DIC.

So, the formula for the sequence of the questions is P = Pregnancy, D = Delivery, N = Neonatal history, D = Developmental history, I = Immunization history, and C = Check-ups.

7.3 Suggested Closure for Pediatric Cases

"Ms. ..., first, let me make sure I understood you correctly. You told me that your child has ... and ..., and you also mentioned that he .... He does not have .... Based on the child's history,

7.1 Medical history strategy for pediatric cases

HPI = history of present illness	1. *Analysis of the complaint.* 2. *Analysis of the possible DD* 3. *Review of local system* 4. *Review of the other systems (i.e., I SAW 2/3 systems).*
Routine information (past medical history)	**PDS** for **PDA** results in fast surgery. *I am going to ask you few questions regarding your child's health:* 　*Does he have any medical diseases?* 　*Has he had any surgeries done?* 　*Did he have a similar condition before?* 　*Is your child taking any medicine on a daily basis?* 　*Does your child have any allergies?* *A couple of questions regarding your child's social life:* 　*Who does he or she live with?* 　*Is he or she safe at home?/Any smokers around him or her?*
Additional Info for pediatric cases	Pediatricians **D**o **N**ot **D**o **I**nvestigations **C**hildishly (or) A **P**regnant woman **D**elivered a **N**eonate who developed **DIC**.

Pregnancy
Was _(name of child) __'s pregnancy full term or preterm?
Did you have any problems with _____ (name of child) __'s pregnancy?
Optional questions:
Did you do the routine checkup visits while you were pregnant?
When you were pregnant, did you smoke? Drink alcohol? Use any street drugs?
... did you have an ultrasound done?
... did you have the routine immunization shots such as influenza?

Delivery
Did you have a natural birth or C-section?
Were there any complications?

Neonatal history
Did your child come out healthy?
Was _____ (name of child) __ a healthy child at birth?
Optional questions:
Did he feed well after delivery?
When did he have the first bowel movement?
Did your child have any yellowish or bluish skin discoloration at birth?

Developmental history: Ask what is relevant to the child's age, Classically, you have to ask about the four major domains for each age: gross motor, fine motor, social and language developmental milestones. However, we chose the most important for the best time management.
At 6 months:
Can your child remain seated with support?
Does your child put things in his mouth when he picks them up?
At 9 months:
Does your child show anxiety when meeting new people?
Can your child remain seated by herself without support?
Can he crawl?
1 y: 1 word:
Can your child say "mom" and "dad"?
Can your child stand up with support?
2 y: 2-word sentence and 2 steps:
Can your child say a sentence of 2 words?
Can your child climb stairs by himself or herself?
Can your child walk? (usually around 15 m)
3 y: 3-word sentence and tricycle + hands:
Can your child say a sentence of 3 words?
Can your child ride a tricycle?
Can your child wash his hands?
Can your child play in a group?
4 y:
Can your child button his/her clothing?
Does your child play with the other kids/tell tales?

Immunization history
Are his or her shots up-to-date? (informal)
What immunizations has he or she had? (formal)

Checkups
Has your child had checkup visits done? When?
What were the results of the last checkup?

it could be … or possibly …. However, I can't rely on the medical history alone. I recommend seeing your child for a PE. So, let's make an appointment where you can bring your child in. Then I can take his pulse, temperature, and other vital statistics, and also take a look at …. Most probably we will need to take a blood sample so we can run a test and take some pictures of …. Now, do you have any questions?"

If the case is serious: *"When can you bring him to the hospital? Once you arrive, just ask someone at the reception to page me. My name is Dr. … and once I know that you've arrived, I'll drop what I'm doing and come to you as soon as possible. How does that sound?"*

7.4 Common Questions in Pediatric Cases and Suggested Answers

Q1. SP: I can't come to the hospital right now. I don't have a car.

Doctor: In **emergency cases,** *"I understand, but your child's condition is serious. Hang up and call 911. They will arrange a ride for you and your child to the hospital. I'll be waiting in the emergency room. Do you have any questions?"*

In **nonemergency cases,** *"Could you call a taxi or get a ride from someone? Your child is not in serious condition, but he or she does need to see a doctor, and the sooner, the better."*

Q2. SP: I have other kids and I can't leave home right now. I don't have any child care.

Doctor: "Well, you're in a difficult situation, and you're concerned about all of your kids, but (child's name)'s health is a priority right now. So, please hold on. I'm going to get one of our social workers to arrange for child care, so you can bring him or her in."

The following cases are common on the CS exam: fever, bedwetting (nocturnal enuresis), yellowish discoloration of the eyes and skin (neonatal jaundice), weight loss, and others (bronchial asthma [BA], FB aspiration, febrile seizures).

Role-Play 28

Opening Scenario

Mrs. Morny David, the mother of Rose, a 1-year-old girl, she calls the office complaining that her child has fever. This is a telephone encounter.

Examinee tasks:

- Take a focused history.
- Explain your clinical impression and workup plan to the mother.
- Write the patient note after leaving the room.

Standardized Patient's Role (▶ Video. 7.2)

You are Mrs. David. Your daughter, Rose, who is 1-year-old, has a fever. You took her temperature at home and it was 101°F. Tylenol brought the fever down, but just by a half degree. She is weak and not playful.

She has had a common cold for 5 days with a runny nose, mild fever, and mild dry cough with some difficulty breathing. She goes to daycare, but you are not quite sure if she came into contact with any sick people there.

You noticed the fever has increased since yesterday, with little response to Tylenol. She has started to pull her ear and has difficulty with breast feeding because it hurts to swallow. She has difficulty sleeping because she wakes up to cough more often. She had a similar episode 3 months ago and that was cured.

She is allergic to amoxicillin. Rose lives with you and her father, and you have BA.

Your pregnancy with Rose was full term, with no problems, and you visited the doctor regularly for checkups. The delivery was a natural birth. Rose was a healthy baby.

Rose can say "mom" and "dad" and can sit without support. You are always punctual with her checkup visits; the last one was 1 month ago, and everything was fine. Her shots and checkup visits are up-to-date (UTD).

At the end of the encounter, ask:

Q1: *Why is my daughter tugging her ear?*

Q2: *I have some antibiotics left over from a prescription I got for her brother when he was sick. Can I just give her some of those?*

Q3: *Is Rose going to be OK?*

Comment 1: If the doctor asks to come to the hospital, tell him that you can't bring your kid in right now because you don't have a car and there's no public transportation around you.

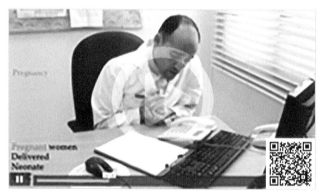

Video. 7.2 This is an example of a telephone encounter. The mother called the clinic because her child who is 1-year-old has a fever. The video follows the up-to-date CS instructions and allocated CS time. https://www.thieme.de/de/q.htm?p=opn/cs/20/3/11450543-4b87d4c3

Please refer to Chapter 13 (Appendix), to review the general instructions for the SP as well as the Doctor roles.

Role-Play 28: Answer Key

Fever is a common case on the CS exam.

History

Analysis of Chief Complaint

Fever:
How long has she had a fever?
Did you check her temperature at home?
What was her temperature when you took it at home?
Did you give her any medicine for the fever such as Tylenol?
When you gave her the medicine, did her temperature drop?

+ Associations:
Does the fever come with sweating or chills?
Is your child alert or sleepy?
Does your child shake as if she were having a seizure?

Analysis of Differential Diagnosis

Remember infections in three systems: (respiratory, gastrointestinal (GI) system, and urinary) + skin and meninges + other infectious diseases.

Upper Respiratory (Ear, Nose, and Throat; ▶Fig. 7.1):
- *Does she tug at her **e**ar?*
- *Have you noticed any discharge coming from her ear?*
- *Does she have a runny **n**ose? Nasal blockage?Any sneezing?*
- *Does she have any difficulty swallowing?* (Throat)
- *Has her voice changed at all?*

Lower respiratory (▶Fig. 7.2):
- *Has she been coughing?*
- *Does she cough up any mucous?If yes, analyze ABC.*
- *Does she have any difficulty breathing?*
- *Does she have any chest wheezing?*

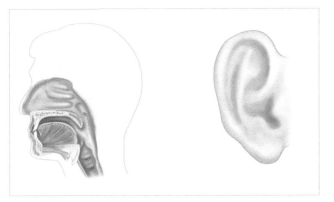

Fig. 7.1 Upper respiratory (ear, nose, and throat).

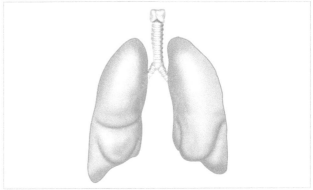

Fig. 7.2 Lower respiratory.

Gastrointestinal (▶Fig. 7.3):
- *Has she vomited? (If yes, analyze **ABC**.)*
- *Has she had any diarrhea? (If yes, analyze **ABC**.)*
- *Did the fever come after eating something* unusual *? In other words, if the fever has been caused by food, I would like to know what she has eaten in the past 24 hours.*
- *Did the fever follow any new medications she took?*
- *If gastroenteritis (vomiting/diarrhea), assess for dehydration.*
- *How much has she been drinking? I'm worried that she might be dehydrated.*
- *Is she thirsty? Does she urinate less often than usual?*

Urinary Tract Infection (▶Fig. 7.4):
- *Does she complain of a burning sensation when she pees?*
- *Has she been going to the bathroom more often than usual?*

Skin (▶Fig. 7.5; measles, rubella, varicella, chicken pox, roseola):
- *Does she have a rash?* If yes, ask more (see Chapter 13, Appendix).

Meningitis:
- *Is her neck stiff?*
- *Does she have any rash? Does she have headache? Did she vomit? Did she seize?* (Meningitis is concerning in her age and it would call for a prompt management.)

Infectious disease:
- *Has she been around any sick person recently?*
- *What can you tell me about her immunizations?*
- *Is she UTD with them?*

Review of the Local System

Based on the system involved.

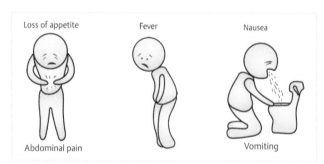

Fig. 7.3 Gastrointestinal.

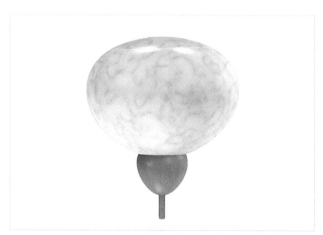

Fig. 7.4 Urinary tract infection (UTI).

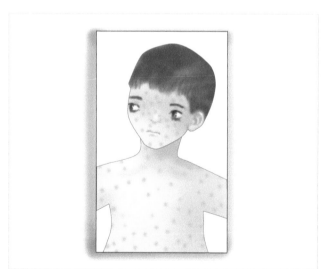

Fig. 7.5 Skin.

Review of Systems

Ask routine questions.

Past History and Others

PDS for PDA results in Fast Surgery.

Additional info unique to pediatric cases:
A Pregnant woman Delivered a Neonate who developed DIC.

Physical Exam

No.

Communication and Interpersonal Skills Component

Suggested Closure

As explained.

Counseling

As a routine.

Suggested Answers to the Standardized Patient's Questions

Q1: *"It's hard for me to answer that question for sure now without having seen your child yet, but based on the history, it seems to me that your child has inflammation in the ear that is common following the flu in young kids. I had better examine Rose to be sure that everything is all right."*

Q2: *"Well, I'm not quite sure if we are going to prescribe antibiotics or not. And even if we do, it may or may not be the ones that her brother took when he was sick. As you know, there are many different kinds of antibiotics and each one works specifically on one kind of bacteria. So, I think it's best if you do not give her any of the antibiotics until I can assess what is causing her illness."*

Q3: *"I understand your concern. Rose's presentation may be due to a simple cause like a viral or a bacterial ear infection or something more serious. I will do a PE and run some blood tests to identify the source of the infection. If the cause is bacterial we will need to use antibiotics, unlike viral infections that may resolve on their own. Do you have any other concerns?"*

Comment 1: *"Could you call a taxi or someone to drive you? If you can't come in right away, please call an ambulance. Do you need my help to do that?"*

Patient Note

History

The mother of a 1-year-old girl who has a fever (is the source of information). The condition started 5 days ago with a common cold and low-grade fever. She has had rhinorrhea and a common cold. The mother noticed that the fever has risen in the last 24 hours and that her child has started to pull at her ear. She took her temperature; it was 101°F. The child is weak and not playful. No discharge from ears, mild rhinorrhea, mild nasal obstruction, difficulty swallowing, no change in voice, persistent dry cough, especially at night, with difficult breathing. No chest wheezing, no vomiting, diarrhea, skin rash, or change in urine. Supple neck with no seizure.
Review of system (ROS): decreased appetite, difficulty sleeping due to nasal obstruction and cough. No recent changes in body weight. She is breastfed, no special formula. Similar episode 3 months ago that was cured. **Med:** Tylenol. **Allergy (All):** Amoxicillin.
Social history (SH): Lives with her parents, mother with BA. She is a product of full-term normal delivery. She can say "mom" and "dad" and stands, Immunizations UTD, regular checkup visits, the last one 1 month ago, showed normal weight, height, hearing, vision, and other developmental milestones.

Physical Exam

Not done.

Differential Diagnosis

History finding(s)	Physical exam finding(s)
1. Otitis media	
Fever	No
Has common cold	
Pulls his or her ear	
Past history 3 mo ago	
2. Lower respiratory tract infection	
Fever	No
Has common cold	
Cough	
Difficult breathing (BA)	
3. Bronchial asthma (BA)	
Persistent dry cough at night	No
Mother has BA	

Diagnostic Studies

Physical and ear exams

CBC (complete blood count) with differential

CXR (chest X-ray)

Consider nebulizer (if wheezes noted while PE)

Role-Play 29

Opening Scenario

Mrs. Lora Smith is the mother of a 6-month-old infant, Tom. She came to the office complaining that her child has a fever and diarrhea.

Standardized Patient's Role

You came to the outpatient clinic, as you are really worried about your 6-month-old infant, Tom. The problem started 2 days ago. You noticed that when he had a bowel movement, the stool was loose and the looseness has worsened since then. Tom has six to eight movements a day, and the stool is yellowish and watery. There is no blood, but his bottom looks reddish.

You feel that he is dehydrated; his mouth is dry, he's always thirsty, and he is not urinating very often, but it's difficult to determine the urine volume since he is having so many bowel movements.

He started vomiting this morning but had not eaten much for breakfast. Now just water and mucous is coming up. He is weak and drowsy and has a mild fever of 100.5°F.

You don't know if it's a coincidence or not, but your sister brought her boy (his cousin) over to visit a few days ago. It turns out that his cousin was sick at the time, and the two children were in close proximity for several hours.

Ask the doctor at this time:

Q1: *Could Tom have caught this from his cousin?*

Tom is healthy and is breastfeeding normally. You introduced some juice for the first time this week. He doesn't have difficulty swallowing, and he hasn't had any of the following recently: upper respiratory tract infection, skin rash, or seizure.

Tom's never been sick before. He doesn't have allergies, his medications are over-the-counter (OTC), multivitamins, and Tylenol, but nothing else. Neither you nor your husband has any major health problems; no genetic diseases run in either of your families. Tom lives in a smoke-free home, and it's a very healthy, safe environment.

As far as you remember, your pregnancy with Tom was completely normal. Moreover, during the pregnancy, you followed the suggested antenatal care instructions, and you didn't smoke or drink. He was delivered by C-section at full term, and there have been no problems since then. He is now able to sit with support and move objects from one hand to the other, but he sometimes expresses anxiety if he sees an unfamiliar face. His immunizations are UTD and the last checkup was 3 months ago and everything was fine.

At the end of the encounter, ask:

Q2: *I've got some antibiotics at home. Can I give them to Tom?*

Role-Play 29: Answer Key

Please refer to Role-play 28.

Communication and Interpersonal Skills Component

Suggested Closure

As routine, but you can add, "*I would advise you not to give Tom any more juice, as it may be contributing to his diarrhea.*"

Suggested Answers to the Standardized Patient's Questions

Q1: Answer as you learned previously.

Q2: "*I understand your concerns. Diarrhea in children is usually caused by a virus called rotavirus. The cure does not usually call for antibiotics that are prescribed in special situations. It's difficult for me to tell you for sure at this moment because I haven't seen Tom yet. So, the best case scenario is for me to examine Tom first so we can figure out exactly what's going on. When can you bring him in?*"

Patient Note

History

The mother of 6-month-old infant is the source of the information. He has had diarrhea for 2 days. At first, it was mild, but it has gotten worse. Now it's six movements per day of yellowish, watery diarrhea with no blood. The mother feels that he is dehydrated, his mouth is dry, he is always thirsty, and he urinates less often than usual. He is weak and drowsy with a mild fever 100.5°F. He was in contact with his cousin who was sick a few days ago. He is breastfeeding, and mother introduced juice this week. Not preceded by new meds. Infrequent vomiting of clear fluid, difficulty swallowing. No recent urinary tract infection, burning urination, skin rash, or seizure.
ROS: ↓ appetite, his weight was normal in the last checkup visit.
PMH: No medical diseases.
Med: Tylenol and vitamins. No known drug allergy (NKDA).
Family history (FH): No medical diseases in the family.
SH: Lives with his parents. He is a product of full-term pregnancy with C-section delivery. He can sit with support, transfers objects from on hand to the other, and expresses anxiety at the sight of strangers. Immunization is UTD. Regular checkup, last one about 3 months ago showed normal weight, height, hearing, vision, and development milestones.
Examination: Not done

Differential Diagnosis

History finding(s)

1. **Viral/bacterial diarrhea**

   Diarrhea

   Dehydrated

   Fever

   Recent contact with sick kid

2. **Malabsorption**

   Diarrhea

   Dehydration

   Recent introduction of juice

Diagnostic Studies

Physical exam

Electrolytes

CBC

Role-Play 30

Opening Scenario

Mrs. Fisher Miller is the mother of Kelci, a 5-year-old girl. She is visiting the clinic because Kelci has been wetting the bed.

Examinee tasks:

- Take a focused history.
- Explain your clinical impression and work up plan to the mother.
- Write the patient note after leaving the room.

Standardized Patient's Role

You are Mrs. Fisher; you came to the clinic because your 5-year-old daughter, Kelci, wets the bed at night. She was successfully toilet-trained when she was 2.5 years old, but since then she has never been continent for long periods of time.

She wets herself one to two times per night, two to three nights a week, and the bed sheets are usually soaking wet. Kelci used to drink quite a lot of soda and juice, but now she is drinking an acceptable amount. You withhold fluids from her a few hours before bedtime, and have her urinate right before bedtime, but these strategies only sometimes prevent bedwetting.

You have recently had to have Kelci sleep overnight at your mother's house a few nights a week as your work schedule has changed; sometimes you have to work the graveyard shift, so you are not at home during the night. You suspect that Kelci's grandmother gets a little bit impatient and upset with Kelci when she is incontinent, but she has never hit or screamed at Kelci.

At this time, ask

Q1: *Do you think that having her sleep at her grandmother's could be making the problem worse?*

You and her father are sympathetic to your daughter's problem. Your husband remembers wetting the bed until the age of 9 years, and he wonders if Kelci could have inherited it from him. Kelci is embarrassed about her bedwetting and avoids sleeping in the same bed, as her siblings.

Kelci is healthy. She is sometimes constipated but other than that, she has no medical problems. She doesn't eat many vegetables or foods with fiber. She eats a lot of cheese. You always take her in for her regularly scheduled checkups. Her last visit was 2 months ago and nothing abnormal was noted.

At the end of the encounter, ask the doctor:

Q2: *I saw a commercial on TV about a bedwetting alarm. Do you think I should buy one? Do you think it will help cure her of this problem, or do you think it's a waste of money?*

Q3: *Could she have inherited this problem from her father? I mean, could she be wetting the bed because her father did when he was a child?*

Role-Play 30: Answer Key

Nocturnal enuresis is involuntary urination while asleep after the age at which bladder control usually occurs. Please—as we always recommend—read more about each topic in your textbooks or notes from medical school before practicing a role-play. Here is a simple way to remember the questions.

Analysis of Chief Complaint

Classify the questions based on daytime, evening, at night, and in the morning (▶Table 7.2).

Psychological impact and others:
Does this problem affect your child in any way? How?
Would you describe her as social or shy?
Have you noticed anything that makes the problem better?
Have you noticed anything that makes the problem worse?

Analysis of Differential Diagnosis

How is your child's sleep? (Sleep apnea)
Does your child have constipation?

Review of the Local System

Does she have any problem passing urine?

Review of Systems

As standard.

Past History and Others (▶Table 7.2)

As routine and ask this question for FH:
Did you or your husband wet the bed when you were children?

Table 7.2 History-taking questions for bedwetting

Suggested questions

Daytime symptoms:
Output:
Is she able to control urine in the daytime?
Does it burn while passing urine?
Does she pee more often throughout the day?
Input:
Does she drink excess cola, tea, or coffee?
Does she eat excess chocolates?

In the evening:
Does she usually drink excessive water or other fluids before going to bed?
How much does she drink?
Does she usually go to the bathroom before going to bed?

At night:
How long has she been wetting the bed?
How many times does she wet the bed per night?
How many days a week does she wet the bed?

In the morning:
Is the bed sheet usually soaked?
Does she feel embarrassed in the morning?
Do you use to shout to or psychologically hurt her?

Physical Exam

Communication and Interpersonal Skills Component

Suggested Closure

As explained earlier.

Counseling

Doctor: *"Ms. Fisher, let me tell you what I'm thinking so far. You told me that your daughter wets the bed. Based on what you have told me, it seems that your child has bedwetting or nocturnal enuresis. However, I can't rely on the history alone... (go ahead as a standard).*
Can I give you some information about nocturnal enuresis?

SP: *Sure.*

Doctor: *Nocturnal enuresis is a common problem in childhood and it doesn't mean your child has any physical or mental problems and it has a high spontaneous cure rate. We usually intervene because it can be embarrassing for kids with subsequent adverse effects. It makes the child feel socially deprived or it may affect her self-confidence."*

SP: *What are the treatment options?*

Doctor: *"Good question!. Let's discuss the treatment options right now, but before discussing the treatment options, I'd like to ask you to keep a **voiding diary**."*

SP: *What is that?*

Doctor: "It is a simple record of various things about bladder function such as the frequency of urination, the volume of urine, and the volume of fluid intake. In addition to *the times your child has urinated/wet the bed."*

SP: *Sure, I will do one.*

Doctor: "Also, I strongly advice for your daughter to follow a **timed voiding** pattern; it is a technique used to empty the bladder on a regular basis. The normal interval between voiding during the day is usually 3 to 4 hours. Simply, it is a kind of simple rehabilitation to the bladder to restore its normal voiding pattern."

*Let's get back to treatment options that can be classified into nonpharmaceutical and pharmaceutical (▶ **Table 7.3**).*

Regarding the pharmaceutical treatment, it is available in pill form. But first, I need to see your child. I need to do a PE and to collect a urine sample. Before we make an appointment, do you have any questions for me?"

Suggested Answers to the Standardized Patient's Questions (▶ Table 7.3)

Q1: *"It's difficult for me to tell you for sure at this moment if this factor may contribute to the problem, but it's well known that any psychological stress may cause nocturnal enuresis, but let me finish taking the history to figure out what other factors could be contributing to the condition."*
Q2: *"A **bedwetting alarm** is a simple device that attaches to the child's underwear. The alarm is activated at the first drop of urine. It wakes the child up so he or she can go to the bathroom. In time, the child learns to wake up when his or her bladder is full, and then he or she can go to the bathroom to urinate. I strongly recommend that you buy it. It usually works well."*
Q3: *"As a matter of fact, nocturnal enuresis has a genetic background, so it's possible that your child has inherited this from his father."*

Table 7.3 Nonpharmaceutical treatment for bedwetting
Nonpharmaceutical treatment
Daytime: *Monitor your child's fluid intake every time he or she drinks*   *Have your kid hold black-colored food and drinks as he or she can like chocolates, cola, tea, and coffee.*
In the evening: *Have her drink a minimal amount of water or fluid 2 h before going to bed*
At night: *Encourage her to go to the bathroom right before going to bed*   *Have you ever used bedwetting alarm? (Q2)*
In the morning: *To be mentioned, studies have shown that positive reinforcement plays a role in increasing the child motivation. Simple things, like keeping a chart, really help.*   *Put a star on the chart every morning whenever he or she has a dry night.*
Finally, I want to tell you something, constipation is a risk factor for voiding dysfunction especially in kids. For this reason, encourage your kid to eat fiber-rich food and less cheese.

Patient Note

History

The mother of a 5-year-old girl is the source of information. Her daughter has been wetting the bed. It occurs one to two times a night, 2 to 3 days a week. She soaks the bed sheet. She is continent during the day, no dysuria or frequency. Mother has withheld fluids, has had her urinate right before bedtime, and has set the alarm clock at 1 a.m. These sometimes help in controlling the problem. The problem is causing distress for the child—she avoids sleeping in the same bed with her siblings, but has never been punished or screamed at for her incontinence.

ROS: occasional constipation and eats lots of cheese with low-fiber diet.
PMH: None.
Med: None. NKDA.
FH: Father wet bed until 9 years old.
SH: She lives with her parents in a happy home. Recently her mother has been leaving her for a few days every week to sleep at her grandmother's. Kelci was a product of full-term normal delivery, toilet trained at 2.5 years, walked at 12 months, compliant with her regular checkup visits, the last one 2 months ago. Immunization is UTD.

Physical Examination

Not done.

Differential Diagnosis

History finding(s)

1. Primary nocturnal enuresis

    He or she wets the bed

    Positive family history (father)

    Continent in daytime

Diagnostic Studies

    Physical exam

    Urine analysis

Role-Play 31

Opening Scenario:

Mrs. Susan Steve calls the office complaining that her child Matthew, a 4-day-old neonate, has yellowish eyes and skin.

Standardized Patient's Role

You are Mrs. Susan Steve. You called the physician on duty because you are very worried about your newborn, Matthew. He is only 4 days old. It was a C-section birth, and he was born healthy. However, 2 days ago, you noticed that his eyes were yellowish, and it has worsened since then. His skin is also becoming yellowish, and his stool is darker than normal.

In all other respects, Matthew is doing fine. He is nursing well, not weak, doesn't have a fever, and you haven't noticed anything unusual besides the yellowish eyes and skin.

Your blood type is A negative and your husband's blood type is A+. Your son is also A+. You remember that you got an injection after the last delivery. The doctor informed you that it was for Rhesus (Rh) negative women.

Matthew's pregnancy was without problems until the last few months when your blood pressure started to rise and doctors decided to induce labor at 8 months by C-section. You don't have any medical problems. You once had C-section to deliver your daughter. She is 4 years old and healthy. Matthew's father has peptic ulcers.

At the end, ask the following:

Q1: *How long will this coloration last?*

Q2: *Why is his stool so dark? I'm so worried about this.*

Role-Play 31: Answer Key

Neonatal jaundice has two types: physiological and pathological.

The first type, **physiological jaundice**, appears a day or two after birth, peaks at 3 to 5 days, and resolves itself by the end of the second week. It is a common cause of neonatal jaundice found on the CS exam, so be ready to discuss it.

Pathological jaundice is the other type of jaundice that you may encounter. The differential diagnoses may include any of the following:

ABO/Rh incompatibility and obstructive jaundice: These types appear at birth.

Breast-feeding jaundice: The baby is not nursing well, and this could be due to a variety of causes. The result is that the child gets dehydrated due to a lack of caloric intake, and jaundice occurs. It most often occurs with the firstborn.

Breast milk jaundice (allergy): It appears in the second week and is treated by temporary cessation of breast-feeding.

Neonatal sepsis: Symptoms include fever, lethargy, and insufficient feeding.

Analysis of Chief Complaint

- *What is his birth date?*
- *When did it start? Did it come on suddenly? Since it started, has it gotten worse?*
- *Could you describe the color of the eyes to me? Now, describe the color of the skin.*
- *Have you noticed any changes in the color of the urine? In the stool?*
- *Was your child healthy at birth?*

Analysis of Differential Diagnosis

ABO incompatibility:
- *What is your child's blood type?*
- *What is your blood type? What is the father's blood type?*

Obstructive jaundice:
- *Did you notice this problem at birth?*

Breast-feeding jaundice:
- *Is he nursing well?*

Neonatal sepsis:
- *Does he have a fever? If yes, analyze.*
- *Is your child alert or sleepy?*
- *Is he coughing?*
- *Does he cough up any mucous?*
- *Does he have any difficulty breathing? Is he wheezing when he breathes?*
- *Is he dehydrated?*

There is no need to ask about the child's development, immunizations, or checkups as he is a neonate (too young).

Communication and Interpersonal Skills Component

Suggested Closure

Mrs. ..., *actually, there are many causes for a yellowish discoloration of the eyes in neonates. Based on what you have told me about your son, it could be physiological jaundice. This situation occurs because our red blood cells undergo cyclic turnover. That means that the old ones die and new ones are formed. The pigments, or colors, of the red blood cells, are filtered out by the liver and the spleen and are released back into the blood stream. In neonates, there is more destruction of the blood cells than in older people, or we can say that there is a higher turnover rate. Since the neonate's liver is too immature to handle the amount of pigments, more pigments are released into the blood. They show up in the eyes and skin. So, this is a normal consequence and nothing to be worried about.*

Suggested Answers to the Standardized Patient's Questions

Q1: *It's difficult for me to tell you for sure at this moment as it depends on the cause, but based on your son's presentation and if it's physiological jaundice as I suspect, the peak usually occurs on the third to fifth day and the coloring usually returns back to normal at the end of the second week.*

Q2: *The release of extra pigments in the blood from blood cell turnover (that we discussed earlier) causes yellowish discoloration of the skin and the eyes contribute to darkness of the stool. Do you have any other concerns?*

Patient Note

History

The mother is the source of information. Her 4-day-old neonate has jaundice. The child was healthy at birth, and had no jaundice. She noticed yellowish discoloration of the skin and the eyes that has started on the second day after birth and has been getting worse. His eyes and skin are yellow. Stool is darker than normal. She has A negative type blood and her baby is A positive. She received an injection after the delivery as she is Rh negative. He is nursing well, doesn't have a fever, cough, or difficulty in breathing. He is alert and playful, sleeps and eats well, hasn't had any loss of weight, nor urinary nor bowel issues. He was born 1 month prematurely (at 8 months), most probably due to preeclampsia. G2P2, both ended by C-section. She did the regular antenatal care. She had neither an infection nor fever while she was pregnant. The home is smoke free, and nobody drinks alcohol.

SH: Lives with parents and home is safe.

FH: Mother has no medical diseases; father has peptic ulcer.

Physical Examination

Not done.

Differential Diagnosis

History finding(s)

1. Physiological jaundice

   Started on the second day

   Healthy, no fever

   Preterm baby

2. RH incompatibility

   Mother is Rh−

   Baby is Rh+

Diagnostic Studies

CBC and blood typing

Bilirubin (total and indirect) and LFTs (liver function tests)

Role-Play 32

Opening Scenario:
Mr. Williams Christopher came to the clinic as his son Scott, an 8-year-old boy, has been losing weight.

Standardized Patient's Role

You are Mr. Williams. You have come to the clinic because you want to talk about your son's recent weight loss. You have a growth chart in your hand (▶ **Fig. 7.6**) that your primary doctor gave to you.

He gave it to you when he informed you that your son has been losing weight lately.

Scott has lost 5 lb in the last 3 months, although he eats a lot. You have noticed that he has been drinking more water than usual, voids urine too often, and he wakes up once or twice a night to pee.

If the doctor asks you about his home situation or with whom your son lives, keep silent for a while and then tell him that you're in a hard situation, as the mother divorced you a year ago and left. Mention, with great sadness, that you have not had enough time to spend with your child, to make sure he is eating properly, getting enough sleep, etc.

At this time, say to the doctor, *"It's really hard for me Doc."* (**Comment 1**)

Your wife has not seen her child, and you are quite busy with work and under a lot of pressure to do well at your job, so you often work late. Tell the doctor that it is very hard on you to raise your child by yourself and that you don't have enough time to adequately take care of your child (**Comment 2**).

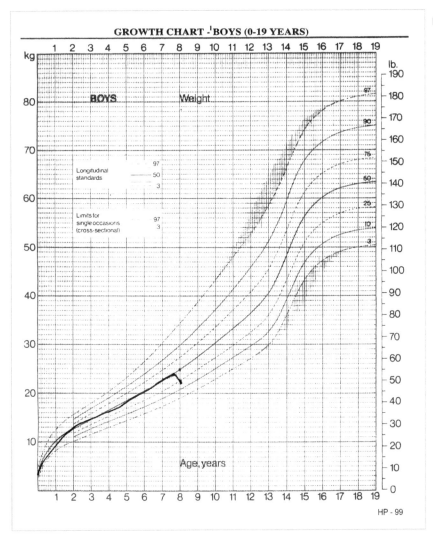

Fig. 7.6 Growth chart.

His mother used to take him to the regular checkup visits, but now you are doing that. You took Scott in 6 months ago and everything was fine. His immunizations are UTD.

Your wife has been diagnosed with diabetes 10 years ago, has hypothyroidism, and a smoker and sometimes smoke around Scott.

Scott was born at 8 months by C-section. He was in the neonatal care unit for some time. He walked at the age of 3 years, was toilet-trained by 3.5 years, and right now all of his developmental milestones are within the norm.

At the end, ask the doctor:

Q1: *"Is there something wrong with his stomach?"*

Q2: *"Is Scott going to be okay?"*

Role-Play 32: Answer Key

Weight loss in pediatrics has a wide range of differential diagnosis. Here are some common causes that may appear in the cases on the CS exam:

- *Diet:* malnutrition, starvation due to child abuse, or neglect.
- *GI problems:* malabsorption, metabolic, or parasites.
- *Chronic diseases:* diabetes mellitus (DM) and tuberculosis (TB).
- *Other:* cancer, immunodeficiency.

Analysis of Chief Complaint

- *How long has your child been losing weight?*
- *How much has your child lost?*
- *Have you noticed anything abnormal besides weight loss?*

Analysis of Differential Diagnosis

Diet:

- *Tell me as much as you can about your child's diet.*
- *Is he on any special formula?*
- *Is he taking any multivitamins?*
- *Whom does he live with?*
- *Is he ever in any danger at home?*
- *Do you suspect or know of any abuse?*

GI tract:

- *Has he been vomiting?*
- *Has he had any stomachaches? If yes, analyze.*
- *Have you noticed if he has any difficulty swallowing?*
- *Have you noticed any change in his stool? Have you noticed any blood?*
- *Does he have any anal itching?*

Infectious diseases:

- *Does he have a fever? If yes, analyze.*
- *Has he been around any sick person recently? If yes, analyze.*
- *Has he traveled outside the country recently?*
- *What about his immunization?*
- *Is he UTD with them?*

Diabetes Mellitus:

- *Has he been drinking more water than usual?/Is he often thirsty?*
- *Has he been urinating more often than usual?*

Communication and Interpersonal Skills

Suggested Answers to the Standardized Patient's Questions

(Comment 1): See similar questions for an answer.

Q1: *Although there could be something wrong with his stomach, I'm leaning toward something else. Scott may have … or …. Based on what you told me, I think that I should check his blood sugar to eliminate the possibility of DM. He is eating, drinking, and urinating a lot, yet he is losing weight. Let me examine Scott first and do a physical exam, and then we'll meet together and I'll give you my final diagnosis and the treatment options.*

Q2: See similar questions for an answer.

Patient Note

History

The father who noticed that his 8-year-old child "Scott" has been losing weight is the source of the information. The child lost 5 lb in 3 months; he has polyphagia, polydipsia, and polyuria. Sometimes, he has to wake up in the night to pee. No special diet, vomiting, abdominal pain, or changes in the bowel movement. No fever, cough, or skin rash. Normal sleep and increased appetite.
PMH: None.
Med: multivitamins, OTC. **All:** penicillin.
FH: Father with DM, mother with hypothyroidism.
SH: Lives with his father after parents divorced, his mother has DM and hypothyroidism, and she is a smoker and sometimes she smokes near Scott. Scott is a product of preterm labor, a C-section, was kept in the neonatal ICU. Delayed walking and potty training. Last checkup visit was 6 months ago and all his developmental milestones are within normal limits. His immunization is UTD.

Physical Examination

Not done.

Differential Diagnosis

History finding(s)

1. **Type I diabetes mellitus**

   Loss of weight

   Polyphagia

   Polydipsia

   Polyuria

2. **Child neglect**

   Loss of weight

   Lives with one parent

   Parents are divorced

   Mother can't take care of him

Diagnostic Studies

Physical exam

FBS (fasting blood sugar) and Hb A1C

Urine analysis and CBC

8 Musculoskeletal System

Keywords: shoulder pain, knee pain, ankle pain, back pain, rheumatic pain

8.1 Introduction

This chapter includes the following cases:
Joint pain that may be:
- *Traumatic:* Shoulder, ankle, and knee pains are the most common on the Clinical Skills (CS) exam. Less commonly, elbow, wrist, and hip pains appear.
- *Nontraumatic (rheumatic) joint pain:* It may be osteoarthritis (OA), rheumatoid arthritis (RA), or systemic lupus erythematosus (SLE).

Spinal pain that may be:
- Lumbar pain.
- Cervical pain.

8.2 History-taking

8.2.1 Analysis of Chief Complaint: Joint Pain

After analysis of **pain**, your first priority in these cases is to determine the nature of the pain, that is, whether it is traumatic or not. Here are some sample questions to begin your analysis:
- *Have you been in an accident recently?/Was the pain preceded by an accident?*
- *Did you hit your knee/ankle/shoulder?*

If yes, ask about specifics:
- *When did that happen?/How long ago did it happen?*
- *What were you doing at the time that it happened?*

Once you have determined if it, in fact, is a case of traumatic pain, ask about the possible **general** and **local** complications/ associations.

General:
- *Did you pass out after the accident?*
- *How did you get to the hospital today?*
- *Do you have any other injuries?*

Local: To help you remember them, here is a mnemonic device—**signs of inflammation + AND** (Artery, Nerve, Disability). Here are some sample questions for the signs of inflammation: It has four parts—swelling, warmness, redness, and sounds.
- *Have you noticed any swelling? Any redness? Hotness? Any cracking or popping sounds?*

Here are the **AND** section questions:
Artery:
- *Have you noticed any bleeding from the affected area?*

Nerve:
Sensation:
- *Have you noticed any numbness in your ___?*

Motor function:
- *Have you had any muscular weakness in your ___?*
- Disability: According to the joint affected
- *Can you move your arm/foot?*
- *Can you bend your elbow?*
- *Can you extend your arm? Can you walk? Run?*
- *Can you put any weight on your ankle/knee?*

8.2.2 Analysis of the Possible Causes: Differential Diagnosis

Note: In most of the circumstances on the CS exam, there are no specific questions for each of the previous differential diagnosis (DD; ▶ Table 8.1).

8.2.3 Symptoms Related to the Local System

Do you have any other complaints besides…?

8.3 Joint Examination (▶ Video 8.1)

No matter which joint is affected, there are a standard set of physical exam (PE) steps that should be followed. Here is a mnemonic device: **IP AND S.**

The letters in the device stand for: Inspection, Palpation, Artery, Nerve, Disability, and Special maneuvers.

Inspection: Start with the contralateral (healthy) joint. Comment on any redness or swelling that you find. Document any abnormal finding, such as erythema or scars.

Palpation: Start by examining the contralateral (healthy) side. Press on certain areas to detect tenderness. Palpate along the joint line.

Artery: Check the pulse at the affected joint and distally.

Table 8.1 Differential diagnosis of joint pain common in CS exam

Shoulder pain	Fractured humerus/clavicle Dislocated shoulder/acromioclavicular (AC) joints Rotator cuff tear
Knee pain	Torn medial meniscus/lateral meniscus Torn medial collateral ligament Torn anterior/posterior cruciate ligament
Hip pain	Hip dislocation or fractured acetabulum Fracture at the proximal femur (neck, intertrochanteric) Avascular necrosis (AVN) of the femoral head (may be nontraumatic)
Ankle pain	Ankle sprain Calcaneal fracture Pott's fracture
Elbow pain	Dislocated elbow Fracture at the elbow joint (lower humerus and upper radius or ulna)

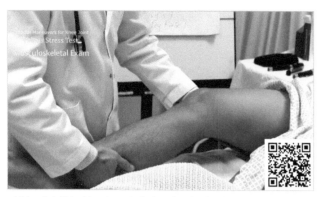

Video 8.1 This video demo is designed and tailored to the lengthy musculoskeletal exam to meet the CS requirements and SPs' checklists. https://www.thieme.de/de/q.htm?p=opn/cs/20/3/11450544-a922c8a8

Nerve:
- Sensation: Test for pinprick and soft touch sensation. Compare the sensation distally to the joint with the sensation proximally, and then compare it with sensation of the other limb.
- Muscle power: Check leg strength. Use the neurological exam method—have the patient kick out, pull back, push out, and pull in against your hand (see Chapter 10, Neurology).
- Deep tendon reflexes (DTRs): For upper limb joints, test biceps and triceps reflexes. For lower limb joints, test ankle and knee reflexes.

Disability:
- There are two ways (active and passive) to test for the range of motion (ROM).
- Whenever the Standardized Patient (SP) cannot move his or her limb or it pains him or her to do so, use the passive method. Have the SP relax completely. Hold his or her limb and move it at the joint.

Use the active way on healthy joints. Ask the SP to move the joint on his own. Test the following at each joint:
- Shoulder, hip: flexion–extension, adduction–abduction, medial/lateral rotation.
- Knee: flexion–extension, medial/lateral rotation.
- Elbow: flexion–extension, pronation–supination.
- Wrist: flexion–extension, ulnar and radial deviation.
- Ankle: dorsiflexion–plantar flexion, inversion–eversion (talocalcaneal joint).

Special maneuvers:
- Knee: anterior drawer test, posterior drawer test, McMurray's test, valgus stress test, varus stress test, and others like Lachman's test.
- Shoulder: Dugas' test, drop arm test, and others (cross arm test, adduction [scarf test], empty can test, Neer's/Hawkin's impingement signs …).
- Carpal tunnel syndrome: Phalen's test, Tinel's sign (see Chapter 12, **Mini Cases**).
- Ankle: Anterior and posterior drawer test.

8.4 Example Dialogue (▶ Table 8.2)

The dialogue below incorporates all of the elements described in the examination for joint pain due to a traumatic injury. Practice it with a friend. After you feel that you have memorized what to ask about, ask the friend to change details of the case. Then do it again, improvising your questions to match the new complaint and new answers. At the end, do not forget to ask the SP: *"Were you able to walk on the joint right after your injury? Are you able to bear weight on it now?"* This will determine if you will order for X-ray.

Table 8.2 Example Dialogues

Doctor	Standardized patient
Hello, Andrew! I understand that your knee is giving you some trouble.	*Yes, that's right, Doctor.*
What happened? And did you pass out when you hurt it?	*I hurt it playing soccer. No, not at all. I remained conscious the whole time, but I had to quit playing after I hurt it.*
How did you hurt it?	*I was running, and then suddenly I changed direction. I felt a sharp pain in my knee.*
How long ago did this happen?	*A couple of days ago.*
Did you walk to the appointment today?	*No, it hurts to bend my knee. My grandfather drove me here.*
Okay, let me give your knee a local exam. Has your knee become swollen or puffy since you hurt it?	*No, not that I have noticed.*
Has it felt hot?	*Nope.*
Has it turned red at all?	*No.*
Has your knee made any snapping, popping, or cracking noises?	*No, it hasn't really made any noises.*
It doesn't look like there's an open wound there, so I assume that the knee hasn't bled.	*No, not a drop of blood.*

Table 8.2 (*Continued*) Example Dialogues

Do you notice any numbness in the knee?	*You mean like a tingling sensation? Yeah. It feels itchy sometimes.*
Does it feel weak?	*Yeah, it sure does. I can't put any weight on it or else a searing pain shoots through it and I have to sit down.*
That leads me to my next question. How is your range of motion affected? Can you bend the knee fully?	*No, I really can't. I have to keep it straight, and it hurts a lot if I try bending it. And I can't put any weight on it.*
Did you strike the knee against anything when this accident occurred? And did anything else get hurt?	*No, I didn't hurt anything else. I was just running, and when I turned, my cleats were dug into the ground, and so when my hips turned, I twisted the knee.*
Okay, let's have a look at your knee. Well, it doesn't look swollen or red. I'll start by pressing on your healthy knee to see what the sensation is in that. Does that hurt?	*No, that doesn't hurt at all.*
Okay, now I will press on your injured knee. Let me know if it hurts.	*Ow! Ouch! Aiieeeeeeeearghhhhhhhh!*
Sorry about that! I am going to check your pulse.	
Okay, now I'll check you for sensation. Does it feel the same on both sides?	*Yes.*
I'll test for your muscle power. *Could you push out against my hand?* *Could you pull in against my hand?*	
Okay, time to check your reflexes. I'll tap your healthy knee.	*Hey, it jerked.*
I am going to do a special exam to test the integrity of the ligaments of your knee. I will be as gentle as I can. Please relax your knee. If at any time it feels painful, let me know.	*Okay.*

Role-Play 33

Mr. Jerry Roberts, a 20-year-old male patient, complains of pain in his **right shoulder**.

Vital signs:
- **Pulse rate (PR):** 86/min, regular.
- **Blood pressure (BP):** 120/80 mm Hg.
- **Respiration rate (RR):** 16/min.
- **Temperature (Temp):** 98.6°F (37°C).

Examinee tasks:
- Obtain a focused history.
- Perform a relevant PE. Do not perform rectal, pelvic, genitourinary, inguinal hernia, female breast, or corneal reflex examinations.
- Discuss your initial diagnostic impression and your workup plan with the patient.
- After leaving the room, complete your patient note on the given form.

Standardized Patient's Role

You are a 20-year-old man, and you have pain in your right shoulder. It started 3 days ago while you were swimming. It was little hot, warm, and puffy. The pain is only in your right shoulder, and has not spread to any other part of your body. You would describe the pain as feeling like a continuous dull ache and would rate it as 5 out of 10. When you raise your arm, the pain worsens. Taking ibuprofen relieves the pain. Putting on a shirt, especially a T-shirt, and combing your hair cause you extreme discomfort as the pain becomes severe. Two years ago, you were diagnosed with a torn rotator cuff.

Ask the doctor at this time:

Q1: *"Do you think it's another tear in my rotator cuff?"*

Your mother has bronchial asthma (BA), and your father has OA.

You are on your university's swim team. You drink socially. You are sexually active exclusively with your girlfriend.

Please put a little rouge on your right shoulder to make the skin look as if it is inflamed. During the exam, as the doctor presses upon your shoulder, say: *"Doc, it hurts so much!"* (**Comment 1**).

Act like your right shoulder is sore. If the doctor raises your right arm, say that it hurts and you cannot raise it above your head. If he pushes it down suddenly, drop your arm suddenly and pretend that this is an involuntarily action. If the doctor asks you about anything other than your shoulder pain, tell him or her that everything else is fine.

As the doctors finishes say:

Q2: *"Tomorrow there is a swim meet. I want to compete. Do you think it's okay if I do?"*

Please refer to Chapter 13 (Appendix), to review the general instructions for the SP as well as the Doctor roles.

Role-Play 33: Answer Key

Right shoulder pain.

History

Ask routine questions following the standard questions in Introduction section of Chapter 8 Musculoskeletal System.

Physical Exam

The standards (VS, ADH, NE, LH) + local (IP AND S) + special maneuvers; remember to test the axillary nerve for any sensory loss.

Dugas' test: This is a test for shoulder dislcoation; ask the SP to place the hand of the injured side on the opposite shoulder; then ask him to lower the elbow to the chest. Pain is indicative of a positive test (▶ Fig. 8.1).

Drop arm test: This is a test for rotator cuff tear. Hold the arm in abduction (at a 90-degree angle). If there is trouble in maintaining this position, the test is positive. Inform the SP that you are going to push the arm down. If the arm drops rapidly, the test is positive (▶ Fig. 8.2).

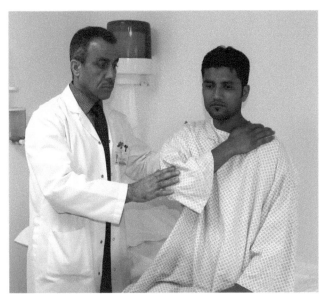

Fig. 8.1 Dugas' test.

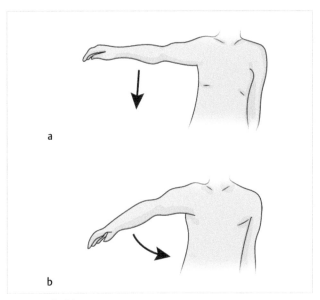

Fig. 8.2 (a, b) Drop arm test.

Communication and Interpersonal Skills

Suggested Closure

Close as routine unless there is severe pain following trauma/accident. In that case, inform the SP that this is an emergency, and so he should stay in the ER until the workup results come back.

Counseling

As routine.

Suggested Answers to the Standardized Patient's Questions

Q1: *"It is definitely a possibility. Allow me to finish taking your medical history and to do a brief physical exam. Then I'll answer your question."*

Comment 1: *"I understand that it could hurt you. Please be patient and relax as much as you can. I'm going to be as gentle as I can."*

Q2: *"I think you may need some rest, but I can't really answer that until I get the results back from the X-rays."*

Patient Note

History

A 20-year-old male patient came to ER with right shoulder pain that started 3 days ago while swimming. Pain is localized to the right shoulder, nonradiating, 5/10, ache, ↓ by Ibuprofen and ↑ by raising the arm. Patient denies loss of consciousness, and head trauma. He noticed erythema, calor, and mild swelling. No bleeding, loss of sensation, or muscle weakness. He can't raise his right arm.

Review of system (ROS): no other injuries or joint pain elsewhere, normal sleep and appetite with no urinary or bowel problems.

Past medical history (PMH): healthy, similar episode of rotator cuff tear 2 years ago. No known drug allergy (NKDA).

Family history (FH): mother has BA and father has OA.

Social history (SH): nonsmoker, drinks socially, sexually active with one girlfriend.

Physical Exam

VS: within normal limit (WNL). Patient has no acute distress.

General exam: no pallor, normal S1 and S2, CTA/BL (clear to auscultation bilaterally). Normal left shoulder. The right shoulder is erythematous, with diffuse tenderness all over, palpable brachial and radial artery pulsations, intact sensation to pinprick and soft touch, muscle power 5/5, DTRs +2. Intact flexion and extension, but cannot abduct his arm over the head. No other joint injury. Positive Dugas' and drop arm tests.

Differential Diagnosis

History finding(s)	Physical exam finding(s)
1. Rotator cuff tear	
Right shoulder pain	Local tenderness
History of redness, hotness, and swelling	Erythema
He cannot move right arm above head	Positive Dugas' and drop arm test
2. Shoulder dislocation (▶ Fig. 8.3)/acromioclavicular joints dislocation	
Right shoulder pain	Local tenderness
History of redness, hotness and swelling	Erythema
He cannot move his right arm	Restricted range of motion and positive Dugas' test
3. Fractured clavicle/scapula/fractured humerus (▶ Fig. 8.4)	
Right shoulder pain	Local tenderness
Redness, hotness and swelling	Erythema
Patient cannot move the right arm	Restricted range of motion
Fell on outstretched hand	
Trauma to right shoulder	

Note: **In axillary nerve** injury, there is loss of sensation over the deltoid.
Wrist drop is one of the presentations of **radial nerve injury**.
We used the copy-and-paste option to save time because the items that support the history and physical exam are the same in both differentials.
These diagnoses can be added especially if the shoulder pain was preceded by motor care accident, injury, or falling on an outstretched hand.

Diagnostic Studies

X-ray of right shoulder (anteroposterior [AP] and lateral views)

X-ray for bilateral shoulders

MRI of the right shoulder

(Continued)

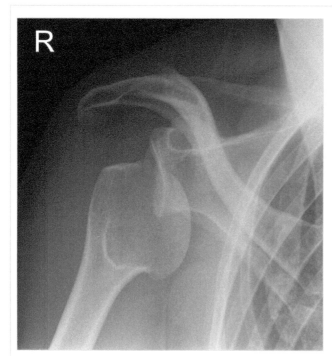

Fig. 8.3 X-ray film showing right shoulder dislocation.

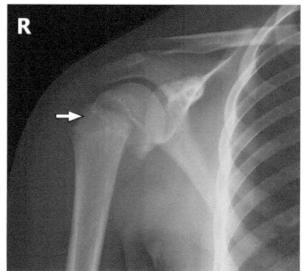

Fig. 8.4 X-ray film showing fracture right humerus.

Role-Play 34

Mr. George Clark, a 55-year-old male patient, came to the clinic with **left knee pain**.
Vital signs:
- **PR:** 90/min, regular.
- **BP:** 100/60 mm Hg.
- **RR:** 16/min.
- **Temp:** 101°F (38.3°C).

Standardized Patient's Role

One week ago while running, you twisted your left knee. The pain was severe, and you stopped running. As you remember, the knee was hot, red, swollen, and tender, but these symptoms have gradually subsided. You took ibuprofen tablets that worked for the pain.

You still have mild pain on the inner side of the knee. It is constant, localized, nonradiating to anywhere else and it's 4 out of 10 in intensity. The pain increases while walking and running and is relieved with rest.

Your mother has RA and your father died from a heart attack. You are retired and stopped smoking 15 years ago; you smoked one pack of cigarette a day for 10 years. You drink socially and don't have sexual partners.

As the physician starts to examine your knee, express tenderness on the inner side of the knee. If he or she performs special maneuvers to examine the integrity of your knee joint, always express tenderness and discomfort on the inner aspect of the knee.

Role-Play 34: Answer Key

History

Follow the standard question.

Physical Exam

On the CS exam, approach traumatic knee pain cases as you would shoulder and ankle pain cases. Focus on the following aspects of the case.

In history-taking for traumatic knee injury, ask the patient if he could resume his activity or sports after the knee injury. If he could, it is mostly a ligament tear. If he couldn't, it likely is a meniscus tear.

Don't forget to perform the following special maneuvers for knee exam GENTLY. Before starting, say: *"I am going to do special exam to test the integrity of the ligaments of your knee. I will be as gentle as I can."*

- **Anterior drawer test** (▶ Fig. 8.5): This test checks the integrity of the anterior cruciate ligament (ACL). While the SP is supine, bend the knee 90 degrees, and gently pull the tibia outward.
- Say, *"Could you bend your knee please; I am going to pull your leg little bit outward. Does it hurt?"*
- **Posterior drawer test** (▶ Fig. 8.6): This test checks the integrity of the posterior cruciate ligament. While the SP is supine, bend the knee 90 degrees, and gently push the tibia inward. Say, *"Now, I will push it inward. Any pain?"*
- **McMurray's meniscus test** (▶ Fig. 8.7): The test checks the integrity of the **men**iscus (remember; **m**edial meniscus, rotate **e**xternally).

While the SP is supine, with flexed hip and knee, hold the foot, and externally rotate the leg. Then extend the leg at the knee joint only. The test is positive if there is pain in the medial meniscus.

Say, *"In this test, I am going to rotate then extend your leg little bit. Does your knee hurt?"*

To test the lateral meniscus, do the same as above, but rotate the leg internally.

Say, *"I will repeat the maneuver again on the opposite side. I so appreciate your cooperation."*

- **Valgus stress test:** This test asses the integrity of the **m**edial collateral ligament. Put your right hand on the inner aspect of the ankle to secure it distally. (**Remember: GMC** car: val**g**us for **m**edial is **c**orrect.)

Put the other hand on the lateral side of the SP's knee and create a valgus stress. Do the test with the knee fully extended (0 degrees).

If you have time, do it again with the knee bent at a 20- to 30-degree angle.

Say, *"I am almost done; I will just put some stress on your knee. Any tenderness?"*

- **Varus stress test** (▶ Fig. 8.8): This test assesses the integrity of the lateral collateral ligament. Do the test in the opposite way. Say, *"I will repeat the maneuver again on the opposite side. Thanks."*

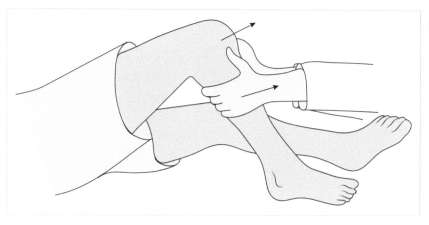

Fig. 8.5 Anterior drawer test.

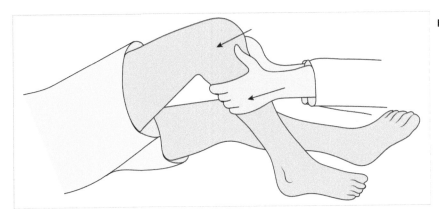

Fig. 8.6 Posterior drawer test.

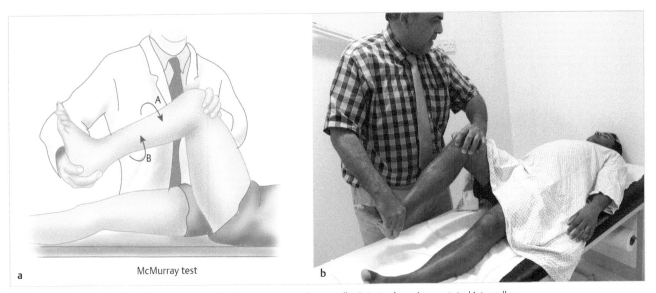

McMurray test

a

b

Fig. 8.7 (a, b) McMurray's meniscus test. A: Medial meniscus rotated externally; B: Lateral meniscus rotated internally.

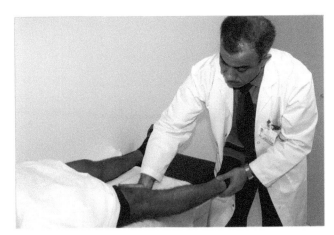

Fig. 8.8 Varus stress test.

Patient Note

History

A 55-year-old man complains of left knee pain that started 1 month ago after he twisted his knee while running. The knee was red, felt hot, and had minor swelling that gradually subsided. Pain on medial side, constant, nonradiating, 4/10, and worsens when exercising, walking. Nonsteroidal anti-inflammatory drugs (NSAIDs) and rest relieve pain. No sensory changes or muscle weakness. He can walk and has no other joint problems.

ROS: no fever, weight change, urinary or bowel problems.
PMH: none, no history of similar episodes.
Med: ibuprofen, NKDA.
FH: father died of heart attack, mother has RA.
SH: retired, ex-smoker 15 years (smoked 1 ppd/10 y). Social drinker and sexually inactive.

Physical Exam

VS: WNL, no acute distress.
General exam: No pallor, normal S1/S2. Normal right knee exam.
Left knee: no erythema, heat, or effusion. The medial side is tender, palpable popliteal and post tibial pulses, intact sensation of pinprick and soft touch, muscle 5/5, DTRs + 2. Full ROM, negative Drawers' and varus stress tests; positive McMurray's test for medial meniscus and valgus stress test.

Differential Diagnoses

History finding(s)	Physical exam finding(s)
1. Medical meniscus tear	
Pain in the medial side of the left knee, increases with walking	Tenderness on the medial side of the knee
Patient twisted his knee	
He noticed redness and swelling	Positive McMurray's test
2. Medial collateral ligament injury	
Pain in the medial side of the left knee, increases with walking	Tenderness on the medial side of the knee
He twisted his knee	
He noticed redness and swelling	Positive McMurray's test

Diagnostic Studies

X-ray for the left knee (AP, lateral views)

X-ray for both knees

MRI for the left knee

Role-Play 35

Doorway Information

Mrs. Luisa Landro, a 27-year-old woman, complains of **ankle pain.**

Vital signs:

- **PR:** 90/min, regular.
- **BP:** 120/80 mm Hg.
- **RR:** 16/min.
- **Temp:** 98°F (36.7°C).

Standardized Patient's Role

You are a 27-year-old woman. You twisted your ankle 2 hours ago. You were ice-skating. Now your right ankle really hurts. The pain does not spread out from the ankle, and is a continuous, aching, agonizing pain, about 9 out of 10. You cannot put weight on your foot, so you cannot walk. Your friends had to bring you to the ER. You have noticed that the ankle is red and swollen. Your last period was 2 weeks ago. You work as an electrical engineer and you drink socially.

If the doctor asks you if anything other than the ankle pain is troubling you, just tell him or her that everything is fine and you are otherwise in good health. Please put a little rouge on your right ankle to make the skin look as if it's inflamed. As the physician finishes his or her exam, pretend that your right ankle is tender. A nice touch would be to put rouge on your ankle to imitate reddened skin.

As he finishes, ask:

Q1: *Do you think that it's a fracture?*

Q2: *What do you think about doing an MRI for my ankle?*

Q3: *Will it require surgery?*

Role-Play 35: Answer Key

Suggested answers for SP's questions:

Q1: *That's a good question. I'll take some pictures of your ankle first to figure out if it's a fracture or not.*

Q2: *Well, MRI is certainly an option. Let's start with an X-ray. If it doesn't tell us anything, I'll order an MRI.*

Q3: *I understand your concern. Based on your history and my physical exam, most probably it's a sprain in your ankle that needs rest, an ankle support or cast, and some meds. Surgery is required in some cases, and for that reason I am ordering a workup: ..., ..., and ....*

Patient Note

History

A 27-year-old woman came to ER after twisting her right ankle 2 hours ago while skating. Pain is localized to the right ankle, constant, severe, agonizing (9/10) with no alleviating factors. Pain increases with movement and is associated with inability to move the right foot. She noticed redness and swelling. She has no bleeding, loss of consciousness, loss of sensation, or muscle weakness. Friends brought her to the ER as she can't walk. **ROS:** no other joint pain or trauma elsewhere. Last menstrual period (LMP) was 2 weeks ago. **PMH and Meds:** none, NKDA. **FH:** none. **SH:** electrical engineer, nonsmoker, drinks socially.

Physical Exam

VS: WNL. Patient is anxious, concerned about pain. **General exam:** No pallor, normal thyroid, normal S1 and S2. Normal left ankle, right ankle is erythematous with diffuse tenderness all over. Palpable posterior tibial and dorsalis pedis arteries pulsation, normal sensation to pinprick and soft touch, muscle is 5/5, DTRs is + 2. Restricted dorsal and plantar flexion, eversion and inversion, no other injured joints.

Differential Diagnosis

History finding(s)	Physical exam finding(s)
1. Ankle sprain	
Ankle pain and she twisted her ankle	Local tenderness
Redness, heat, and swelling	Erythema
She cannot move the right foot	Restricted range of motion of the right foot
2. Pott's fracture (▶Fig. 8.9)	
Ankle pain and she twisted her ankle	Local tenderness
Redness, heat, and swelling	Erythema
She cannot move her right foot	Restricted range of motion of the right foot
3. Calcaneal fracture	

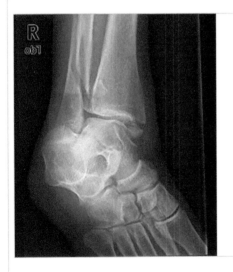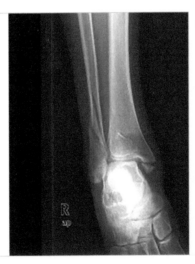

Fig. 8.9 X-ray films showing Pott's fracture.

Diagnostic Studies

X-ray of the right ankle (AP, lateral view)

X-ray for bilateral ankles

CT right ankle/MRI right ankle

Rheumatic (Nontraumatic) Joint Pain

As a general rule, joint pain in rheumatic diseases is either mechanical or inflammatory.

Mechanical pain or usage-related pain: Pain is worse by movement and relieved by rest. This occurs in OA and periarticular diseases.

In periarticular conditions (e.g., medial and lateral epicondylitis) and although the condition is usually inflammatory, the rhythm of pain tends to be "mechanical"—that is, made worse by movement and relieved by rest without joint stiffness (Bijlsma JWJ, Hachulla E, eds. EULAR Textbook on Rheumatic Diseases. 2nd ed. Eular: Kilchberg (Zürich), Switzerland; 2015).

Inflammatory pain: Pain is worst in the morning (i.e., after prolonged rest) and is relieved as patient gets up and starts to move his or her joints.

Fever in the doorway information with joint pain usually refers to nontraumatic rheumatic joint pain.

In these cases, joint pain usually is not caused by trauma; to be sure, ask:
- *Did you injure your …?* (name the joint)
- *Were you involved in an accident?*
- *Have you had any trauma to your…?* (name the joint)

Possible DDs: For each disease in the list, there are specific questions to be asked (▶ Table 8.3).

Table 8.3 Specific questions to be asked for each disease in the list.

Disease	Questions
Osteoarthritis (OA)	*Does the pain get worse when you walk?* *Does the pain lessen when you rest?* *Do you feel or hear any cracking of your joints?*
Rheumatoid arthritis (RA)	*Do you feel stiff in the morning?* *Is it difficult to get out of bed?*
Systemic lupus erythematous (SLE)	*Have you noticed any hair loss?* *Have you had any facial rashes?* *Have you noticed any sores on your tongue?* *Do you have any chest pain?* *Have you noticed if your urine is darker than usual?* *Do you have any abdominal pain?* *Have you had any miscarriages? (Female SP)*
Septic arthritis	*Have you had any fevers recently?* *Do you have any STDs?* *Have you noticed any vaginal or cervical discharge? (in female SPs)*
Gout	*Have you had any swelling in your big toe?*
Others	
Reactive arthritis	*Have you had an upper respiratory tract infection recently?*
Lyme disease	*Have you gone camping or hiking recently?* *Have you spent time outdoors, in a forest, or a park?*
Psoriatic arthritis	*Do you have psoriasis?*
Hemophilic arthritis	*Have you noticed any skin rashes?*

Role-Play 36

Mrs. Nancy Chuck, a 35-year-old female patient, came to the clinic with **joint pain**.

Vital signs:
- **PR:** 90/min, regular.
- **BP:** 120/70 mm Hg.
- **RR:** 16/min.
- **Temp:** 100.5°F (38°C).

Standardized Patient's Role

You have had pain in your hand and knee joints for 3 months. As you remember, it came on gradually and has gotten worse since then. It wasn't preceded by trauma. The pain is mild all night and in the daytime. In early morning, you feel stiff for about 30 minutes, and you can't move. Your movement improves as you get up and move. The pain doesn't travel to anywhere else and is an aching pain. On a scale of 1 to 10, it's probably 4.

You have noticed a few tongue sores in the last few weeks. You have lost about 8 lb over the last 6 months; you got pregnant once, and that ended with C-section. You smoke 10 cigarettes daily and drink socially. You are sexually active with your husband. Your mother has RA.

Please put rouge on your knees to make the skin look as if it's inflamed. As the physician examines you, express tenderness on your knees and act as if you can extend your fingers but with a little stiffness.

Role-Play 36: Answer Key

As mentioned at the beginning of the role-plays, your priority is to determine if the case is traumatic or not, as the DDs will be completely different for the two. Rheumatic joint pain is nontraumatic.

History

Analysis of Chief Complaint

Conduct a normal analysis for pain and fever.

Analysis of Differential Diagnosis

A detailed analysis of the differential diagnosis is presented in ▶ Table 8.3.

Review of the local system

Fever, skin rash, loss of weight, other joint pain.

Past History and Others

D (RA, SLE, sexually transmitted diseases [STDs]), P (usually there was a previous episode), D (NSAIDs, steroids), F (family history), ±S (STD for septic arthritis).

Physical Exam

VS: fever? H: Hair, face (malar flush), pallor, tongue; E: Pallor, Raynaud's phenomenon; LH (auscultation only).

If you suspect STDs/gonococcal urethritis, ask for pelvic and vaginal exams and counsel for safe sex precautions.

Patient Note

History

A 35-year-old woman complains of pain in the hand and knee joints for 3 months; it wasn't preceded by trauma. It had a gradual onset, progressive, and is a nonradiating dull aching pain (4/10). She feels stiff early in the morning for nearly 30 minutes, and better as she gets up, moves, and takes NSAID. The right knee feels hot and red but not swollen. She has not heard any cracking sounds in the joint, has not seen any skin rash, and she has not experienced any chest or abdominal pain. She recalls having a few tongue sores. She has no history of miscarriage or STDs, no recent URT infection, and she has not been camping or hiking recently.

ROS: mild fever, lost 8 lb/6 mo, no change in bowel movements, and no urinary symptoms. G1P1.

PMH: C-section once.

Med: NSAID, NKDA.

FH: mother has RA.

SH: smokes 0.5 ppd/d for 10 years, drinks socially.

Sexual history: She is sexually active, monogamous with her husband.

Physical Exam

VS: Temp: 100.5°F, others WNL, no acute distress, alert and oriented ×3.

Head and Neck: no pallor, cyanosis, malar flush, hair loss, or tongue ulcers.

Chest and heart: normal S1, S2, CTA/BL.

Abdomen: soft, non tender (NT), bowel sounds +.

Ext: no Raynaud's phenomenon.

Joint: Both knees showed erythema and tenderness with no swelling. Finger joints showed restricted ROM. Other joints were not inflamed or tender. Intact sensation and muscle 5/5.

Differential Diagnosis

History finding(s)	Physical exam finding(s)
1. Rheumatoid arthritis (RA)	
Knee pain, morning stiffness	Tenderness over knees and finger joints showed restricted range of motion (ROM)
Family history of RA	
Fever	Fever (100.5°F)
2. Systemic lupus erythematosus	
Knee pain, morning stiffness	Tenderness over right knee and finger joints showed restricted ROM
Fever	Fever (100.5°F)
Loss of weight	Weight loss (8 lb/6 mo)
Tongue ulcers	

Diagnostic Studies

CBC with diff, ESR, CRP

RF assay, ANA, anti-dsDNA, anti-CCP

Culture for cervical secretion (septic arthritis)

X-ray of the hands (AP and lateral views)

MRI knees

Aspiration of the joint for synovial fluid analysis

Cervical and Lumbar Pain

Back and neck pains are common cases in medical practice. However, the vast majority of cases will escape a precise etiological diagnosis even after meticulous investigation. This is owing to the anatomic complexity of the spine, muscles, ligaments, nerves, and supporting soft tissues in the area, which leads to a multiplicity of potential causes (Reference: http://www.uptodate.com/contents/evaluation-of-low-back-pain).

The DDs for this category are as follows:
- *Muscles:* muscle strain and ligament sprain.
- *Bones:* spinal fracture (▶Fig. 8.10), osteoporosis, and spondylosis.
- *In between the bones (intervertebral disk):* degenerative arthritis and herniated disk.

History

Analysis of Chief Complaint

Pain as standard.

Signs of inflammation + AND (Artery, Nerve, Disability).

Disability, for cervical pain: *Are you able to get dressed by yourself? Are you able to firmly grasp things in your hand?*

Disability, for lumbar pain: *Can you walk? Do you have drop foot? Are you incontinent for urine?*

Have you ever had an accidental bowel movement?

Analysis of Differential Diagnosis

Does movement make the pain get worse? (checking for muscle strain)
Did you hit your back? Were you in a car wreck? (checking for spinal fracture)
Are you taking any calcium pills? Do you have osteoporosis?

Have you been diagnosed with cancer or an infection lately? (metastasis and infection)

Review of the Local System

Do you have any problems in the other joints?

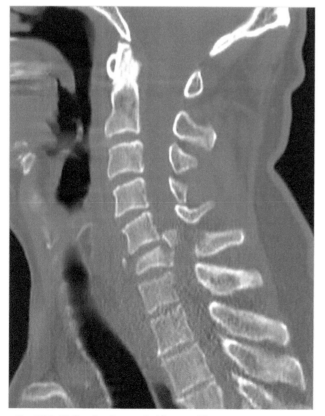

Fig. 8.10 CT film showing cervical fracture (C).

Physical Exam

Spinal Examination

As a part of communication and interpersonal skills (CIS) and good bedside manner, don't forget to say the magic word "Please" when you ask SPs to do something for you. Of course, it's also a good idea to thank them after they do what you tell them. This also signals that you are done with that procedure.

Below is a chart offering tips and sample questions about conducting a spinal exam. After you finish the exam, if you feel that you need to investigate further, order an X-ray in the patient note, specifying an AP and a lateral view. You can also order an MRI. Document this in the workup.

Just as when you examine joints affected by traumatic pain, you use the **IP AND S** formula. The components and order remain the same—inspection, palpation, artery, nerve, disability, and special maneuvers—but the questions are modified and tailored to the spine. As always, tell the SP what you are going to do. It's also a good idea to fill him or her in on why you are doing it and what you see or don't see.

Inspection:
- Tell the SP: *"I need to examine your neck/back, so may I untie your gown? I'm looking for anything out of the ordinary."* Document for any erythema or scar.

Palpation:
- Say something like *"I'm going to press on your …. Does it hurt here? What about here?"* Start by pressing on the paravertebral muscles, away from the painful area. Then press on the spine, going from the top to the bottom, asking the SP if it hurts.

Artery:
- Tell the SP: *"I'm going to check your pulse."* For cervical pain, take the pulse in the upper limbs (radial and brachial). For lumbar pain, take the pulse in the lower limbs (popliteal and posterior tibial).

Nerve:
- Sensation: Ask the SP, *"Does it feel the same on both sides?"* Upper limbs for cervical pain, legs for lumbar pain. Test the unaffected arm for comparison purposes. See Chapter 13, Appendix at the end of the book for the most common dermatomal areas tested.
- Muscle power: For cervical pain, ask the SP: *"Could you spread your fingers out? Can you bring them together? Please hold my fingers; squeeze them as hard as you can."* Then, test the muscle strength at the wrist, elbow, and shoulder. For lumbar pain, test the muscle strength in the lower limb. Use the same method described in the neurological exam (see Chapter 10, Neurology).
- DTRs: For cervical pain, test biceps and triceps reflexes. For lumbar pain, test ankle and knee reflexes (see Chapter 10, Neurology).

Disability:
- Remember that if the SP is not in severe pain, do the active ROM test. You can act out these actions to make it easier for the SP to know what you are directing.
- In cases of cervical pain, examine the neck, saying, "Could you please look down? Now look up. Please look to your left…now to your right…and make your right ear touch your right shoulder…now your left ear to your left shoulder."
- In cases of lumbar pain, examine the back, saying: "Could you bend down and touch your toes? Can you lean backward? Could you twist your body from side to side?"

Note: If you find the SP is in severe pain and can't move, say: *"It is preferred not to do any active movements for your spine because that may worsen the problem."*

Special tests:
- Perform straight leg raise test for lumbar pain and Spurling's test for cervical pain (see the individual cases).

Role-Play 37

Mr. Smith, a 65-year-old man, has **low back pain.**
Vital signs:
- **PR:** 96/min, regular.
- **BP:** 120/70 mm Hg.
- **RR:** 16/min.
- **Temp:** 98°F (36.7°C).

Standardized Patient's Role

When the doctor enters the room, act like you are in extreme pain, and immediately ask:
Q1: *Could you prescribe me some painkillers right now? My back is killing me.*

You came to the ER with severe low back pain that started a few hours ago. The pain began right after you lifted a heavy box at work. You also feel the pain in your left leg. This feels like an electrical shock, and is constant. You would rate it about 4 out of 10 in intensity, but any movement makes the pain increase to 8 out of 10. Your left leg sometimes feels numb and weak. Taking NSAIDs helps relieve the pain. You have no problems in controlling your urination and defecation.

Over the last month, you have lost about 10 lb. Your urine stream is weak, and you have difficulty in passing urine. Four years ago, you were diagnosed with prostate cancer and you have finished a radiotherapy course. Three months ago, you experienced a similar pain and it went away after you rested and took NSAID.

You have smoked 1 ppd for 25 years. You are not currently sexually active.

During the exam:

Pretend that your lower back is extremely tender.

If the doctor asks you to raise your left leg, act like it hurts badly when you raise it to about 30 to 40 degrees.

Ask your doctor when he or she examines the leg:
Q2: *Can you tell me why my leg is hurting?*

Role-Play 37: Answer Key

The SP will often be in a great deal of pain, so you should be prepared to be supportive and gentle. Since this is a lower back pain case, remember to do the straight leg raise test.

Past History and Others

D (Primary spine cancer or secondary like prostate cancer, TB, osteomalacia), **P** (previous episode), **D** (calcium, HRT [hormone replacement therapy]), **F** (osteoporosis).

Physical Exam

Straight leg raise test (▶ **Fig. 8.11**): While the SP is lying down, raise the leg up, knee extended, leg straight. Normally, there is no pain till 80 degrees. The test is positive if the SP's leg begins to hurt when it is moved past 30 degrees. Pain indicates nerve root stretching. If the test is positive, repeat it on the other leg to compare. Sometimes, positive leg raise can be due to a tight hamstring—although rare to be simulated by SPs in the CS exam—drop the leg by 10 degrees and dorsiflex the ipsilateral foot; if still positive, you have a tight hamstring and a negative straight leg test.

Communication and Interpersonal Skills

Suggested Closure

Assure the SP if he is in severe pain. Inform him that you will return as soon as the test results come back. To do pelvic exam to test the sensation in the saddle area, inform the SP that you will call the nurse to prepare him for a pelvic exam.

Suggested Answers to the Standardized Patient's Questions

Q1: *"I'm so sorry to see you in pain. Please give me a few minutes to ask you a few questions regarding your medical history and do a physical exam. Then I'll prescribe the proper meds. So please hang in there just a bit more. Help will be on the way."*

Q2: On a paper, draw while explaining to the SP: *This is the spine, and as you know it has a number of vertebrae and there is a small piece of cartilage that acts as a cushion between the vertebrae. If this cartilage moves, it puts pressure or stress on the nerves there. Those nerves control your leg, and for this reason your leg hurts. I'm going to give you a handout. It gives a simple explanation for back pain that was prepared for patient education. You can read it at home, and I will be happy to address your concerns at your next visit."*

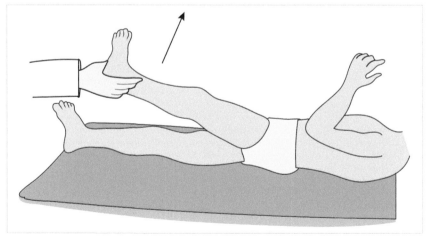

Fig. 8.11 Straight leg raise test.

History

A 65-year-old man came to the ER with lower back pain that started a few hours ago immediately after he lifted a heavy box at work. The pain in the lower back radiates to the left leg, feels like electric shock, constant, 4/10, and movement makes it worse 8/10. It is ↓ by rest and NSAID, and ↑ by movement. Associated with tingling in the back of the left leg and difficulty walking. Not preceded with trauma, pain doesn't change with position.

ROS: no fever, recent weight loss 10 lb/6 mo, good urine and bowel control.

PMH: prostate cancer; on radiotherapy. A previous episode 3 months ago, was relieved with rest and NSAID.

FH: father died from prostate cancer.

SH: smokes 1ppd/25 y, is not sexually active.

Physical Exam

VS: WNL, the patient was lying down on the bed in pain. No deformities noted, no erythema of the back. Mild tenderness over the lower paraspinal muscles.

Lower limb exam: palpable pulsation, intact sensation for pinprick and soft touch, muscle power 5/5, DTR + 2 (+) straight leg raise on left side and negative Babinski's sign.

Differential Diagnosis

History finding(s)	Physical exam finding(s)
1. Lumbar disk herniation (▶ Fig. 8.12)	
Low back pain, after lifting a heavy object	Tenderness over the lumbar spine
Radiates to left leg	
Pain relieved by NSAID and rest	Positive straight leg raising test
2. Metastatic prostate cancer (pathological fracture)	
Low back pain	Tenderness over the lumbar spine
Has prostate cancer on radiation therapy	
Loss of weight	Lost 10 lb/6 mo
3. Back muscles strain	
Lower back pain	Tenderness over the paraspinal muscles
Pain increases with movement	

Abbreviation: NSAID, nonsteroidal anti-inflammatory drug.

Diagnostic Studies

Pelvic and rectal exam

PSA (prostate-specific antigen)

X-ray of lumbosacral spine (AP and lateral views) and MRI

Bone scan

(Continued)

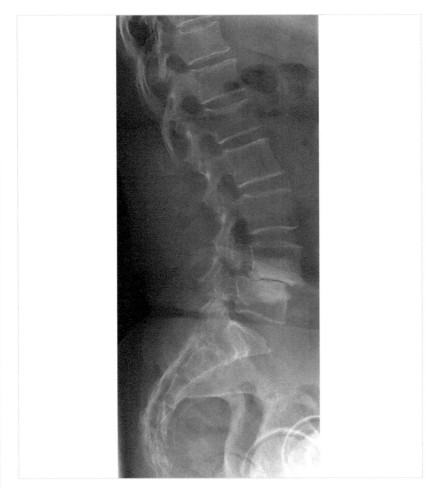

Fig. 8.12 X-ray spine showing herniated disk L4–L5.

Role-Play 38

Mr. Jerry Roberts, a 60-year-old male patient, complains of **neck pain**.

Vital signs:
- **PR:** 86/min, regular.
- **BP:** 120/80 mm Hg.
- **RR:** 16/min.
- **Temp:** 98.6°F (37°C).

Standardized Patient's Role

You have had neck pain for 3 months; it started gradually and has gotten worse with time. The pain travels to the left arm and feels like an electric shock; on a scale of 1 to 10, you would rate the intensity as 6. It feels better with an over-the counter (OTC) pain-killer (ibuprofen). You feel tingling and numbness in your left arm, and it becomes weak when grasping things with your hand. A few years ago, you fell off a horse. After X-rays, you were told that you had a fracture in one of your neck bones.

At this time, ask your doctor:

Q1: *Do I have the same fracture?*

You retired few years ago, do not smoke, and drink socially. Your mother has OA.

As the doctor examines you, express tenderness over the cervical spine. Act as if the sensation of your left arm is less than the right one and that the left arm is weak.

If the doctor presses on your head while doing special maneuvers to test your neck, say that there is a shooting pain that travels along your left arm.

Role-Play 38: Answer Key

Cervical pain is best examined in the same way that back pain is dealt with. This will also make it easier for you to remember the procedure.

Spurling's test (▶**Fig. 8.13**): While the neck is flexed toward the affected side, press the head gently down. A positive test is when the pain arising in the neck radiates in the direction of the corresponding ipsilateral dermatome.

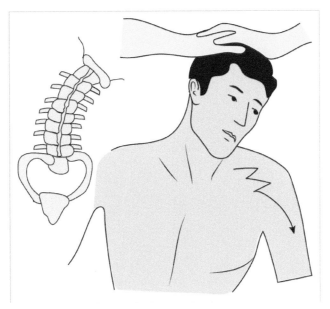

Fig. 8.13 Spurling's test.

History

A 60-year-old man came to the clinic with complaint of cervical pain. The pain came on gradually and got worse as time passed. It radiates to the left arm, feels like an electrical shock, is constant, 6/10, and is partially relieved by OTC painkiller. It is associated with tingling, numbness, and a weak hand grasp. Movement does not affect the pain in any way. He has no other joint problems.

ROS: no fever or loss of weight, and urinary and bowel functions are normal.

PMH: patient fell off a horse a long time ago. He was diagnosed with a minor fracture of the neck bones.

Med: ibuprofen, NKDA.

FH: mother has OA.

SH: he is retired, does not smoke but drinks socially.

Physical Exam

VS: WNL, the patient with no acute distress.

General exam: no pallor or skin rash, normal S1 and S2.

Local exam: normal right arm exam.

Left arm: no erythema or swelling. Tenderness over the cervical spine area, palpable brachial and radial pulse. Impaired sensation in the left arm, muscle power 4/5. DTR +2, intact ROM of the left shoulder, Spurling's test is positive.

Differential Diagnosis

History finding(s)	Physical exam finding(s)
1. Cervical disk herniation	
Cervical pain (electrical shock)	Tenderness over paraspinal muscle
Tingling, numbness in the left arm	Impaired sensation in the left arm
Weak hand grip	Muscle power 4/5
	Spurling's test is +ve
2. Fractured cervical spine	
Cervical pain	Tenderness over the cervical spine
Past history of fractured neck bones	Impaired sensation in the left arm
	Muscle power 4/5

Diagnostic Studies

X-ray of the cervical spine (AP and lateral views)

MRI cervical spine

9 Psychiatry

Keywords: panic attack, anxiety, depression, post-traumatic stress disorder, schizophrenia

9.1 Introduction (▶ Audio 9.1)

On the Clinical Skills (CS) exam, psychiatric cases have a special concern compared to the other cases. Problems are rarely found in the diagnosis, history-taking, or physical exam; the greatest difficulties are found in the Communication and Interpersonal Skills (CIS) components. The Standardized Patients (SPs) are well trained to act very professionally, as if they are real psychiatric patients. They intend to create realistic circumstances to test how you are going to handle such cases. As they are good actors, you should be one, too. **Maintain your sensitive and supportive behavior** when you enter the room, while taking history and doing the exam. You should leave at least a couple of minutes for counseling. Don't forget to determine the **home situation** and **safety** for these patients .

9.2 A Quick Review

To be best prepared for the CS exam, refresh your knowledge of psychiatry, and then read the following snapshots for common psychiatric cases on the CS exam.

Panic attack: A condition characterized by sudden onset of intense fear during which the following physical and mental symptoms might occur: physical like, sweating, palpitation, tremors, chest pain, dyspnea, and choking sensation, and mental symptoms like losing of control and feeling of impending death. The patient is persistently concerned and worried about

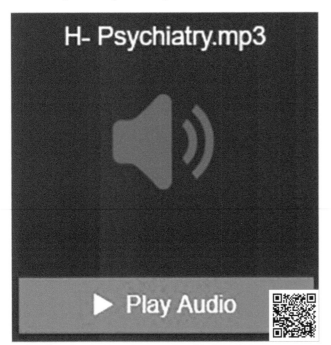

Audio 9.1 The audio contains the core of psychiatry and can be used as a quick review before the exam https://www.thieme.de/de/q. htm?p=opn/cs/20/3/11453117-801f2a3b&t=audio

having an attack and may have behavioral changes to evade future attacks. This case could be represented on the doorway information as chest pain.

Post-traumatic stress disorder (PTSD): A triad of symptoms: intrusive re-experiencing of a traumatic event, avoidance, and hyperarousal. Symptoms last for more than 1 month and can last longer.

*In **acute stress disorder (ASD):*** Symptoms are similar to PTSD but only last between 2 days and 4 weeks.

Adjustment disorder: It is a maladaptive reaction to an identifiable psychological stressor (e.g., moving, divorce, etc.). This usually occurs within 3 months of the stressor and lasts less than 6 months. Symptoms include anxiety, mild depression, and interpersonal stress, and conduct problems.

Anxiety: A condition characterized by fear and apprehension. Physical and psychological symptoms occur in response to minor events or unknown sources. Examples of symptoms include the following:

- *Physical symptoms:* Restlessness, disturbed sleep, sweating, and palpitation.
- *Psychological:* Worry and apprehension that are difficult to control.

Grief/bereavement: A condition characterized by a group of symptoms that come after loss of a loved one or loss of a body part. They are minor in comparison to the symptoms of depression and can be mitigated with good grooming and hygiene and a return to a normal routine.

Symptoms revolve around the loved one and include sadness, sleep disturbance, and guilt; they usually subside within 2 months.

Schizophrenia: On the CS exam, the SP usually exhibits two or more of the following:

- *Delusions:* Beliefs with no evidence that cannot be corrected by reasoning.
- *Hallucinations:* False perceptions without external stimuli; they may be auditory, hallucinatory, or olfactory.
- Disorganized speech.
- Disorganized behavior.

The symptoms usually last more than 6 months and are accompanied by impairment of the ability to function socially and at work.

The SP usually presents with some negative symptoms such as slow speech or flat affect.

Two conditions you might encounter that are similar to schizophrenia include the following:

- *Brief psychotic disorder:* symptoms occur for 1 month.
- *Schizophreniform disorder:* symptoms occur for 1 to 6 months.

Major depressive disorder: On the CS exam, the SP usually exhibits the following symptoms as described in the DSM-IV (Diagnostic and Statistical Manual of Mental Disorders - 4)

Criteria for Major Depressive Disorder (MDD) (Project Safety Net. Diagnostic Criteria for Major Depressive Disorder and Depressive Episodes. Available at: http://www.psnpaloalto.com/wp/wp-content/uploads/2010/12/Depression-Diagnostic-Criteria-and-Severity-Rating.pdf):

- Depressed mood or a loss of interest or pleasure in daily activities for more than 2 weeks.
- Mood represents a change from the person's baseline.
- Impaired function: social, occupational, educational.
- Specific symptoms, at least five of these nine, present nearly every day:

1. *Depressed mood or irritable* most of the day, nearly every day, as indicated by either subjective report (e.g., feels sad or empty) or observation made by others (e.g., appears tearful).
2. *Decreased interest or pleasure* in most activities, most of each day.
3. *Significant weight change* (5%) or change in appetite.
4. *Change in sleep:* insomnia or hypersomnia.
5. *Change in activity:* psychomotor agitation or retardation.
6. Fatigue or loss of energy.
7. *Guilt/worthlessness:* feelings of worthlessness or excessive or inappropriate guilt.
8. *Concentration:* diminished ability to think or concentrate, or more indecisiveness.
9. *Suicidality:* thoughts of death or suicide, or has suicide plan.

You can use the **SIG E CAPS** mnemonics (Sleep, Interest, Guilty, Energy, Concentration, Appetite, Psychomotor agitation and Suicidal thoughts) to help you remember the symptoms.

Bipolar disorder:
- Bipolar 1 (manic-depressive disorder): episodes of both mania and depression.
- Bipolar 2: recurrent attacks of depression with episodes of hypomania.

Mania:
- Elated or irritable mood longer than 1 week with disturbed social and work life.
- Increased activity and energy.
- Pressured speech.
- Feeling of high creativity and mental efficiency that can lead to grandiose ideas.
- Sexual disinhibition/exhibitionism.
- Reduced need to sleep.

Handling difficult situations with psychiatric SPs: SPs experiencing psychiatric distress may require you to adjust your behavior and manner. Here are some common situations that can occur with psychiatric cases on the CS exam and the appropriate behavior for each.

If the SP doesn't respond after introducing yourself: stop smiling and soften your tone and say, *"It seems that you have a lot of emotional stress; would you like to share with me your trouble? Why are you feeling this way?* Or, *it seems that something is bringing you down. Is there any way that I can help you?"*

In most of the cases, the SP will start to speak; if not, say, *"Mrs./ Miss …. Life is sometimes hard for everyone, so we should have someone to speak with. I'm your doctor and I am here to assist you. Please tell me what is going on."* After that, in the majority of the cases, the SP will respond.

9.3 General Instructions for History-Taking

Analysis of the chief complaint:
- *How long have you been feeling this way?*
- *Was it sudden?*
- *Since it started, has it gotten worse?*
- *What makes it better?*
- *What makes it worse?*
- *Is it constant or does it come and go?*
- *What symptoms do you have besides …?*

Analysis of the differential diagnosis:
- *Do you have any idea what might be causing your symptoms?*
- *Do you have any kind of stress at your job? In your family?*
- *Have you had recent financial troubles? Any psychiatric trauma? Any emotional stress?*

Note: Don't forget to ask questions for possible hypothyroidism.

Symptoms related to the local system:
- *Do you feel sad?*
- *Do you feel depressed?*

If the SP answers yes, go through questions for possible depression.

Review of systems:
Ask routine questions.

9.4 General Instructions for Physical Examination

In psychiatric cases, do a short exam, as more time is usually needed for counseling. It may include the following:
- Quick general exam.
- Checking the thyroid.
- Listening to the heart and lungs.
- A few steps of a neurological exam.
- Do MMSE (Mini-mental status exam) if the SP has a problem with memory.

Role-Play 39

Mrs. Carol Roberts, a 35-year-old woman, came to the ER with chest pain.

Vital signs:
- **Pulse rate (PR):** 86/min, regular.
- **Blood pressure (BP):** 120/80 mm Hg.
- **Respiratory rate (RR):** 16/min.
- **Temperature (Temp):** 98.6° F (37°C).

Examinee tasks:
- Obtain a focused history.
- Perform a relevant physical examination. Do not perform rectal, pelvic, genitourinary, inguinal hernia, female breast, or corneal reflex examinations.
- Discuss your initial diagnostic impression and your workup plan with the patient.
- After leaving the room, complete your patient note on the given form.

Standardized Patient's Role

For a long time, you have had personal conflicts and arguments with your husband about many issues regarding the future of your children. In the last 2 to 3 weeks, you have had episodes of intense chest pain, in the center part of the chest, and not appearing anywhere else. The episodes last for half a minute. When it comes, you feel tightness in your chest, have difficulty breathing, a rapidly beating heart, and sweating. These episodes also come when you are in crowded places, and you feel like you are going to die. Recently, your sleep has become difficult, and it takes up to a couple of hours to fall asleep.

You have visited many doctors. Unfortunately, they haven't reached a final diagnosis.

Your last menstrual period was 2 weeks ago; you had a pap smear done 2 years ago, and it was normal. You are taking contraceptive pills.

You have irritable bowel syndrome and overactive bladder. You take oxybutynin tablets. Your mother has thyroid problems. You work as a physician assistant, drink coffee, 4 to 5 cups/d, and have smoked one pack of cigarettes per day for 10 years and drink socially. You are sexually active with your husband.

As the doctor finishes his or her exam, ask the following question:

Q1: *Do I have any problem with my heart?*

Role-Play 39: Answer Key

Chest pain

Please refer to the answer key in Chapter 4, Chest (Cardiology and Respiratory), Role-Play 5. We also put chest pain case in this chapter to show that this complain can appear in different system-area scenarios.

Please refer to Chapter 13 (Appendix), to review the general instructions for the SP as well as the Doctor roles.

Role-Play 40

Miss Dana Weiss, a 30-year-old female patient, feels sad.
Vital signs:
- **PR:** 84/min, regular.
- **BP:** 110/80 mm Hg.
- **RR:** 16/min.
- **Temp:** 98.6°F (37°C).

Standardized Patient's Role

Three weeks ago, you were hiking with your friends and saw one of them drown. You did your best to save your friend, but it was to no avail.

Tell your doctor: *"I'm so sad, I couldn't save my friend, and she was the best friend to me!"* (**Comment 1**)

You feel sad, tired, can't concentrate, and have less interest in your daily activities. Sometimes you have flashbacks and nightmares about the event. You work as an accountant and most of your colleagues have noticed how your performance has been affected. You also have difficulty falling asleep, and your appetite has decreased recently.

You are sexually active with multiple male partners, don't usually use condoms, and had two occurrences of sexually transmitted diseases last year. Your last period was 2 weeks ago. Your last Pap smear was 2 years ago, and it was normal. You also drink two beers a day.

Q1: *Do I have depression?*

Role-Play 40: Answer Key

Communication and Interpersonal Skills Component

As you read "feels sad" from the doorway information, stop smiling and soften your voice. Be responsive to the SP's mood in your facial expression and tone of voice. Consider depression among the differential diagnosis (DD).

Suggested Closure

"Miss…, as you told me you have …, …, …. My preliminary diagnosis is ASD or PTSD. Your symptoms are mostly related to the bad experience and the psychiatric trauma that you had 3 weeks ago. You don't have any suicidal thoughts and are not feeling guilty, but I couldn't eliminate other possible causes of sadness and tiredness. You are sexually active with occasional use of condoms with multiple sexual partners. When was your last HIV test? We can do one here. May I ask our nurse to prepare you for local and vaginal exams?"

Suggested Answers to the Standardized Patient's Questions

Answer as given in the previous examples.

History

A 30-year-old female patient complains of fatigue following an unsuccessful attempt to save her friend from drowning 3 weeks ago. The fatigue exists during the day; she has flashbacks and nightmares about the event. She feels sad, tired, with decreased ability to concentrate. She has less interest in her daily activities and the condition has started to affect her job as an accountant. She has decreased appetite and disturbed sleep. She denies feeling guilty, has no suicidal thoughts, no cold intolerance, or recent changes in her weight. She has normal urinary and bowel movements. LMP was 2 weeks ago, last pap was smear 2 years ago that was normal. **Past medical history (PMH):** STD twice last year, abortion, no known drug allergy (NKDA), 2 beers/d, no street drugs. Sexually active with multiple male partners, occasional condom use, never tested for HIV.

Physical Exam

Vital signs (VS): within normal limit (WNL). The patient is alert and oriented ×3. **Head:** PERRLA, mouth without erythema, no pallor. **Neck:** normal thyroid. **Extremities (Ext.):** no peripheral edema, palpable peripheral pulse, no tremors. **Lung:** CTA/BL (clear to auscultation bilaterally). **Heart:** normal S1 and S2 with no murmurs. **Neuro:** intact sensation.

Differential Diagnosis

History finding(s)	Physical exam finding(s)
1. Acute stress disorder	
Fatigue, sadness, ↓ concentration	
Flashbacks, nightmares	Free physical exam
Comes after stressful event	
2. Human immunodeficiency virus	
Fatigue	
Multiple sexual partners	
History of sexually transmitted diseases (STDs)	

Diagnostic Studies

Pelvic exam

Complete blood count (CBC), thyroid-stimulating hormone (TSH)

HIV virus load, CD4 count

Role-Play 41

Doorway Information

Mrs. Sabrina Armstrong, a 35-year-old woman, is feeling sad.

Vital signs:

- **PR:** 84/min, regular.
- **BP:** 120/80 mm Hg.
- **RR:** 16/min.
- **Temp:** 98.6°F (37°C).

Standardized Patient's Role

Be sad during the entire encounter. Speak slowly and, if possible, try to put bluish or greenish makeup on your face, shoulders, back, and legs to replicate bruises.

You have been married for 10 years, and for the last 6 months, your husband has been drinking heavily and has started to beat you. He was fired from his job and has placed all the financial issues on you. Two weeks ago, he returned home very late, and because you were angry with him, he beat you. The beating left multiple bruises on your body. You left with your two kids to stay at a nearby hotel, but you are no longer able to pay for it.

You don't have any other injuries. He didn't use a gun or knife. He didn't hurt your kids, and they are with you in the hotel. You haven't informed anyone, including your friends or family or the police.

You feel sad, depressed, and guilty as you haven't disclosed this abusive relationship since it began. You thought about ending your life twice, but every time you think about your children and decide not to hurt yourself. You are healthy and your last menses was 2 weeks ago, you use oral contraceptive pills, and your last pap smear 2 years ago was normal. You have difficulty sleeping and use over-the-counter (OTC) sleeping pills. You are a nonsmoker, drink socially, and have no other sexual partners. You work as bus driver.

Your mother has hypothyroidism and depression.

As the physician examines you, express little tenderness over the bruises.

At the end of the encounter, tell the doctor: *I'm in a hard situation and I need a small apartment for me and my kids, and I can't pay the rent* (**comment 1**).

Role-Play 41: Answer Key

In such sensitive cases, you should be gentle and supportive during the encounter. Speak slowly, sit beside the SP, and express your concern in your tone of voice. Finally, give 2 to 3 minutes of counseling. Try not to touch the patient or appear physically threatening/imposing in any way.

The complaint can vary in these cases. It may be bruises (with bluish makeup), feeling sad or depressed, or even crying.

If it is bruises, ask directly, *"I notice some bruises. Could you tell me what happened to you?"*

In the cases when the SP appears sad, depressed, and doesn't disclose violence, you can ask in this way, *"Are you currently in a relationship with someone who hurts you?"*

History

Analysis of Chief Complaint

Use mnemonic device (**A**ssault happened when **He** hurt **Her** at **Home**) to complete the analysis.

Assault
- *When did it happen?*
- *Where did it happen?*
- *How long have you been in this abusive relationship?*
- *Has it ever happened before?*
- *Do you worry it may happen again?*
- *How did he hurt you?*

Physical abuse:
- *Did he hit you?*
- *Do you have any injuries?*

Sexual abuse:
- *Were there any sexual assaults?* **If yes:** *Did he use condoms?*
- *When was your LMP?*
- *Are you using any contraception?/Is there any chance you could be pregnant?*

He (assailant)
- *Do you know him?* **If yes:** *Are you financially dependent on him?*
- *Was he drinking?*
- *Does he use any street drugs?*
- *Did he have a gun?*

She (victim)
- *Did you inform anyone in your family? Any of your friends?*
- *Did you inform the police?*
- *Do you have a plan to leave your home?*
- *Do you feel sad? Do you feel depressed?*
- *Do you feel guilty?*
- *Have you ever thought about ending your life?*

Home
- *Do you have kids?* **If yes:** *Did he hurt your kids?*
- *Are they safe at home?*
- *Do you have a place to stay?*

Review of Systems

As routine.

Physical Exam

Exam bruises with a quick general exam.

Communication and Interpersonal Skills Component

Suggested Closure and Counseling

"Miss ..., I'm so sorry for what happened to you; it's really sad and very difficult for anyone. I want to emphasize two things. First of all, it was not your fault, and secondly, you should not feel guilty about what happened. You know that violence may vary over time, but it usually never ends on its own unless you get away from the abuser. So let me know how I can help you. I'm here to do everything possible to maintain your safety.

Have you thought of informing the police? The police have the authority to act appropriately.

How does that sound to you? Even if you don't want to talk to the police, would you mind if I call one of our social workers? They have more experience and more options to help you, for example, safety resources for women as well as places you can go.

Do you have any concerns? Do you have any questions?"

Patient Note

History

A 35-year-old-female patient who feels sad. she was beaten by her husband 2 weeks ago and left home with her kids to stay at a nearby hotel. She has multiple bruises on her body, no other injuries, or sexual abuse. Her husband is a heavy drinker and was fired from his job and left her without money. She hasn't informed family, friends, or the police of violence. She feels sad, depressed, and guilty, has tried suicide twice. **Review of systems (ROS):** insomnia, good appetite, feels like she has lost weight, no urinary or bowel problems. **PMH:** none. **Med:** OTC sleeping pills, NKDA. **FH:** mother with hypothyroidism and depression. **SH:** bus driver, nonsmoker, and drinks socially and monogamous with her husband.

Physical Exam

VS: WNL. The patient appeared sad, depressed, and spoke slowly, alert and oriented ×3.
Head and neck (H&N): PERRLA, normal thyroid.
Ext.: no tremors.
Lung: CTA/BL.
Heart: normal S1 and S2 with no murmurs.
Neuro: intact sensation, muscle 5/5. There are multiple bruises on the face, shoulder, left flank and thigh, greenish blue, and little tender.

Differential Diagnosis

History finding(s)	Physical exam finding(s)
1. Domestic violence	
Feels sad	Multiple bruises in the face, shoulder, left flank, and thigh
Admitted domestic violence by her husband	
2. Depression	
Feels sad and depressed	
Guilt and insomnia	
Attempted suicide twice	

Diagnostic Studies

CBC

Role-Play 42

Doorway Information

Miss Alana Murphy, a 60-year-old woman, does not feel well.

Vital signs:

- **PR:** 84/min, regular.
- **BP:** 120/80 mm Hg.
- **RR:** 16/min.
- **Temp:** 98.6°F (37°C).

Standardized Patient's Role

Throughout the conversation, express sadness, depression, and with decreased attention and concentration. Please speak slowly.

Since your husband's death 3 months ago, you have been very sad and depressed. You feel hopeless and like life no longer deserves to be lived because your late husband was so lovely to you.

Tell the doctor: *Doc, it's hard to live alone in my house. It's really hard.* Try to cry at that time. (**Comment 1**)

Your appetite has decreased, but you feel that you are gaining weight at the same time. You also feel tiredness with decreased concentration and memory.

Your husband was sick for the last year, and you feel guilty as you were very busy at work and couldn't help him as much as you wanted. You have a gun at home, and you tried to hurt yourself once a few weeks ago.

You feel cold intolerance and constipation. You are taking a medicine named L-thyroxine for your thyroid gland and insulin for your diabetes. You got more weight, about 8 lb in the last 3 months.

Your mother has Alzheimer's disease, and now you are living alone at the home you shared with your late husband.

Tell the doctor: *"I'm feeling guilty. I can't forgive myself as I didn't take care of my husband when he was sick. Is there anything I can do to make him forgive me?"* (**Comment 2**)

Role-Play 42: Answer Key

Depression is common on the CS exam; the complaints may be direct (depression) or indirect (feeling sad, depressed, not feeling well, after violence...). It's really a challenging case as the SP intends to put you under stress to test how you will react in such cases. The SP usually appears sad with blunt affect and speaks slowly. Don't worry, they have been informed to do that.

In such cases, take the history as routine; do a focused physical exam leaving more time for closure and counseling. You should address the SP's needs and be sure of his safety.

History

Analysis of Chief Complaint

Ask routine questions to analyze depression and then ask about symptoms of depression: SIG E CAPS (Sleep, Interest, Guilty, Energy, Concentration, Appetite, Psychomotor agitation and Suicidal thoughts). Ask for all and observe for psychomotor agitation.

- *How is your sleep?*
- *Could you tell me about your daily routine?*
- *Could you tell me about your hobbies and interests?*
- *Have you lost your interest in doing that?/Do you enjoy them?*
- *Do you feel guilty about anything?*
- *Do you feel tired?* Energy
- *Do you have trouble concentrating on what you are doing?*
- *How is your appetite?*
- *Have you ever felt life is not worth living?*
- *Have you ever thought about ending your life?* Suicide
- *Do you have guns or pills at home?*

Predisposing factors of depression (before depression):
- *Do you have any kind of stress at your job?*
- *Do you have any problems at home?*
- *Have you had recent financial troubles? Any psychiatric trauma? Any emotional stress?*

The impact of depression (after depression):
- *How is your performance on your job?/Does this problem affect your performance at work?*
- *Can you still perform your daily activities?*
- Ask questions for hypothyroidism.

Communication and Interpersonal Skills Component

"Miss.... you told me ...,..... You also told me .... Based on your history and my physical exam, it seems that you have depression after your husband's death. Also, you told me you attempted suicide. I'm worried that you may attempt it again. For that reason, I do recommend hospital admission for you. I need to be sure that you are safe; you may also need some psychotherapy that can be done while you are in the hospital. Is that OK with you? Do you have any questions for me?"

Suggested Answers to the Standardized Patient's Questions and Comments

Comment 1: Try to calm the SP and respond as you learned.

Comment 2: *"This must hard for you, and I'm going to do everything possible to make you feel better. We have a good support group; do you have interest to join it?"* or *"Feeling guilty is a part of the disease; all is going to be cured with medications. We are going to do everything possible to make you feel better."*

Patient Note

History

A 60-year-old-female patient who does not feel well since the death of her husband 3 months ago. She feels hopelessness and that life is not worth living. She has disturbed sleep and lost interest in daily activities, feels guilty as she couldn't help her husband, tired, and has trouble concentrating, decreased appetite, and attempted suicide once at home. She feels cold intolerance and has constipation. **ROS:** recent weight gain, 8 lb/3 mo. **PMH:** diabetes mellitus (DM) and hypothyroidism. **Med:** insulin and L-thyroxine. **FH:** mother with Alzheimer's disease. **SH:** lives alone after her husband's death.

Physical Exam

VS: WNL. The patient is alert and oriented ×3. The patient appears sad, depressed with slow speech, with blunt affect, and is inattentive to the interviewer. **H&N:** PERRLA, normal thyroid. **Ext.:** no tremors. **Lung:** CTA/BL. **Heart:** normal S1 and S2 with no murmurs. **Neuro:** intact sensation, muscle 5/5.

Differential Diagnosis

History finding(s)	Physical exam finding(s)
1. Major depressive disorder	
Depressed mood, sad	Blunt affect
↓ appetite, concentration	Inattentive to the interviewer
Guilty, suicide attempt	
2. Hypothyroidism	
Depressed mood, sad	
Constipation	
Weight gain	

Diagnostic Studies

CBC and TSH

Role-Play 43

Miss Pat Johnson, a 20-year-old woman, is feeling nervous and irritable.

Vital signs:
- **PR:** 84/min, regular.
- **BP:** 120/80 mm Hg.
- **RR:** 16/min.
- **Temp:** 98.6°F (37°C).

Standardized Patient's Role

Act like you are nervous and irritable.

For the last 2 weeks and since you moved to a new college and left your parents, you've felt nervous and irritable and have sleeping difficulties. You feel irregular beats in your heart and are sweating more than usual. Sleeping in the college dormitory is difficult, taking more than one and a half hours to fall asleep. However, you feel refreshed in the morning.

You attend your classes regularly, and your overall performance is good.

You have loose stool and go to the toilet often. You know that you have an overactive bladder.

You take OTC sleeping pills and oxybutynin. You had a tonsillectomy performed many years ago. You smoke two packs of cigarettes a day and drink socially. You used marijuana in high school and have had only one boyfriend.

Role-Play 43: Answer Key

Patient Note

History

Write your note following the instructions given in the previous cases.

Physical Exam

Write you note following the instructions given in the previous cases.

Differential Diagnosis

History finding(s)	Physical exam finding(s)
1. Adjustment disorder	
Nervous, mild depression	Free physical exam
Insomnia	
In response to recent stress	
2. Anxiety	
Nervous, palpitation, sweating	Free physical exam
Insomnia	
Overactive bladder	
Heavy smoker, used marijuana	

Diagnostic Studies

TSH

Toxicology screen

Role-Play 44

Doorway Information

Mr. David Mark, a 25-year-old man, was brought to the clinic by relatives because he was not acting normal and had disorganized speech.

Vital signs:
- **PR:** 84/min, regular.
- **BP:** 100/70 mm Hg.
- **RR:** 16/min.
- **Temp:** 98.6°F (37°C).

Standardized Patient's Role

In this case, act like a patient who has psychosis. That means you are out of touch with reality and behave in an odd manner. Don't put on any hospital drapes; instead stay in your street clothes.

As the doctor enters the room, look at the wall, and act as if you are listening to someone who is telling you that the Earth is in danger and giving you a plan to save it. Inform the doctor that this person comes to you two to three times a day to tell you that.

Then tell him or her that you are very worried because one of your friends follows you, and you think he wants to harm you.

You work at a grocery store, and you haven't gone to work for a couple of weeks. You have difficulty sleeping and are getting only a few hours a night.

You smoked one package of cigarettes a day for 10 years, drink three beers daily, and use cocaine (crack). You don't drink early in the morning, and you want to cut down your drinking. You are annoyed by people's comments about your drinking, but you don't feel guilty about it.

If the doctor asks you for blood tests say, *"I don't want any tests to be done. I don't want you to implant me with any monitoring devices."* (**Situation 1**)

Role-Play 44: Answer Key

This is not a common case on CS exams. You may have an SP who is wearing street clothes; in this case, don't do physical exam as he won't be wearing a gown.

Analysis of Chief Complaint

- *How long have you been feeling this way?*
- *Did it come on suddenly? Since it started, has it gotten worse or stayed the same? Is this constant or does it come and go?*
- *Do you remember anything in particular that happened before this started?*
- *Are you still going to your work?*
- *Have you been treated for this problem before? Where?*

Depression symptoms:
- *Do you feel sad? Do you feel depressed? If yes, ask SIG E CAPS.*

Hallucinations:
- *Do you hear things that other people don't? If yes, what do you hear?*
- *Do you see things that other people don't? If yes: What do you see?*
- *Do you smell anything unusual?*
- *Do you have any other experiences?*

Delusions:
- *Have you ever received any special message? If yes: What?*
- *Have you ever informed that you have been selected as a special person?*
- *Do you feel that you are being followed or controlled by the others?*
- *Have you ever felt threatened from anyone?*
- *Have you ever thought to harm yourself? Do you think about harming yourself?*

Analysis of Differential Diagnosis

- *Have you had any recent trauma to your head?*
- *Did you ever lose your consciousness?*
- *Have you had any abnormal jerky movements?*
- *Do you have headache? Any blurry vision?*
- *Do feel tingling or numbness anywhere in your body? Any muscle weakness?*
- *Have you had any recent exposure to irritating chemicals or toxins?*

Communication and Interpersonal Skills component

Situation 1: *"I understand your concern. I'm here to try and help you. I won't hurt you. Please give me a minute to call the counselor and he is going to speak to you. Does that sound good?"*

Patient Note

History

The patient is a 25-year-old man who is out of touch with reality. As I entered the room, he was speaking while staring at the wall. When asked who he was speaking to, he informed that somebody was telling him a plan to save the earth. These auditory hallucinations come to him two to three times a day. He also has delusional thoughts; he thinks that one of his friends follows him. He has not been at work for 2 weeks. He is not depressed or sad and sleeps a few hours a day. **ROS:** normal appetite, no urinary problems. **PMH:** none. **SH:** works at a grocery store, smokes 1 ppd/10 y, drinks 3 beers/d. CAGE 2/4, and uses crack. Not sexually active, denies suicide attempts.

Physical Exam

VS: WNL, patient appears dirty and staring at the wall. MMSE: alert, oriented to time, place, and persons, spells backward, intact memory. Elated mood, agitated affect, and delusional thoughts; the physical exam could not be done as the patient was not draped.

Differential Diagnoses

History finding(s)	Physical exam finding(s)
1. Brief psychotic disorder	
Auditory hallucination	Agitated affect
Delusion	Disorganized speech
	Out of touch with reality
2. Substance-induced psychosis	
Using crack	
Auditory hallucination	

Diagnostic Studies

Physical exam

Urine toxicology screen

CBC with differential

Appendix: Your assessment for psychiatric cases and plan should contain five components:
- *Bio:* medications to prescribe (SSRI [selective serotonin reuptake inhibitor], antipsychotic, etc.).
- *Psycho:* psychotherapy, CBT (cognitive behavioral therapy), behavioral therapy, etc.
- *Social:* changes in the home or community that should be made (e.g., moving from a house to a group home).
- *Admission or not?* Admit all patients expressing suicidal/homicidal intention or are dangers to themselves.
- *Additional workup:* thyroid function, ammonia, brain MRI, etc.

10 Neurology

Keywords: neurology for USMLE CS, headache, syncope, dizziness, insomnia, hemiplegia

10.1 Introduction

Neurology cases on the Clinical Skills (CS) exam may include headache, dizziness, passing out/fainting/syncope, difficulty in falling asleep/insomnia, memory loss, stroke, causing weakness in the limbs, and tremors.

10.2 Medical History (►Audio. 10.1)

When getting the neurologic history, remember this mnemonic that will help in accomplishing this task quickly on the CS exam:

Neurological patients with **M**ini-**C**ranium may **S**ense, **M**ove, and **W**alk with **S**pecial senses.

10.2.1 Memory

Do you have any problems with your memory?
Have you been forgetting things more than usual lately?
Do you have any problems in managing your business or household affairs?

10.2.2 Concentration/Consciousness

Do you have trouble concentrating on what you are doing?
Does your mind wander, and you forget what you're doing?
Have you ever passed out?/Have you fainted recently?

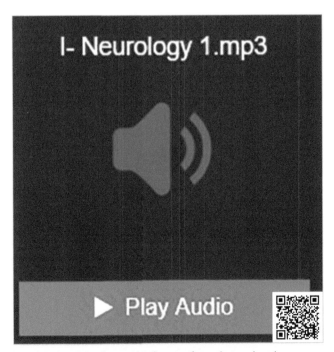

Audio 10.1 The audio contains the core of neurology and can be used as a quick review before the exam. https://www.thieme.de/de/q. htm?p=opn/cs/20/3/11453118-5ca80234&t=audio

10.2.3 Sensory

Have you noticed any tingling in your ...?
Have you noticed any numbness in your ...? (left arm, right leg)
Have you noticed any changes in your ability to sense touch?

10.2.4 Motor

Motor: General
- *Have you noticed any weakness in your arms or legs? Any stiffness?*
- *Have you been unable to grasp things firmly?*

Motor: Larynx and Pharynx
- *Do you have any difficulty speaking?*
- *Do you have any difficulty swallowing?*

Motor: Sphincters (Bladder and Bowel)
- *Do you have to rush to the bathroom when you urinate?/Do you have any urinary incontinence?*
- *Have you ever had any bowel movement unintentionally?*

10.2.5 Walking: Coordination/Gait

Do you have a tendency to fall while walking?

10.2.6 Special Senses

Hearing: *Have you had any hearing difficulties?*

Vision: *Do you have any blurry vision?/Any problems in your vision?*

In addition, ask about symptoms suggestive of increased intracranial pressure (ICP) such as headache and/or vomiting.

10.3 Neurological Examination

Remember the same mnemonic with adding maneuvers for exam: Neurological patients with **M**ini **C**ranium may **S**ense, **M**ove, and **W**alk with **S**pecial maneuvers:
- Mini-mental status exam.
- Cranial Nerves.
- Sensory System.
- Motor Control System.
- Cerebellar Functioning and Gait and Balance.
  - Special maneuvers.

10.3.1 Mini-Mental State Examination (MMSE)

This exam assesses the patient's awareness to time, place, and persons. Memory is also tested. Do the Mini-Mental State Examination (MMSE) only for those neurological cases in which the memory has been affected (e.g., forgetfulness, stroke, severe depression, etc.; see Role-Play 51).

10.3.2 Cranial Nerves

I—Olfactory: Not done on CS exam.

II—Optic: The visual acuity can be examined simply by having the Standardized Patient (SP) count your fingers (▶ Fig. 10.1). There is no time for a Snellen chart.

III, IV, and VI: The extraocular muscles can be examined together simply by asking the SP to trace your finger (follow the shape of the letter H; ▶ Fig. 10.2). Pupillary light reflex assumed to be done as a part of the general exam.

V—Trigeminal:
Sensory part: You can do this quickly just by using your hands. Put your hands on both sides of the SP's face, starting at the temples. Ask the SP if they feel equal sensation on both sides. Examine in the three areas of the trigeminal nerve (ophthalmic, maxillary, and mandibular).

Motor Part (▶ Fig. 10.3): Test the strength of the temporalis and masseter muscles with gentle palpation after asking the SP to clench their teeth.

VII—Facial (motor part): To test the orbicularis oculi (▶ Fig. 10.4), ask the SP to close their eyes firmly, and try to open their eyes. For the orbicularis oris, simply ask the SP to show their teeth, or ask them to smile.

VIII—Vestibulocochlear:
Cochlear part: Ask the patient to close their eyes. Then, close to their ear, snap your fingers, and ask the SP on which side they hear the sound (▶ Fig. 10.5).

You can repeat this on the other side.

Special tests (such as Rinne's and/or Weber's test) should only be done in the cases that involve hearing loss or dizziness (see the corresponding cases).

IX—Glossopharyngeal nerve: Gag and palate reflex tests are not allowed on the CS exam.

X—Vagus: Test this by asking the SP to open their mouth and to say "Ahh."

XI—Accessory:
Sternomastoid muscle: Put your hand on the right side of the SP's jaw, and then ask them to turn their head to the same side. Repeat the test on the other side (▶ Fig. 10.6).

Trapezius muscle: Ask the SP to **shrug one shoulder**. Repeat on the other side (▶ Fig. 10.7).

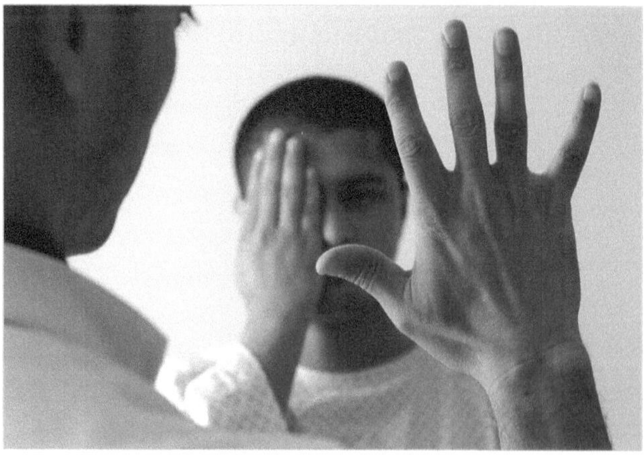

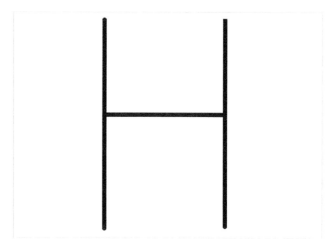

Fig. 10.1 Simple examination of the visual acuity by counting fingers.

Fig. 10.2 Letter H: extraocular muscles exam.

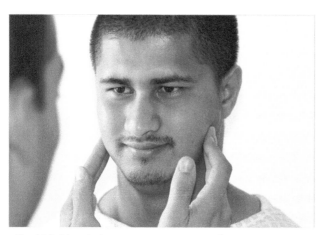

Fig. 10.3 Trigeminal nerve exam: masseter muscle.

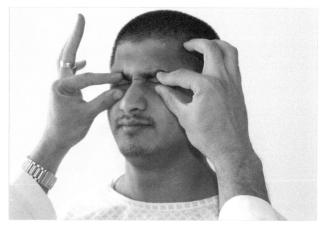

Fig. 10.4 Fascial nerve exam: orbicularis oculi muscle.

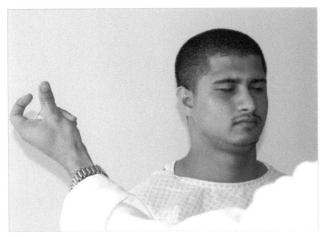

Fig. 10.5 Examining the cochlear part of vestibulocochlear nerve.

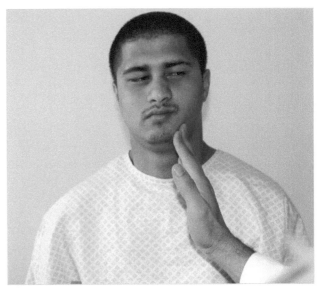

Fig. 10.6 Examining the sternomastoid muscle.

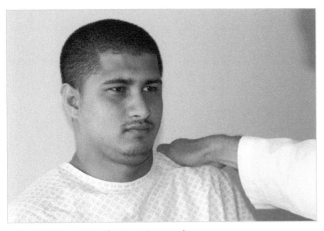

Fig. 10.7 Examining the trapezius muscle

XII—Hypoglossal nerve: By testing the shape and the movement of the tongue, ask the SP to **stick the tongue out** and to move it from side to side.

If you have time, test for ability to feel dull and sharp sensations on the face. Use a Q-tip with a sharp and a blunt end (will be provided for you in the examination room). Inform the SP which one is the sharp end and which one is the dull end. Then ask them to close their eyes and ask again.

Remember this scenario while practicing for cranial nerves:

"I'm going to examine your nerves; I'll start with your eyes. Please cover your right eye. Now, count the fingers that I am holding up. Could you count them again? Cover your left eye. How many fingers am I holding up?

Without moving your head, follow my finger with your eyes.

Does it feel the same on both sides?

I'm going to examine the muscles of your face. Could you clench your teeth firmly?

Could you show me your teeth?

Please close your eyes firmly, and then I'll try to open them. Resist. Try to keep them closed while I try to move your eyelids.

Please keep your eyes closed; from which side do you hear the sound?

Could you open your mouth? Can you say 'Ahhh'? Could you stick your tongue out? Please move it from side to side.

Could you turn your head to the right, against my hand? Please move it in the opposite side.

Please shrug your right shoulder. Shrug your left shoulder. Thank you."

10.3.3 Sensory System

You can test for sensitivity to touch simply by gently and loosely pinching the SP's leg or arm with your fingers and letting the skin slip through your grasp (▶ Fig. 10.8).

Ask the SP: *"Does it feel the same on both sides?"*

Inform the SP first, while their eyes are open: *"This is sharp and this is the dull."*

Note: Sensory deficits are expected in the following cases (cerebral stroke, diabetic patients, carpal tunnel, or shoulder dislocation on the lateral aspect of the deltoid muscle). It is recommended to use Q-tip in such cases.

Ask them to close their eyes and then press the ends of the piece of wood several times at different points on each limb.

Ask the SP: *"Is it sharp or dull? Sharp or dull? What about this one?"*

10.3.4 Motor System

Muscle tone: Gently flex and extend the SP's joints, starting with the elbow, and then the wrist, the knee, and finally the ankle.

If your time is limited, skip the tone test, and instead examine only the muscle power and reflexes.

Note: In describing the muscle tone in the patient notes (PNs), use one of these three descriptions: normal, spastic or flaccid.

Muscle Power

Upper Limb: Ask the SP to hold your fingers, and ask them to squeeze firmly (▶Fig. 10.9).

Press your hand against the outside of their forearm, and tell the SP to push out. Then put your hand on the inner side of the forearm, and tell the SP to pull their forearm inward (▶Fig. 10.10).

Shoulder: Ask the SP to put their arms up like a boxer. Then put your hand on the inside of their arm; say: *"Please pull me in, against my hand."*

Then, put your hand on the outside of their arm; say: *"Please push outward, against the pushing of my hand."*

Lower Limb: Put your hand on the shin, and ask the SP to gently push outward while you are pushing inward (▶Fig. 10.11). Then, put your hand on the calf. Ask the SP to pull their leg in,

against the pressure of your hand. Test the muscles at the hip joint. If you have time, examine the muscle power at the ankle joint by asking the SP for dorsal and plantar flexion.

Put your hand on the top of the thigh, and ask the SP to push their thigh up, against your hand. Then, put your hand on the bottom of their thigh (hamstring) and have them push against your hand.

Deep Tendon Reflexes (DTRs)

Tell the SP that you will check their reflexes.

In most cases, checking only the reflexes of the biceps (▶Fig. 10.12) and triceps (▶Fig. 10.13; for the upper limb) and the knee (for the lower limb) is enough. If you have time, add the ankle jerk test.

10.3.5 Cerebellar Functioning and Balance

Do the finger-to-nose (▶Fig. 10.14) and finger-to-finger (▶Fig. 10.15) tests.

Ask the SP to extend their arm, and then to touch their nose with their index finger. Then they have to touch your index

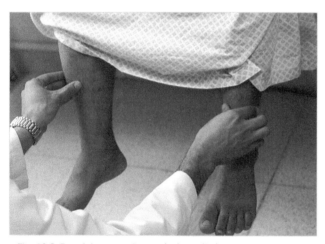

Fig. 10.8 Examining sensation on the lower limbs.

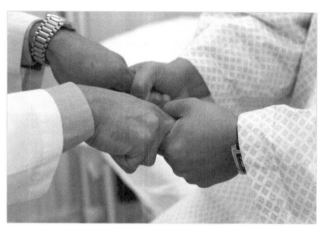

Fig. 10.9 Examining muscle strength at fingers.

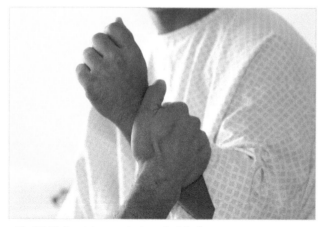

Fig. 10.10 Examining muscle strength at the forearm.

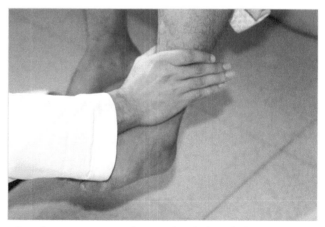

Fig. 10.11 Examining muscle strength at the lower limb.

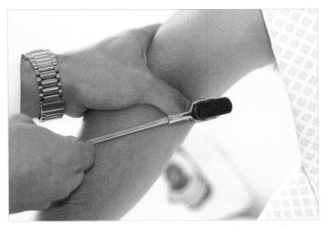

Fig. 10.12 Checking the deep tendon reflex of the biceps muscle.

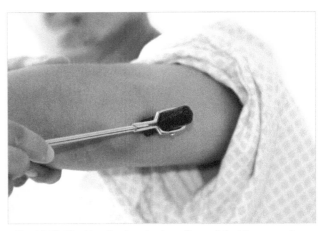

Fig. 10.13 Checking the deep tendon reflexes of the triceps muscle.

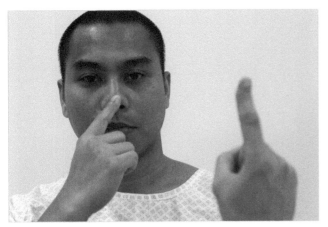

Fig. 10.14 Finger-to-nose test.

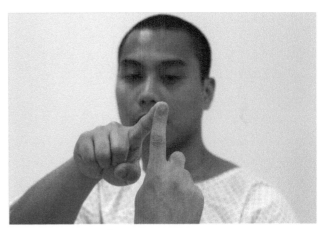

Fig. 10.15 Finger-to-finger test.

finger. Move your index finger to different places, and have them continue to touch it with their index finger.

Balance and gait: Ask the SP to stand up and walk in a straight line.

10.3.6 Special Tests

Romberg's test, neck stiffness, Brudzinski's sign, and Babinski's sign (see the individual cases in this chapter).

Please review the Muscle Power Scale and the Reflex Scale and important sensory levels in the body. They are provided in the Appendix in the end of the book.

Remember this scenario for neurological exam while practicing:

"I'm going to examine the nerves of your arms and legs.

Does the sensation feel the same on both sides? Is it sharp or dull? Sharp or dull? What about this one?

I'm going to examine your muscle tone. Please relax.

Now let's see if the muscular power of your arms and legs is normal. Hold my fingers and try to gently squeeze them.

Move your limb against my hand. Resist just a little.

Please pull inward, against the pulling of my hand. Please push outward, against the pushing of my hand.

Could you push your thigh up? Please push it down?

Could you please kick out? Please pull in?

Could you push your foot up against my finger?

Could you push your foot down against my finger?

I would like to check your jerks. I'll start with your arms. Please relax for me.

Let me check the jerks in your legs. Please relax your muscles.

Using your index finger, please touch my finger and then touch your nose.

I'm going to examine your balance and then we'll be almost done.

Please stand up. Just step down carefully. I'd like for you to walk over here a few steps in a straight line to the wall. Please turn around.

Hold your arms out in front of you. Close your eyes. Don't worry, I will catch you if you lose your balance. Okay, that's all; you can put your arms down now. Thank you."

10.4 Patient Note

Here is a sample draft of a normal neurological exam:
The patient is alert and oriented ×3. Cranial nerves II–XII are apparently intact. Sensations to pinprick and soft touches are intact. Muscle power is 5/5 throughout. DTR is +2 and symmetric. Gait and finger-to-nose test are both normal.

End your report with the results of any special tests, such as Romberg's, Babinski's, Brudzinki's, or Kerning's.

Note: To avoid missing data while typing the PN, write in the same sequence as you did the exam using the same mnemonic.

The Glasgow Coma Scale is an integral part of the neurological exam, but it is not on the syllabus of the CS exam.

Role-Play 45

Mr. Charles Roberts, a 35-year-old man, came to the ER complaining of severe **headache**.

Vital signs:
- **Pulse rate (PR):** 98/min, regular.
- **Blood pressure (BP):** 140/100 mm Hg.
- **Respiratory rate (RR):** 20/min.
- **Temperature (Temp):** 98.6°F (37°C).

Examinee tasks:
- Obtain a focused history.
- Perform a relevant physical examination. Do not perform rectal, pelvic, genitourinary, inguinal hernia, female breast, or corneal reflex examinations.
- Discuss your initial diagnostic impression and your workup plan with the patient.
- After leaving the room, complete your PN on the given form.

Standardized Patient's Role

Before the doctor enters the room, lie back in the bed and cover your eyes with your hands as if the light annoys you. Wait for the doctor to speak first. (**Comment 1**)

You came to the ER with a severe headache that started last night while you were visiting your girlfriend. The pain is getting worse with time. The pain is located in the back of the head and is sharp 9/10, and nothing alleviated the pain.

Tell the doctor: *"My head feels like it's going to burst. Am I going to die?"* (**Comment 2**)

The pain is nonradiating, and you feel that your head is going to burst, and that it is the worst headache you have ever had in your life. Light makes the pain worse and nothing makes it better.

You work at the train station, smoke 1 pack per day (ppd), drink 2 beers or more a day, sometimes first thing in the morning. The doctor may ask you a few questions about alcohol drinking; inform that you get annoyed by people's criticism about your drinking. Otherwise, answer the other questions by no.

You use cocaine and the last time was yesterday while you were with your girlfriend. Your mother is healthy, but your father died from kidney failure. The doctor said he had cysts in his kidneys.

You are sexually active with multiple female partners. You use condoms most of the time, but have never been tested for HIV or for STDs.

When the doctor examines you, express neck stiffness and if he or she bends the neck, bend your legs at the hip. If he or she raises one of your legs and bend it at the knee, express severe pain.

Please refer to Chapter 13 (Appendix), to review the general instructions for the SP as well as the Doctor roles.

Role-Play 45: Answer Key

Headache

Headache is a common case on CS exams. Although the differential diagnosis is broad, migraines and subarachnoid hemorrhages (SAHs) are common cases on CS exam. Even knowing this, while taking the SP's history, do not neglect to ask questions about the other possible causes of the SP's headache (▶ Table 10.1).

Table 10.1 Differential diagnosis of headache and questions provided for medical history

Differential diagnosis (DD)

Cranial	Extracranial
• 3 recurrent headaches: migraine, tension, and cluster	Sinusitis, tooth, or eye problems
• Positive symptoms of ↑ICP: brain tumor, pseudotumor cerebri (idiopathic intracranial HTN)	Rare in CS:
	Temporal arteritis: temporal headache, fever, pain in jaw when chewing, tenderness and sensitivity on the scalp
• Positive signs of meningeal irritation: with fever (meningitis and encephalitis); without fever (SAH)	*Trigeminal neuralgia*: episodes of intense facial pain

Analysis of DD

Migraines	
• Unilateral, recurrent	*Before the migraine comes on, are there any warning signs? Do you see a flashing light?*
• Preceded by aura	*Have you had migraines before?*
• Family history of migraines	*Does anyone of your family suffer from migraines?*
• ↑ with light and ↓ with dark and NSAIDs	

Tension	
• Bandlike or viselike	*Does it feel like a band around your head?*
• No aura	*Does the headache get worse when you feel stressed? After heavy drinking? With smoking?*
• ↑ by stress, alcohol, smoking	*Do your muscles spasm?*
• Associated with muscle spasm and neck stiffness	*Does your neck feel stiff when you have a headache?*

Cluster headache	
• Unilateral	*Are your eyes watery?*
• Headache free interval (occur in clusters)	*Do you have a runny nose?*
• Eye tears and rhinorrhea	*How frequent do you have this headache?*

Symptoms indicating an increased ICP	*Have you been vomiting?*
	Do you have blurry vision?
	Have you noticed any numbness in your limbs? Any changes in sensation? Any muscle weakness?

Symptoms indicating meningeal irritation	*Is your neck stiff?*
	Did you use any street drugs?
	Does anyone in your family have kidney disease, like cysts?
	Do you have a fever?
	If there is fever, then ask:
	Have you been around any sick person?
	Have you traveled outside the United States recently?
	Are your immunizations up-to-date?

Extracranial causes	*Do your sinuses feel tender?*
	Do you have any toothache?
	Do you have any problems in your vision?

Abbreviations: CS, Clinical Skills; HTN, hypertension; ICP, intracranial pressure; NSAIDs, nonsteroidal anti-inflammatory diseases; SAH, subarachnoid hemorrhage.

Note: If the headache was preceded by trauma—although not common on CS exam—always ask for any loss of consciousness (passing out). In this scenario, causes of the headache other than the ones listed above should be taken into consideration in the differential diagnosis. Examples to consider include intracranial bleeding (subdural, epidural, SAH, or intraparenchymal hemorrhage).

The flowchart illustrates how you can approach the differential diagnosis of headache on the CS exam (▶ Fig. 10.16).

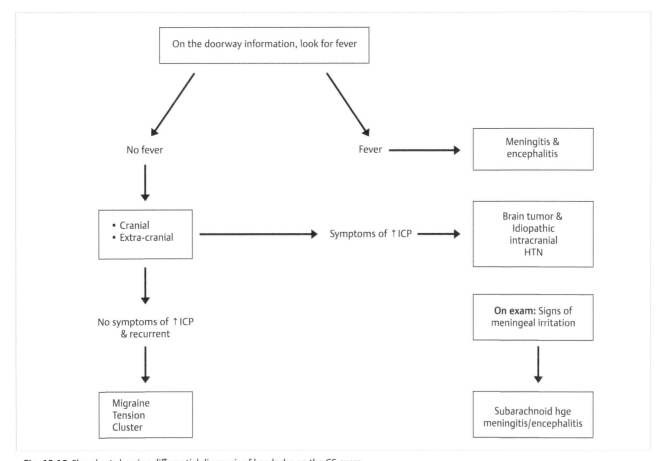

Fig. 10.16 Flowchart showing differential diagnosis of headache on the CS exam.

Answer Key

History

Ask standard questions as explained in the introduction.

Past History and Others

Past medical history (PMH): D, S, P: previous episodes; **D:** NSAID as OTC; **A, F:** migraine, brain tumor, renal cystic disease (berry cerebral aneurysm); **S:** stress, smoking, alcohol, and cocaine use in SAH.

Physical Exam

Vital sign (VS): fever (meningitis), high blood pressure (BP) (cocaine-induced SAH); **A:** pain and photophobia; **D:** lying back on bed; **H:** do full HEENT (Head, eyes, ears, nose, and throat) exam. **N:** look for neck stiffness; E, lung and heart (LH): quick auscultation. **Local exam:** focal neurological exam. **Special signs:** neck stiffness, Brudzinski's sign, and Kerning's test (Knee).

Neck stiffness: While the SP is lying on his back, flex the neck gently. As a sign of meningeal irritation, you will notice resistance and neck stiffness.

Brudzinski's sign: Upon flexion of the neck, there may be flexion of patient's hips and knees (▶ Fig. 10.17).

Kerning's test (Knee): While the SP is lying on his back and with flexed hip and knee, try to extend the knee only. Discomfort or pain indicates a positive test (▶ Fig. 10.18).

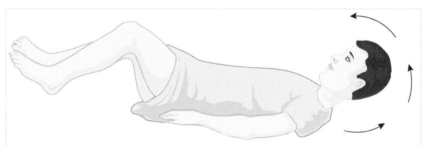

Fig. 10.17 Brudzinski's sign.

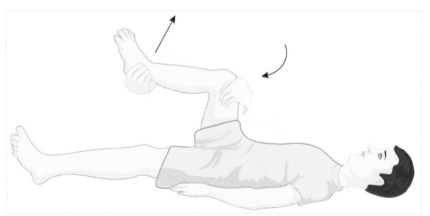

Fig. 10.18 Kerning's test.

Communication and Interpersonal Skills Component

Suggested Closure

Done as emergency cases.

Counseling

Advice on quitting cocaine.

Suggested Answers to the SP's Questions and Comments

Comment 1: Given that the SP has photophobia, you should dim the light after you enter the room. Start your encounter with the light dimmed, after a few minutes, you can ask him if you can switch on the light.

Comment 2: *"Sounds hard for you. I'm so sorry to see you in pain. We are going to do everything possible to make you feel better."*

History

A 35-year-old male patient complains of occipital headache, started last night and getting worse, sharp, 9/10, and constant. It is aggravated by light, alleviated by ibuprofen, accompanied by photophobia and neck stiffness. No previous episodes, denies fever, no symptoms suggestive of increased ICP (no projectile vomiting or blurry vision), no numbness, tingling sensation, or muscle weakness elsewhere. **Review of system (ROS):** normal urinary as well as bowel habits. **PMH and Meds:** N/D. NKDA (no known drug allergy). **Family history (FH):** father died from PCKD and mother healthy. **Social history (SH):** smoker 1 ppd/10 y, 2 beers/d, CAGE: 2/4. Uses cocaine; the last time was last night. Sexually active with multiple female partners with occasional condom use.

Physical exam

VS:BP: 140/100 mm Hg, PR: 98/min, RR: 20/min, Temp: 98.6°F, alert ×3, lying supine in pain. **Head and neck (H&N):** atraumatic (AT), normocephalic (NC), PERRLA (pupils equal, round, reactive to light and accommodation), EOMI (external ocular muscle intact), no papilledema, nose without rhinorrhea, throat without erythema, but with neck stiff. **Extremities (Ext):** palpable peripheral pulse bilaterally. **Neuro:** cranial nerves II–XII apparently intact, intact sensation to pinprick and soft touch, motor 5/5 throughout, DTR +2 on both sides, and positive Brudzinski's and Kerning's tests.

Differential Diagnosis

History finding(s)	Physical exam finding(s)
1. Subarachnoid hemorrhage (cocaine induced)	
Occipital headache	Photophobia
Intense headache	Neck stiffness
Recent cocaine use	Positive Brudzinski's and Kerning's tests
	High ABP=140/100 mm Hg
2. Subarachnoid hemorrhage (ruptured berry aneurysm)	
Occipital headache	Photophobia
Father with autosomal dominant polycystic kidney disease	Neck stiffness
Possible ruptured berry aneurysm	Positive Brudzinski's and Kerning's tests

Diagnostic Studies

Complete blood count (CBC), with diff
CT head

Role-Play 46

Miss Jasmine Lee, a 30-year-old woman, came to the ER complaining of headache.

Vital signs:
- **PR:** 86/min, regular.
- **BP:** 120/80 mm Hg.
- **RR:** 16/min.
- **Temp:** 98.6°F (37°C).

Standardized Patient's Role

You came to the ER with a severe headache that started 1 hour ago on the right side of your head. It's nonradiating; before it started, you saw flashing lights. The pain is sharp, 7/10, and is constant. It is aggravated by light, and is alleviated by sitting in a dark room and taking a couple of ibuprofen tablets.

You have had this kind of headache for many years, just like your mother had.

The last time you got a headache was 2 months ago. Sometimes it gets worse during menstruation and when you are under emotional stress.

You have allergic rhinitis, take Claritin, and last week you had a common cold, which was complicated by acute sinusitis. Your sinuses still feel tender, and there is the sensation of pressure in them.

Your father died of a brain tumor, and your mother suffers from migraine headaches.

Ask the doctor:
Q1: *Is it possible that I have migraines because my mom does?*
Q2: *Do migraines run in families?*

Role-Play 46: Answer Key

History, Physical Exam, and Communication and Interpersonal Skills Component

Follow the standards as previously answered.

Patient Note

History

Write your note following the instructions given in the previous cases.

Examination

Write your note following the instructions given in the previous cases.

Differential Diagnosis

History finding(s)	Physical exam finding(s)
1. Migraine headache	
Unilateral headache	No fever
↑ by light, noise	Supple neck
↓ by dark and rest	Free neurological exam
Family history and previous episodes	
2. Sinusitis	
Headache	Tenderness over the sinuses
Common cold and sinusitis	

Diagnostic Studies

CBC, with differential

Role-Play 47

Doorway Information

Mr. Randal Ross, a 24-year-old man, passed out yesterday.

Vital signs:

- **PR:** 98/min, regular.
- **BP:** 140/100 mm Hg.
- **RR:** 20/min.
- **Temp.:** 98.6°F (37°C).

Standardized Patient's Role

You are a 24-year-old man in excellent health. You passed out yesterday while playing basketball. Your friends told you that you fell on the ground suddenly and were out for less than a minute. You didn't suffer any head injury from the fall. You recall that your heart was beating like a racehorse's, and there was mild chest pain.

Nobody told you that you had any shaking movements, you didn't bite your tongue, and you regained your conscious quickly. You didn't notice any urine in your clothes.

You are pretty healthy, apart from allergic rhinitis, and you take Claritin. Nobody in your family has had any major health problems, except your older brother. He died suddenly when he was 28 years old. Only after the autopsy did you learn that he had heart problems and had died of a heart attack.

You are a professional basketball player. Your sex life is active, and you are monogamous with your wife.

At the end of the encounter, ask:

Q1: *Doc, could there be something wrong with my heart like there was with my brother?*

Q2: *We have a big game tomorrow. My team really needs me. Can I play?*

Role-Play 47: Answer Key

Syncope is the clinical term for passing out or fainting; they are often used interchangeably.

History

Analysis of Chief Complaint

When did it happen?/How long ago did it happen?
How long were you out?
What were you doing when you passed out?
Has it ever happened before? **If yes, then ask:** *How often do you pass out? How long does it usually last?*

Analysis of Differential Diagnosis

For the CS exam, focus on the following differential diagnoses:
- Vasovagal attack.
- Medication side effects.
- *Cardiovascular system (CVS):* arrhythmia, valvular heart disease, hypertrophic cardiomyopathy (HCM).
- *Neuro:* transient ischemic attack (TIA), stroke, seizure (tonic-clonic seizure).

Organize your questions into three time periods: **before the syncope, at the time of syncope, and after syncope.**

Before the syncope:

I'm going ask you few questions to understand more what happened before you passed out. Try to remember what you were doing and how you felt beforehand.

Vasovagal attack:
- *Did you feel light headed or blackout?*
- *Were you sweating?*

Medication side effects:
- *Have you started a new prescription recently?*

Cardiac:
- *Was your heart beating fast?*
- *Did you have any chest pain?*

Neurological:
- *Had you hit your head?*
- *Had you been in an accident?*
- *Did you have a headache?*
- *Did you feel any numbness in your arms or legs?*
- *Did you feel any weakness in your arms or leg?*
- *Do you have tendency to fall while walking?*

At the time of syncope:

- *Was there anyone around you at that time?*
- *Did they tell you that you were shaking, as if you were having a seizure?.(pause) Did you bite your tongue?*
- *How long did it last?*

After syncope:

- *After you came to, did you notice that you had wet your pants?*
- *Did you feel tired?*

Review of the Local System

If the SP's answers warrant further investigation, ask more questions relating to the CVS or neurology.

Review of Systems

As the routine.

Past History and Others

As the routine.

Physical Exam

General exam + local (cardiac or neurology), according to the analysis of the possible causes and special maneuver such as Romberg's test.

Communication and Interpersonal Skills Component

Suggested Closure

Just use thestandard closure (see Introduction for a sample Standard Closure).

Suggested Answers to the Standardized Patient's Questions

Q1: *"I understand your concern; it's hard to tell you what might have caused you to faint for certain. We should…."*

Alternative answer: *"I understand your concern. Although you seem to be in good health and don't smoke, or drink, I am worried about what you told me about your brother. Since he died suddenly from a heart attack, we should take genetics into consideration. At this point, I strongly recommend taking some pictures of your heart and doing some blood test."*

Q2: *"Mr. …, your health is our main concern right now, but I'm little bit worried that you may have this problem again. I strongly recommend that you skip the game tomorrow till we know for sure what's going on."*

Patient Note

History

A 24-year-old man came to the clinic because he had passed out yesterday while playing basketball. His friends told him he suddenly collapsed. The incident was not preceded by trauma. They did not notice any seizures or any shaking movement. He did not bite his tongue and had no headache, numbness, tingling, or muscle weakness at that time. He recalled nonradiating chest pain on the left side of the chest with palpitation. He recovered after 30 to 60 seconds; no urinary incontinence. **ROS:** no fever, good appetite, pretty healthy, no urinary or bowel movement problems, nor recent loss of weight. **PMH:** allergic rhinitis. **Med:** loratadine tablets, NKDA. **FH:** brother died of heart disease. **SH:** basketball player, denies smoking, alcohol or illicit drug use, sexually active, monogamous with his wife.

Examination

VS: within normal limit (WNL) and alert, oriented ×3. **Head:** NC, AT, PERRLA, EOMI. **Neck:** supple, +2 carotid pulses. **Ext:** +2 symmetric brachial, radial and post tibial on both sides. **Lung:** CTA/BL (clear to auscultation bilaterally). **Heart:** normal S1 and S2 with no murmurs. **Neuro:** cranial nerves II–XII intact, intact sensation, muscle power is 5/5, DTRs is +2, normal gait, negative Romberg's test.

Differential Diagnosis

History finding(s)	Physical exam finding(s)
1. Hypertrophic cardiomyopathy	
Passed out, came without warning	Free neurological exam
Young and athletic	
Positive family history	
2. Cardiac arrhythmia/valvular heart disease	
Passed out	Free neurological exam
Chest pain with palpitation	

Diagnostic Studies

CBC and electrolytes

Echocardiography

Electrocardiogram (ECG), 24-h Holter monitoring

Note: For neurologic causes, the following are to be documented: CT, MRI, electroencephalogram (EEG), and carotid Doppler.

Role-Play 48

Mr. Mark Thompson, a 65-year-old male patient, is complaining of syncope.

Vital signs:
- **PR:** 98/min, regular.
- **BP:** 140/100 mm Hg.
- **RR:** 20/min.
- **Temp.:** 98.6°F (37°C).

Standardized Patient's Role

You are a 65-year-old man. Yesterday, after you finished shopping with your wife, you passed out on the ground. Your wife told you that it was for about 30 seconds. You remember and just before the event, you felt a racing heart, mild chest pain in your left side, and lightheadedness. You and your wife didn't notice any injuries after you recovered.

You have heart problems, have to stop after four to five blocks to catch your breath and rest because of difficulty breathing. A cardiac angiography was done a couple of years ago and you were told that there was a narrowing in the coronaries. You had a cerebral stroke 3 years ago and after treatment and physiotherapy, you still have some weakness in your right arm and leg.

You take lisinopril and hydrochlorothiazide (HCTZ) for high BP that you have had for 20 years.

Your father died from a heart attack, and your mother has depression. You are retired and stopped smoking 10 years ago.

When the doctor performs a physical exam on you, act as if the previous stroke has affected your right side. In comparison to the left side, make the right side weaker in its muscle strength and power, and in response to the tendon reflexes or jerks.

Also, if the doctors tests for sensation, act like your right side feels sensation less than the left.

Role-Play 48: Answer Key

History

This case is quite similar to the previous case; remember to take note of the following while taking the SP's history.
- Analysis of the complaint:
  - Before syncope.
  - At the time of syncope.
  - After syncope.
  - Quick review of systems.

Physical Exam

Perform a quick general exam, followed by a local exam. Focus on the cardiovascular and neurological systems (include gait).

Communication and Interpersonal Skills Component

Follow the standard.

Patient Note

History

Write your note following the instructions given in the previous cases.

Physical Exam

Write your note following the instructions given in the previous cases.

Differential Diagnosis

History finding(s)	Physical exam finding(s)
1. Transient ischemic attack (TIA)	
Passed out	Right side: muscle power is 3/5, DTR is +1
History of stroke 3 y ago	
Cardiac arrhythmia	Impaired sensation
Passed out	
Palpitations and chest pain	
Cardiac angiography revealed coronary artery stenosis	

Diagnostic Studies

CBC and electrolytes

CT head and echocardiography

ECG and Holter monitoring

EEG

Role-Play 49 (▶Video. 10.1)

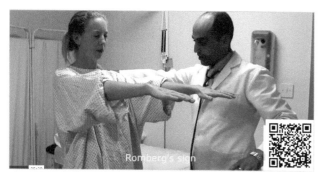

Video 10.1 Dizziness is a common case on the CS exam. At the end of the video, a live demo is introduced to teach you how to type the PN within the CS time frame. https://www.thieme.de/de/q.htm?p=opn/cs/20/3/11450550-dba01e13

Doorway Information

Mrs. Kim Miller, a 55-year-old female patient, came to the clinic complaining of dizziness.

Vital signs:

- **PR:** 98/min, regular.
- **BP:** 140/100 mm Hg.
- **RR:** 20/min.
- **Temp.:** 98.6°F (37°C).

Standardized Patient's Role

You have had dizzy spells for a month now, but you haven't really cared because they were not frequent. Recently, however, the episodes have increased, occurring two to three times a day, and this bothers you, and the last one was this morning. The dizziness lasts for 20 to 30 seconds and increases when you stand up suddenly. When the dizziness comes on, sometimes you feel that the room is spinning around you. You remember that it started when you began taking a new prescription, HCTZ, that your family doctor had added to your medications.

Q1: *Doc, What about stopping these new pills?*

You had a chest infection a few weeks ago. You have high BP and take HCTZ and lisinopril. You had an appendectomy 30 years ago. You don't smoke, and you drink only two to three beers a week.

While the doctor examines you, obey the doctor's orders; don't express any abnormal signs.

Role-Play 49: Answer Key

History

Analysis of Chief Complaint

Dizziness:
- *How long have you had this problem?*
- *How often do you get dizzy?*
- *How long did/does it last?*
- *What makes it worse?*
- *What makes it better?*
- *Do you have warning signs beforehand?*
- *Have you passed out?*

Analysis of Differential Diagnosis

Vasovagal and medication induced:
See the syncope case.

Paroxysmal positional vertigo:
- *When you change position, do you get dizzy?*
- *Do you feel the room spinning around you?*

Ear causes:
- *Do you hear any noise or buzzing sound in your ear? (tinnitus)*
- *Have you noticed any hearing loss?*

More questions:
- *Have you had an ear infection? Do you have any discharge or fluid leaking from your ear?*

Vestibular neuritis:
- *Have you had a recent upper respiratory tract (URT) infection?*

Cardiac:
- *Did you have chest pain?*
- *Does your heart race sometimes, for no apparent reason?*

Vertigo (others):
- *Do you have a tendency to fall while walking?*

Review of the Local System

As routine.

Review of Systems

As routine.

Past History and Others

As routine.

Physical Exam

General exam includes focused ENT (ear, nose, and throat) exam. **LH:** auscultate the lung only, do a local heart exam, focal neurological exam and **Special signs as** Romberg's sign, finger-to-nose test. Ask the patient to walk and examine the gait. If the SP has hearing problems and if you have time, do Rinne's and Weber's tests.

Romberg's test (▶**Fig. 10.19**): This primarily tests position sense. Ask the SP to stand with the feet together; ask him to hold the arms out in front of him, and wait for few seconds. Then ask him to close his eyes. Assure the SP that you are close and will support

him. If the SP maintains a steady position while opening his eyes, but he couldn't with closed eyes, that is considered a positive test.

Communication and Interpersonal Skills

Suggested Answers to the Standardized Patient's Questions

Q1: Answer as explained earlier, after closure, answer the SP's question: *"Okay, let's look at your hypertension (HTN) prescription. The dizziness you have been experiencing could be a side effect of the medication, but on the other hand, it could be due to something else. Because of that, I need to do a workup like … and …. When the results come back, I will discuss this issue with your family doctor. How does that sound to you?"*

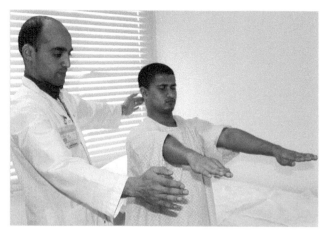

Fig. 10.19 Romberg's test.

Patient Note

History

A 55-year-old woman complains of dizziness that started 1 month ago. It was infrequent, but now it occurs two to three times a day. The last one was this morning. It lasted less than a minute, no warning signs beforehand, and never passed out. She does not feel lightheadedness, nor associated sweating or palpitation. It started when the patient began taking a new prescription (HCTZ) for HTN. She feels like the room is spinning around her and increases with sudden change of position. No hearing loss or ear discharge. She had URT infection a few weeks ago. No dyspnea, orthopnea, or peripheral edema, no headache or blurry vision. **ROS:** postmenopausal for 1 year; others irrelevant. **PMH:** HTN, appendectomy. **Meds:** HCTZ and lisinopril. NKDA. **FH:** N/D. **SH:** nonsmoker, two to three beers a week, no illicit drugs.

Examination

VS: WNL and alert, oriented ×3. Head: AT, NC, PERRLA, intact red reflex, no tenderness over the mastoid, nontender ear pinna, clear TMs. Rinne's test (air conduction > bone conduction) on both sides. **Weber's test:** no lateralization.
Neuro: Cranial nerves II–XII otherwise intact, intact sensation all over, muscle power is 5/5, DTRs is +2, normal gait, and negative Romberg's test.

Differential Diagnosis

History finding(s)	Physical exam finding(s)
1. Benign paroxysmal positional vertigo	
Feels dizzy	
Brief intense episode, room spins around	Free neurological exam
↑ with change in position	No facial weakness
No hearing loss	Normal Rinne's and Weber's tests
2. Vestibular neuritis	
Feels dizzy	
Recent upper respiratory tract infection	Free neurological exam
No hearing loss	No facial weakness
	Normal Rinne's and Weber's tests
3. Medication side effect (diuretic)	
Feels dizzy	
Recent use of diuretic	
It comes when getting up	

Diagnostic Studies

Dix–Hallpike maneuver

Audiometry

MRI brain

Role-Play 50

Mrs. Mary Wilson, a 24 year-old woman, has difficulty sleeping.

Vital signs:

- **PR:** 98/min, regular.
- **BP:** 140/100 mm Hg.
- **RR:** 20/min.
- **Temp.:** 98.6°F (37°C).

Standardized Patient's Role

You have had difficulty falling asleep for 3 weeks now, and it's getting worse as the date of your university final exams nears. You usually go to bed around 10 p.m. and wake up around 6 a.m. However, you usually don't get to sleep until midnight, as it takes you about 2 hours to fall asleep. Moreover, you no longer feel refreshed in the morning when you awake, as you used to before this problem started. You find that you need to take a nap during the day to catch up on sleep. You notice that you have been sweating and your heart races.

Your last period was 2 weeks ago.

You also feel that you have lost some weight, but have not actually weighed yourself.

The symptoms that you are experiencing happened once last year. It was at the same time of the year, just before the final exams.

You have bronchial asthma (BA), take an albuterol inhaler, and have just started to use over-the-counter (OTC) sleeping pills. You are allergic to penicillin and pollen.

You are a college student, smoke 2 ppd/5 y, seldom drink during the week, but you drink more on the weekends, and you are sexually active with your boyfriend. When the doctor examines you and ask to stretch your hands, please induce fine tremors on your fingers.

Ask the following:

Q1: *Doc, I'm worried that I won't pass my exam. I really feel stressed about it.*

Q2: *Doc, sometimes my heart beats as fast as a racehorse. Do you think there is something wrong with my heart?*

Q3: *Could you prescribe me some more powerful sleeping pills?*

Role-Play 50: Answer Key

Difficulty in falling sleep (insomnia) has a wide range of differential diagnoses. In addition, it also requires an in-depth, long-term counseling in order for treatment to be successful. Please be aware when it is listed on the doorway information. Make an allowance of time for this accordingly.

Analysis of Chief Complaint

- *How long have you been having this problem?*
- *Did it come about suddenly, or did it gradually become a problem?*
- *Since it started, has it gotten worse?*
- *Does anything make your sleep better?*
- *Does anything make it worse?*
- *How does this problem affect your work or daily life?*
- *Do you have any problems besides difficulty in sleeping?*
- Determine the sleep patterns and habits, environment (▶ **Table 10.2**).

Analysis of Differential Diagnosis

Analysis of possible causes includes:
- Psychiatric: anxiety, posttraumatic, adjustment disorder, and depression.
- Circadian rhythm sleep disorder.
- Caffeine and medication induced.
- Medical diseases: chronic cough, GERD and for older age consider CHF and BPH.

Psychiatric causes:
- *Are you sad?/Do you feel depressed?*
- *How is your mood?*
- *Do you have any kind of stress at work? At home?*

If yes:
- *What do you have?*
- *Have you had any recent psychiatric trauma? Complete the questions for SIG E CAPS (See Chapter 9, Psychiatry).*

Circadian rhythm sleep disorder:
- *Has your schedule changed?*
- *Has your work shift schedule been changed recently?*

Stimulant induced:
- *Do you use any street drugs?*
- *Do you use speed (amphetamines)?*
- *How much do you smoke?*
- *Do you chew tobacco?*
- *How much coffee/tea do you drink a day? When do you drink it?*
- *What about energy drinks or soft drinks that contain caffeine, for example, Coca-Cola and Red Bull?*

Table 10.2 Questions to determine the sleep patterns and habits, environment.

	Suggested questions
In the evening	*I am going to ask you a few questions about your sleep patterns and habits:* *Do you work out in the evening?* *Before going to bed, do you smoke a lot? Do you drink heavily?* *Do you watch TV in bed? Do you go to bed on a full stomach?* *Do you use your bedroom only for sleeping?*
At night	*When do you usually go to bed?* *How much time does it take to fall asleep?* *Do you have a problem falling asleep or staying asleep?* *Do you wake up during the night? How often?* *When you wake up, do you fall asleep again immediately, or do you stay awake for a long time?*
Questions about daytime symptoms	*When do you usually wake up in the morning?* *When you wake up in the morning, do you feel refreshed?* *Do you feel sleepy during the daytime?* *Do you have to take a nap during the daytime?*

(**Note:** The classification is similar to a nocturnal enuresis case.)

Medical diseases:
- Has anyone in *your family noticed that you snore?* (Sleep apnea)
- *Have you ever had any episodes of difficulty breathing at night?*
- *Do you have trouble breathing while lying back?* (CHF)
- *Do you have to wake up at night to pee?* (BPH) Complete the questions for SIG E CAPS (See Chapter 9, Psychiatry).
- *Have you ever woken up with heartburn? Coughing?* (GERD)
- Ask questions of hyperthyroidism.

Physical Exam

Do a quick general exam, and for a specific complaint, do a local exam.

Communication and Interpersonal Skills

Suggested Closure

"It seems that the symptoms that you have are caused by anxiety. You have …, …, and you had these symptoms the same time last year close to the exam. However, I want to to eliminate the possibility of the symptoms being caused by something else, so I need to run some tests. Next visit, after we have the results, I will sit with you again to discuss them.

I have some recommendations for you that will help improve your sleep patterns:
- *First of all, try to quit or limit your caffeine, nicotine, and alcohol intake (if you have time, you can counsel more regarding smoking and drinking).*
- *Do not use the bed as a place to think; use the bedroom only for sleeping. Don't eat or watch TV in the bedroom.*
- *Keep regular hours—go to bed and wake up at around the same time every day.*
- *Exercise regularly, but preferably not at the end of the day.*
- *Get regular exposure to sunlight."*

Suggested Answers to the Standardized Patient's Questions

Q1 and Q2: Answers as given previously.

Q3: *"I really shouldn't prescribe any meds for you without having a definitive diagnosis. For that reason, let's forgo the sleeping pills until we run some tests and get the results. Then we can meet again. I'll give you my diagnosis, and then we'll see what treatment options we have. So, for the lab tests, I will need to get a urine sample, and a blood draw."*

Patient Note

History

A 24-year-old female student complaints of difficulty sleeping for 3 weeks, gradual onset and worsening with time, ↓ by OTC sleep pills, but nothing makes sleep come any easier. She has also been sweating, and has palpitation. She usually goes to bed at 10 o'clock and takes around 2 hours to fall asleep. She usually wakes up at 6 o'clock in the morning, does not feel refreshed, and is sleepy during the day. This problem interferes with university studies. She is stressed about upcoming exams. She denies snoring, coughing, or heartburn. **ROS:** last menstrual period was 2 weeks ago, good appetite, feels a recent weight loss. **PMH:** BA; previous episode was last year. **Med:** albuterol inhaler and OTC sleeping pills. NKDA. **FH:** N/D. **SH:** college student, smoker 2 ppd/5 y, drinks (especially on the weekends), no illicit drug use. Sexually active with one boyfriend; uses condoms.

Examination

VS: WNL. Appears anxious and restless, alert and oriented ×3. **Head:** PERRLA, throat without erythema, nose without rhinorrhea. **Neck:** normal thyroid. **Ext:** no excessive sweating, fine tremors visible on outstretched hands.
Heart: normal S1 and S2, no murmurs. **Abdomen:** soft, non-tender, non-distended. **Neuro:** intact cranial nerves, muscle 5/5, and intact sensation.

Differential Diagnosis

History finding(s)	Physical exam finding(s)
1. Anxiety	
Worries about exam, recent onset	Free neurological exam
Insomnia, irritability, and sweating	Normal thyroid exam
Similar episode last year	Hand tremors and palpitation
2. Adjustment disorder	
Worries about exam, recent onset	Free neurological exam
Insomnia, irritability, and sweating	Normal thyroid exam

Diagnostic Studies

Thyroid-stimulating hormone (TSH)

Urine toxicology screen

CBC with differential

Role-Play 51

Mrs. Freddi Miller, a 65-year-old woman, has forgetfulness.

Vital signs:
- **PR:** 98/min, regular.
- **BP:** 140/100 mm Hg.
- **RR:** 20/min.
- **Temp.:** 98.6°F (37°C).

Standardized Patient's Role

Since the death of your husband, you have been living with your daughter. Recently, you have had problems with remembering important things such as the date, telephone and bank account numbers, appointments, and other things. This has started to seriously impact your daily life: you forget that you have put something on the stove and it burns. You have forgotten to turn off the faucet, and the sink overflowed. You have had trouble managing your bank and email accounts, and your daughter has had to check to make sure you have balanced things correctly and responded to all emails. Last week, you got lost while returning home from the grocery store.

You can no longer live independently without the aid of your daughter.

You are postmenopausal for 15 years.

You have high BP. You had a stroke on your right side, and are surprised that you can't remember how many years ago it occurred. You also had an angiography done for your heart, but can't recall when.

Your medications are lisinopril, aspirin, and nitrates.

Your mother had Alzheimer's disease and you drink socially.

During the exam:

When the doctor asks you to remember three names and then repeat them, act as if you cannot recall them. When he or she examines your right arm and leg, mention that your right side has been feeling a little weak. When he or she tests your reflexes, pretend that your right side is weaker than your left.

Ask the doctor the following:

Q1: *Is it possible that I have Alzheimer's?*
Q2: *Do you think I should abstain from having sex?*

Role-Play 51: Answer Key

Often due to senility, memory loss or forgetfulness is common with elderly SPs. Amnesia, the loss of memory, is not commonly found on the CS exam.

History

Analysis of Chief Complaint

Ask about onset, course, duration, and quality of life.
- *When did it start?/Since it started, has it gotten worse?*
- *What things do you usually forget?*
- *Who is concerned about this problem, are you or your family?*
- *Do you have any idea what may have caused this?*
- *How does this problem affect your life?*

Analysis of Differential Diagnosis

Alzheimer's disease:
- *Do you need help while going to the toilet? With bathing? With getting dressed?*
- *Do you need help with preparing your food? With taking your medicine?*
- *Do you have any problems with driving to the supermarket? With returning back home?*
- *Are you still able to manage your bank/email account?*

Vascular (multi-infarct) dementia:
- *Have you had a stroke?*
- *Do your feel any tingling or numbness anywhere in your body?/Any weakness?*

Normal-pressure hydrocephalus:
- Wacky (cognitive changes): dementia.
- Wet: *Do you leak urine unintentionally?*
- Wobbly (gait instability): *Do you have a tendency to fall while walking?*

Depression:
- *Do you feel sad/depressed?*
- **If yes:** Ask the questions for depression (Chapter 9, Psychiatry).

Hypothyroidism: Ask questions as a standard.

Review of the Local System

Neurological system.

Review of Systems

Ask standard questions.

Past History and Others

D (cerebral stroke), S (cardiac angiography), D (lisinopril, aspirin, and nitrates), F (Alzheimer's disease), S (home situation), ±S (one question).

Physical Exam

As routine; don't forget to do fundus exam, carotid bruit, and jugular venous distension (JVD). Auscultate the lung and the heart only. **Local exam:** do brief neurological exam. MMSE: Ask the following:
- *Could you tell me your first and last name?*
- *Who is the president of the United States?*
- *What year is it?*
- *Where are we now?*
- *Can you spell the word CAT backward?*
- *Please repeat these three words: roof, wall, and floor. Later, I will ask you to repeat them again.*

Note: World is probably a standard word in MMSE for the patient to spell, and three words/objects preferably not to be related. Roof, wall, and floor are 3 simple words that can be remembered easily while you are in the the room. However, what is mentioned was intended for simplification.

Communication and Interpersonal Skills Component

Suggested Closure

Do the standard closure. However, if you suspect Alzheimer's disease, provide a little information regarding this disease.

Counseling

Do counseling for HTN. You should assess the **SP's safety** at home by asking: *"With whom do you live? Are you safe at home? Please tell me if there is anything I can help you with."* Offer nursing or senior home, if in need.

Suggested Answers to the Standardized Patient's Questions

Q1: *"As just explained, based on your family history and my physical exam, Alzheimer's disease is a possibility. But let's not jump to conclusion since we really should run tests to eliminate other treatable causes of your forgetfulness. I need to do … and …. When the results come back, we'll make an appointment and discuss them. My receptionist will give you a call when the lab sends us the results."*

Q2: *"I see no reason why that would be unhealthy or unwise to do, unless there's a problem that I don't know about. Have you had any troubles or discomfort with your sexual life before? Don't be afraid to give me a call anytime if something comes up.*

Now if you have no further questions, let's call the nurse to prepare you for a pelvic exam."

Note: If you see the SP's memory is greatly affected, and making it difficult to remember, ask for permission to contact one of the relatives to explain more.

Patient Note

History

A 65-year-old woman complains of forgetfulness for 6 months, gradual onset, getting worse. She and her family are concerned about this matter, as it has started to affect their daily lives. She is forgetting things on the stove, forgetting to turn off the tap water, etc. She is no longer able to manage either her bank or her email accounts. Last week, she couldn't return from the nearby grocery. She lives with her daughter, who helps her with bathing and going to the toilet. She has weakness in her right arm and leg. No urinary incontinence or bowel movement problems. No depression. **ROS:** irrelevant, postmenopausal for 15 years. **PMH:** HTN, cardiac angiography, and stroke (but can't remember when). **Med:** lisinopril, aspirin, and nitrates. **FH:** mother had Alzheimer's disease. **SH:** she is a widow, lives with her daughter, doesn't smoke, but drinks socially.

Physical Examination

VS: BP: 140/100 mm Hg; others WNL. **Head:** PERRLA, intact red reflex. **Neck:** no carotid bruit. **Ext:** palpable peripheral pulse. **Neuro: MMSE:** alert, oriented ×3. Spells backward, couldn't recall three objects. Cranial nerves II–XII are intact; muscle power is 4/5 on the right side, others 5/5; intact sensation throughout. DTRs is + 1 on the right side, normal gait, and Romberg's test was negative.

Differential Diagnosis

History finding(s)	Physical exam finding(s)
1. Alzheimer's disease	
Forgetfulness	MMSE: couldn't recall three objects
Affects her daily activities	
Family history	
2. Vascular dementia	
Forgetfulness	MMSE: couldn't recall three objects
Muscle weakness on the right side	Muscle power is 4/5 on the right side, DTRs is +1
Past history of stroke	

Diagnostic Studies

CBC and electrolyte panel

Serum B12, TSH

MRI brain

Role-Play 52

Mrs. Debbie Pascal, a 65 year-old woman, experiencing weakness in her right arm and leg.

Vital signs:
- **PR:** 104/min, irregular.
- **BP:** 160/110 mm Hg.
- **RR:** 22/min.
- **Temp.:** 98.6°F (37°C).

Standardized Patient's Role

During the encounter, you will be lying on the bed. As the doctor enters the room, pretend to be sad and worried.

Say to the doctor: *I can't move my right arm and my right leg! Please help me.* (**comment 1**)

The weakness in your arm and in your leg came on suddenly 1 hour ago. You felt and you still feel tingling and numbness on the right side with inability to raise your arm and leg.

You had heart attack 5 years ago with open heart surgery done 2 years ago, and you have had high BP for 15 years and have high cholesterol.

You are postmenopausal for 15 years, you are taking atenolol, aspirin, and Zocor.

Your mother died of heart disease, and your father died of a stroke. You have lived alone since the death of your husband. You quit smoking 5 years ago; you had smoked 2 ppd/35 y.

If the doctor examines you, express muscle weakness on the right arm and right leg; also, express impaired sensation. If the doctor tests for muscle jerks, exaggerate your response a little bit on this side.

Ask your doctor:
Q1: *Am I having a stroke?*
Q2: *Doctor, do you think that I'll regain the use of my arm and leg?*

Role-Play 52: Answer Key

Stroke is not a common diagnosis on the CS exam, however, this is an example of a case that requires a comprehensive neurological examination and plenty of emotional support from the attending physician. The SP usually lies in bed and complains of weakness of one arm and leg on one side. He or she may also express difficulty with speech. As you have learned, express great concern for his or her situation, and always be supportive during the encounter. Recommend hospital admission at the end, and be sure of home safety.

History

Analysis of Chief Complaint

Weakness of one side.
- *When did it start?/Did it come on suddenly?*
- *Do you have any weakness in your arm? Any weakness in your leg?*
- *Do you have any tingling or numbness in your arm? In your legs?*
- *Do you have difficulty swallowing? Any difficulty speaking?*

Analysis of Differential Diagnosis

TIA, stroke: hemorrhagic (▶ Fig. 10.20) or ischemic (▶ Fig. 10.21). **Others:** conversion disorder, seizures, Guillain–Barré syndrome, and complex migraine.

"I'm going ask you a few questions to understand more what happened before you has had weakness. Try to remember what you were doing and how you felt beforehand."
- *Did you have any chest pain?*
- *Was your heart beating rapidly?*
- *Did you have a headache? Was your vision blurred? Did you vomit?*
- *Had you hit your head?*
- *Had you been involved in any accident?*
- *Have you had a recent psychiatric trauma?*
- *Have you had any recent respiratory tract infection?*

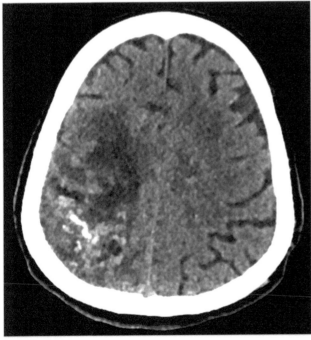

Fig. 10.20 CT of the head showing cerebral hemorrhagic.

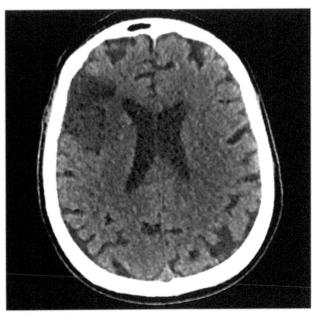

Fig. 10.21 CT of the head showing cerebral infarction.

Review of the Local System

As routine.

Review of Systems

As routine.

Past History and Others

D (HTN, hypercholesterolemia, heart disease), **S** (open heart), **P** (any previous history?), **D** (atenolol, aspirin, and Zocor), **F** (stroke), **S** and skip asking about sexual history.

Physical Exam

VS: high BP, tachycardia. **A** (anxious), **D** (lying back, can't move her arm nor leg), **H** (examine the head carefully including fundus exam), **N** (carotid bruit, JVD), **E** (peripheral pulse). **LH:** auscultate the heart only, cancel or do a quick lung exam. Please do the general exam quickly since the neurological exam is long.

Local exam: Neurological exam in detail, do planter reflex (Babinski's sign) gently as shown in ▶ **Fig. 10.22 (a, b)**.

Communication and Interpersonal Skills Component

Suggested Closure

Inform the SP that it's an emergency case that requires inpatient admission while expressing great concern. Inform the SP that you will start the workup immediately.

Counseling

Counseling for HTN and assess the home situation.

Suggested Answers to the Standardized Patient's Questions

As previously answered.

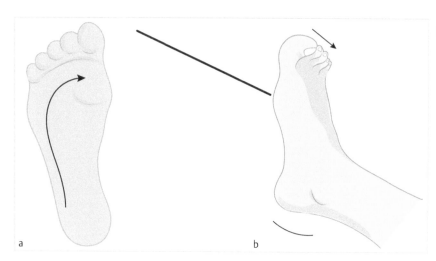

Fig. 10.22 (a, b) Planter reflex (Babinski's sign).

Patient Note

History

A 65-year-old female patient complains of weakness of the right arm and leg, which started 1 hour ago suddenly and is getting worse. She felt loss of sensation and tingling in the right side together with weakness and inability to move the right side, headache 5/10 all over the head, not preceded by any head injury. No chest pain or palpitation, no dysarthria or dysphagia, no urine or fecal incontinence, or seizures. **ROS:** postmenopausal for 15 years. **PMH:** no history of stroke, history of heart attack 5 years ago, HTN for 15 years, hyper-cholesterolemia, CABG (coronary artery bypass grafting). **Med:** atenolol, aspirin, and Zocor. NKDA. **FH:** mother died of heart attack and father of stroke. **SH:** lives alone since the death of her husband. Ex-smoker, quit 5 years ago (2 ppd/35 y).

Examination

The patient was lying down, couldn't move the right arm and leg. She is oriented ×3. **VS:** Temp., 98.6°F; PR, 104/min, irregular; RR, 22/min; BP, 160/110 mm Hg. HEENT; NT, AT, NC, PERRLA, the neck is supple with no carotid bruit or JVD. Heart is regular in rate and rhythm (RRR) with no murmurs or gallop.

Neuro: cranial nerves II–XII otherwise normal. **Right side exam:** muscle power is 3/5 and impaired sensations; DTRs is +3. **Left side exam:** WNL. Cerebellar function and gait can't be assessed as the patient can't stand or walk.

Differential Diagnosis

History finding(s)	Physical exam finding(s)
1. Cerebral stroke	
Sudden weakness in the right side	Decrease sensation on the right side
Long Hx of HTN, hypercholesterolemia	Muscle power is 3/5
Family Hx	DTRs is +3
2. Transient ischemic attack	
Sudden weakness on the right side	Decreased sensation on the right side
Long Hx of HTN, hypercholesterolemia	Muscle power is 3/5
	DTRs is +3
3. Conversion disorder	
Sudden weakness on the right side	
Lives alone since the death of her husband	

Abbreviations: DTRs, deep tendon reflexes; HTN, hypertension; Hx, history.

Diagnostic Studies

Basic electrolytes

CT brain

ECG and carotid Doppler ultrasound (US)

11 Miscellaneous

Keywords: diabetes mellitus, hypertension, hearing loss, fatigue

11.1 Introduction

Checkup visit/medication refill cases include the following:
- Diabetes mellitus.
- Hypertension (HTN).
- Human immunodeficiency virus (HIV)/acquired immunodeficiency syndrome (AIDS).
- Bronchial asthma (BA).

11.2 Strategy for Medical History

For medical history in such cases, and in addition to the basic questions in the history, there are specific ones to those cases. We developed an easy-to-recall general scheme that will help you in handling them: questions about the **disease** and **its complications**, then questions about **medication** and **its side effects** (▶Video. 11.1).

11.2.1 Specific Questions

Questions about the Disease

- *When were you first diagnosed with (diabetes, high blood pressure [BP], HIV…)?*
- *Are you seen regularly by a physician? If yes: When was your last checkup?*
- *What did the doctor tell you during your last visit?*
- *Is your … under control? What is the usual range of your ….? What was the last reading of …?*

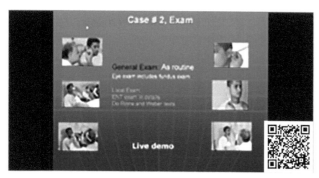

Video. 11.1 This is a special lecture that collects unclassified cases. Examples are checkup visits/medications refill for D.M, hypertension and more. https://www.thieme.de/de/q.htm?p=opn/cs/20/3/11450547-fff1bf64

Questions about Complications of the Disease

Look at individual cases.

Questions about the Medication

- *Are you currently taking any medicine for …? If yes: What do you take? Do you remember the dose? How often do you take …?*
- *Do you take the medications on a regular basis?*
- *Do you think that your medicine is controlling your disease effectively?*

Questions about Side Effects of the Medication

Do you have any problems that may be related to your medicine? Do you have any complaint that you think is a side effect of your medicine?

11.2.2 Basic Questions

As standard.

Note: If the standardized patient (SP) doesn't have a specific complaint, you can ask an open-ended question like: *"I appreciate that you came for your checkup visit. Do you have any issue specifically that you want to tell me about?"*

11.3 Communication and Interpersonal Skills Component

11.3.1 Appropriate Closure and Counseling

Appropriate closure and counseling are important in these cases, so give it at least 2 to 3 minutes to provide a bit of information regarding the disease. Give the SPs some recommendations regarding diet, exercise, checkups visits, and medications.

11.3.2 Medication Refill

Medication refill via phone is acceptable, but your response depends on the patient's condition. If the patient's condition is stable, he or she doesn't have medical problems, and has had no apparent medication side effects, respond to his or her request, and offer an appointment for a physical exam just for the Clinical Skills (CS) exam.

You can say something like, *"I'll go ahead and refill your medicine today, but I'm interested in seeing you for a physical exam, just* to be sure that everything is fine. Could you tell me about your schedule?/What about an appointment next week?"

If the patient has complaints from uncontrolled HTN (headache, chest pain, etc.), uncontrolled diabetes mellitus (DM; visual problems, peripheral neuropathy, etc.), or side effects to medicine (dry cough from angiotensin-converting enzyme inhibitors [ACEIs], dizziness from propranolol, etc.), postpone the medication refill, and advise the patient to come to the hospital.

> You can respond with, "Mr. .... You told me that you have ..., ..., and .... It seems to me that your medicine doesn't control your disease well, and what you complain about may be one of the side effects of your medication. I prefer for you to come to the clinic to do a physical exam, and we

may need to do ... and ... then we are going to review your medication again."

11.3.3 A Common Question That May Be Asked by SPs in These Cases

Q1: *Doc, I came here to refill my medicine. Why are you asking me all of these questions?*

Doc: *"I understand your concern, Mr./ Mrs. .... Although your meds refill is your concern, your health in general is my concern, too, and I need to make sure things haven't changed from the clinical perspective. Please give me few minutes to ask you few questions and to do a brief physical exam to figure out what is going on. I need to be sure that everything is fine."*

Role-Play 53

Mr. Douglas Jackson, a 55-year-old man, came to the clinic for a diabetes checkup.

Vital signs:

- **Pulse rate (PR):** 86/min, regular.
- **BP:** 140/100 mm Hg.
- **Respiratory rate (RR):** 16/min.
- **Temperature (Temp):** 98.6°F (37°C).

Examinee tasks:

- Obtain a focused history.
- Perform a relevant physical exam. Do not perform rectal, pelvic, genitourinary, inguinal hernia, female breast, or corneal reflex exams.
- Discuss your initial diagnostic impression and your workup plan with the patient.
- After leaving the room, complete your patient note on the given form.

Standardized Patient's Role

You are a 55-year-old man, and came to the clinic, as you feel that your diabetes isn't as well controlled as it used to be. You have had diabetes for 15 years, and used to be compliant to checkup visits every 6 months. However, you haven't gone for a checkup visit for the last year because of some financial issues with the medical insurance company.

You are sad because your blood sugar was 300 mg/dL last week, and it never goes above 200. Say, *"I'm so worried about my blood sugar."* (**comment 1**)

You drink more water, go to the bathroom more often, and you have lost more than 6 lb since the last checkup for your weight 6 months ago, despite eating more than usual.

You feel that the sensation has decreased in your legs.

You have abdominal pain in the upper part of your abdomen, and you would rate it as 4 out of 10, with distension and bloating. It increases greatly with meals.

You have taken metformin 500 mg once daily for 15 years, and insulin (Humulin 70/30) was added 3-years ago. You remember that you have got sick and sweaty once, after taking insulin, when you missed your meal. You have had high BP for 10 years taking lisinopril, and lovastatin for high cholesterol.

Recently, your sleep has become difficult as you have to wake up to pee once or twice at night.

Your mother has diabetes, you live alone, and your brother expects a call from you every morning.

You work for a business, smoke (1 pack per day [ppd] for 25 years), drink socially, and you are not sexually active. When the doctor examines you, pretend that the sensation in the legs in comparison to the arms, otherwise, react normally.

At the end, ask your doctor: **Q1:** *"Is the numbness and the pins that I feel in my legs related to diabetes?"*

Please refer to Chapter 13 (Appendix), to review the general instructions for the SP as well as the Doctor roles.

Role-Play 53: Answer Key

History and Specific Questions

About the Disease

DM, as explained.

Complications of the Disease

DM.

General

Do you drink more water than usual?
Do you go to the bathroom to urinate more often than usual?
How is your appetite?
Have you noticed any recent weight loss? **If yes:** *How much did you lose?*

Specific

Retinopathy (▶ Fig. 11.1): *Do you have blurry vision?*

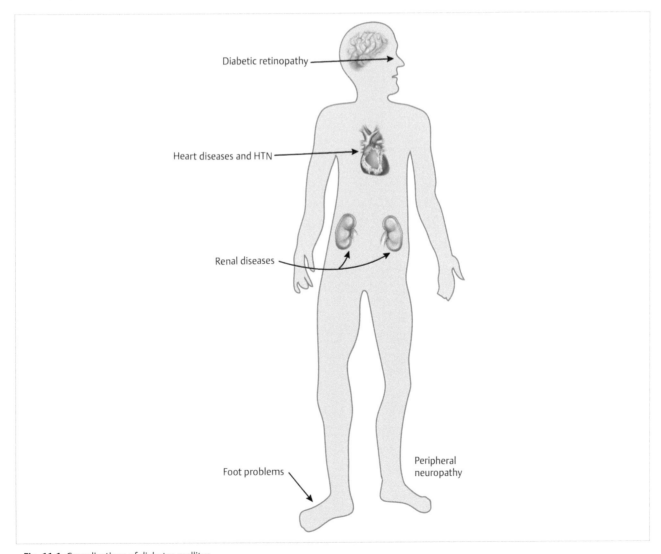

Fig. 11.1 Complications of diabetes mellitus.

Diabetic gastropathy: *Do you have any abdominal pain? Any heartburn?*
Do you have any problems with your bowel movements?

Coronary: *Do you have chest pain? Do you feel tired while walking upstairs?*

Sexual: *Are you sexually active?* **If yes:** *Do you have any problems in your sexual life?*

Peripheral neuropathy: *Do you have any tingling or numbness in your legs? Any pinprick sensation in your feet?*
Have you noticed any changes in your ability to sense touch?
Have you noticed any infections in your feet? Any sores?

Diabetic coma: *Have you ever been hospitalized for diabetic complications?*

Medication

General questions: As explained.

Specific: *Have you ever taken insulin?*

Side Effects of the Medication

Have you ever had any complications that related to insulin therapy? (If he takes insulin)

Basic Questions

Ask routine questions.

Physical Exam

Vital signs (VS), head; visual acuity by counting fingers and fundus exam), **N** (carotid bruit), **E** (lower limb sensation, peripheral pulsation, foot exam in detail), **Lung and heart (LH):** If there is no chest pain, do auscultation only.

Lower limb exam (AND: Artery, Nerve, Diabetic foot).

Artery: Feel the peripheral pulse in the posterior tibial artery and dorsalis pedis artery.

Nerve: For sensory, test for touch sensation and vibration sense (see below). For deep tendon reflexes, check for knee and ankle jerk.

Test for vibration sense (▶ **Fig. 11.2**): First, try a nonvibrating tuning fork (156 Hz) on a bony prominence of the hand of the arm while the patient opens his or her eyes. Ask him or her if he or she feels the vibration, then stop it by your hand and ask him or her again. Then, ask the patient to close his or her eyes and put the tuning fork on the base of the big toe. Then ask the SP: *"Do you feel anything from this device?"* Ask him to inform you as the sound stops, and stop it with your hand. If the vibration sense is impaired at the level of the big toe, move proximally on the medial malleolus.

Foot exam: Examine the foot carefully, along with inspection of toes. If the SP wears socks, ask him or her to take them off. If the SP has sexual complaint, ask for a pelvic and genital examination.

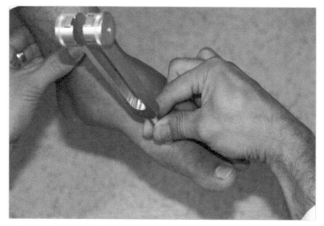

Fig. 11.2 Test for vibration sense.

Communication and Interpersonal Skills Component

Give 2 to 3 minutes for closure and counseling.

Suggested Closure

Provide information: *"Mrs./Miss ..., you told me .... First of all, I want to give you some information about diabetes. Diabetes is a disease that is associated with a problem in a hormone named insulin, a hormone that is secreted by a group of cells from the pancreas. The insulin hormone is responsible for glucose uptake by the tissues. Diabetes may either result from a deficiency of insulin secretion from the pancreas or from insensitivity of the peripheral tissue to this hormone. Subsequently, some problems result, not only from carbohydrates, but also from fat and protein metabolism. Our objectives are to keep your blood sugar close to its normal range. Uncontrolled diabetes may hurt the eyes, heart, and kidneys. For more information, I have here a wonderful handout. Please read it at home, write down any questions or concerns, and I'll be glad to address anything at the next visit."*

Counseling: Recommendations for Better Control of Diabetes

General Recommendation

See the Communication and Interpersonal Skills part (triple 2 formula).

Specific Recommendations

Diabetic foot care: *"I have some recommendations for better foot care: Dry your feet every time you wash it, always wear socks, and cut your nails on a regular basis. Check your feet from time to time for any infections or any sores; if those go missed, you can get a deeper infection."*

Eye clinic: *"Do you do eye clinic visits?"* If yes, *"When was your last visit?"*

If no: *"What about me scheduling an appointment for you?"*

Suggested Answers to the SP's Questions, Comments

As previously explained.

History

A 55-year-old male diabetic patient who came to the clinic because his diabetes isn't well controlled. He has had DM for the last 15 years. He hadn't had checkup for the last year due to financial troubles. He discovered that his blood sugar level rose to 300; the average reading used to be 200. He has polyuria, polydipsia, polyphagia, epigastric pain 4/10, nonradiating, with dyspepsia and abdominal distension. He also noticed decreased sensation in both legs. No blurry vision or chest pain, never hospitalized for diabetic complications. **Review of systems (ROS):** Difficult sleep, increased appetite, and lost 6 lb/6 mo. **Past medical history (PMH):** HTN 10 y. **Medication (Med):** metformin, Humulin 70/30, lisinopril, and lovastatin. **Family history (FH):** mother with DM. **Social history (SH):** He is a businessman, smokes 1 ppd/25 y, drinks socially, lives alone, but his brother expects a call every morning, not sexually active.

Physical Exam

VS: Bp: 140/100 mm Hg; others within normal limit (WNL), no acute distress. **Head:** PERRLA (pupils equal, round, reactive to light and accommodation), visual acuity 6/6, intact red reflex. **Neck:** no carotid bruit or jugular venous distension (JVD). **Extremities (Ext):** palpable peripheral pulse in four limbs. **Chest:** CTA/BL (clear to auscultation bilaterally). **Heart:** normal S1 and S2. **Abdomen:** mild epigastric tenderness.

  Lower limb: palpable peripheral pulsation, impaired touch sensation bilaterally, normal vibration sense. **Feet:** clean with no ulcers.

Differential Diagnosis

History finding(s)	Physical exam finding(s)
1. Diabetic gastropathy	
Diabetes mellitus (DM) for 15 y	
Noncontrolled DM	
Epigastric pain	Epigastric tenderness
2. Peripheral neuropathy	
DM for 15 y	
Noncontrolled DM	
Impaired lower limb sensation	Impaired sensation to fine touch

Diagnostic Studies

Genital exam

Fasting blood sugar, Hb A1c

Urinalysis, serum creatinine

Complete blood count with differential and lipid profile

Role-Play 54

Opening Scenario: Mr. Paul Black, a 55-year-old man, calls the clinic to refill his medication for high BP.

Standardized Patient's Role

You are a 55-year-old man. You are calling the clinic to refill your medications, as you have high BP.

As you start the conversation with the doctor, say, *"I've been waiting on phone for a long time."* (**comment 1**).

You have had high BP for 10 years; you are calling your doctor to refill your medication (lisinopril, 20-mg tablet). You take it once daily. You check your BP from time to time at home; the range is 130 to 140 for the upper reading and 100 to 110 for the lower one.

The doctor may ask you many questions regarding your BP and your health in general. Inform him or her that you have to sleep on two pillows; otherwise, you have trouble breathing. Also, you have noticed mild cramps and pain in your legs, especially if you walk for 4-5 blocks. There is a mild cough without sputum that doesn't disturb your daily activity.

You take Zocor (simvastatin) for high cholesterol, and your father died from a stroke.

You work in the food industry, don't exercise regularly, are a smoker (1 ppd/25 y), and drink two or three cups of wine in a party. You are sexually active with your wife with no problems.

(**Comment 2**): *"Doc, I'm so worried. My father's BP was not controlled, and he had a stroke."*

Role-Play 54: Answer Key

History and Specific Questions

About the Disease

(HTN): standard.

Complications of the Disease

(HTN; ▶ **Fig. 11.3**).

Ask about any passing out, headache, blurry vision, and bleeding from the nose.

Cardiovascular system (CVS) symptoms: chest pain, angina, paroxysmal nocturnal dyspnea (PND), orthopnea. See Chapter 4, Chest (Cardiology and Respiratory).

Peripheral vascular disease: *Do you have any pain/cramps in your legs upon walking?*

Side Effects of the Medication

Determine what the SP takes, and ask accordingly about the side effects of the medications.

B-blockers: Ask about dizziness, asthma, and sexual impairment.

ACE inhibitors: Ask about dry cough.

If the SP takes statin, ask about any muscle ache and order liver function tests (LFTs) in the workup.

Refer to the medication list in the Chapter 13, Appendix.

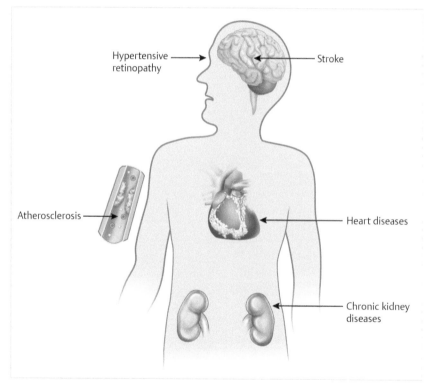

Fig. 11.3 Complications of hypertension.

Basic Questions and Other Components of the History

As routine.

Review of System

CVS symptoms (refer to Chapter 4, Chest (Cardiology and Respiratory)).

Physical Exam

Standard, but stress on visual acuity (counting fingers), fundus exam, carotid bruit, and JVD. **Ext:** examine for peripheral pulsation and edema. Do cardiac exam in detail.

Communication and Interpersonal Skills Component

Suggested Closure and Counseling

> *"Mr. Black, let me make sure that I understand what you said correctly. You told me that you are calling to refill your medicine (lisinopril) for high BP. You have … and … and you don't have …, …, and …. Am I right? You also told me that you have had to sleep on two pillows recently and … and …. Your BP reading is 140/100. Really, I can't refill your medication today for many reasons: you have mild swelling in your legs and trouble breathing, especially during the night. It seems to me that your medicine isn't working well; moreover, you have a dry cough that may be a side effect of lisinopril. I prefer for you come to the clinic to review your medicine, do a physical exam, and to take pictures for your chest and heart. How does that sound to you?"*

> *"I would also like to speak with you in person about improving your diet, exercise, smoking cessation, and other issues that will help in controlling your BP."*

Do you have any questions? Any other concerns? Thanks for your time, and have a good day."

Provide information if needed: *"Mrs./Miss …. High BP is a systemic disease. In most cases, it results from some changes in the vessel walls. They become less elastic and more rigid than normal; subsequently, the BP increases inside. HTN is a leading cause of cerebral stroke, heart attack, and many other diseases. HTN is a lifelong disease. We are aiming to keep your BP under control and as close to normal as we can."*

"I have some general recommendations to you" (refer to the Chapter 2, The Basics, Component 2, Communication and Interpersonal Skills, Communication and Interpersonal Skills Component section for triple 2 formula).

For more information, I can give you a wonderful handout about high BP. I will be glad to address all your questions or concerns at the next visit. How does that sound to you? Do you have any questions? Do you have any concerns?

Thanks for your time. Have a good day."

Suggested Answers to the SP's Questions and Comments

As explained in the previous cases.

Patient Note

History

A 55-year-old male patient who called the clinic to refill his medication, lisinopril 20 mg oral every day. He was diagnosed with HTN 10 years ago; he used to check his BP at home; it ranges from 130 to 140/100 to 110 mm Hg. He denies headache, nosebleed, blurry vision, chest pain, or palpitation. He has to sleep on two pillows recently (? Orthopnea), no PND, mild lower limb edema, and no limb claudication. Has mild dry cough and denies chest wheezes or dizziness. **ROS:** normal appetite, difficult sleep, no recent changes in his weight, no urinary or bowel problems. **PMH:** hypercholesterolemia. **Med:** Zocor (simvastatin) 40 mg orally at bedtime, no known drug allergy (NKDA). **FH:** father had HTN and died from stroke. **SH:** works in food industry, and has no stress, smoker (1 ppd/25 y) no alcohol use, sexually active, monogamous with his wife.

Physical Exam

None.

Differential Diagnosis

History finding(s)	Physical exam finding(s)

1. **Essential hypertension (HTN)**

   History (Hx) of HTN for 10 y

   BP ranges from 140/110 to 130/100

2. **Heart failure and lower limb ischemia**

   Hx of HTN

   Orthopnea

   Lower limb claudication after 4–5 blocks

3. **Lisinopril-induced cough**

   Takes lisinopril and has dry cough

Diagnostic Studies

Physical exam

Urinalysis, complete blood count, lipid profile, alanine transaminase (ALT), and aspartate transaminase (AST)

Echocardiography, chest X-ray

Electrocardiogram

Note: Here is a suggestion for documenting the physical examination if the SP attends. **VS:** Bp 140/100 mm Hg; others WNL. Patient is with no acute distress, alert, and oriented ×3. **Head and neck (H&N):** PERRLA, normal fundus exam. No pallor, cyanosis, JVD, or carotid bruit. **Ext:** equal peripheral pulsation bilaterally. **Chest:** no chest deformities, normal tactile vocal fremitus (TVFs), air or fluid per percussion, CTA/BL, no wheezes or crepitation. **Heart:** PMI not displaced. Normal S1 and S2, no gallop or rub.

Role-Play 55

Doorway Information

Mrs. Erena Johnson, a 30-year-old woman, came to the clinic to refill her medication for BA.

Vital signs

- **PR:** 90/min, regular.
- **BP:** 130/90 mm Hg.
- **RR:** 16/min.
- **Temp:** 98.6°F (37°C).

Standardized Patient's Role

You have had BA for many years that is well controlled with medicine, and you came to the clinic to refill your asthma medications.

This appointment was supposed to be a couple of weeks ago, but you were in Canada visiting your daughter. It was so cold there, with lots of snow, and you had a cold that has improved on over-the-counter (OTC). You still have a little dry cough.

During your trip, unfortunately, your medications ran out. You had difficulty breathing, and chest wheezes a few times last week.

Your medications are albuterol MDI (metered-dose inhaler) and a beclomethasone inhaler. You take them on a regular basis. You remember you were hospitalized twice only, in your entire life, for asthma exacerbation.

You don't take any other medications. You had an appendectomy done many years ago. You are allergic to pets, pollens, and dust.

Your mother also has BA.

You work as a landscape gardener. You stopped smoking 5 years ago (smoked 10 cigarettes for 10 years). You are sexually active and monogamous with your husband.

Role-Play 55: Answer Key

History and Specific Questions

About the Disease

BA: ask standard questions.

Complications of the Disease

BA:
Do you have any trouble breathing during the daytime? **If yes**: *How often?*
Do you have any trouble breathing at night? **If yes**: *How often?*

For asthma exacerbation:
Have you been exposed to any allergens?
Have you ever been hospitalized for any acute or severe asthmatic episodes?

Ask for symptoms that may be suggestive of chest infection, such as fever, chest pain, cough, and sputum. If yes, analyze as **ABC**.

Side Effects of the Medication

Because it may include albuterol MDI and/or steroid inhaler, ask: *Have you noticed any white patches on your tongue, or any throat infection?*

Basic Questions: Analyze Chest Wheezes and Dyspnea

Ask about respiratory tract symptoms (Chapter 4, Chest (Cardiology and Respiratory)) and take allergic history in detail (food, pollen, medicine) and occupational hazards at work (Chapter 2, The Basics, Component 2, Communication and Interpersonal Skills).

Physical Exam

As standard and please refer to Chapter 4, Chest (Cardiology and Respiratory) for chest exam.

Communication and Interpersonal Skills Component

Provide information if needed: *"BA is a hyper-reactive airway disease. As you may know, in our lungs, there are tubes that conduct the air inside the lungs, named bronchi. In some patients, like you, those tubes become hypersensitive to some allergens, like pollen, dust, and cold weather. Upon contact with any allergen, those tubes respond more than usual, secreting chemical materials, named mediators, that result in narrowing of the tubes. For that reason, we can hear wheezing. BA comes in episodes, but taking your medicine in between the episodes makes them less frequent.*

I have some recommendations to you: Keep yourself away from any known allergens. It may be really hard for you, as a gardener, but do your best to take safety precautions.

Please be compliant with your medicine, and take them on a regular basis."

Patient Note

History

A 30-year-old female patient came for BA medications refill. She has had BA for many years. She has had dyspnea, had chest wheezes last week, and dry cough. She is compliant with her meds, and her symptoms are well controlled, but exposure to cold weather, recent flu, and running out of medications may explain these infrequent exacerbations. **ROS:** good appetite, normal sleep, no recent weight loss, and normal urinary and bowel habits. **PMH:** appendectomy many years ago; she was hospitalized twice for asthma exacerbations. **Med:** albuterol MDI, beclomethasone inhaler. **Allergy (ALL):** pets, pollens, and dust. **FH:** mother with BA. **SH:** landscape gardener, ex-smoker 5 years ago (smoked 10 cigarettes/10 y), drinks socially, and sexually active, monogamous with her husband.

Examinations

VS: WNL. Patient is with no acute distress, alert, and oriented ×3. **H&N:** no pallor or cyanosis, mouth without erythema, nose without rhinorrhea, no tenderness over the sinuses. **Ext:** no pallor, cyanosis, clubbing, or palpable peripheral pulse. **Chest:** no chest deformities, normal TVFs, and percussion, CTA/BL, no wheezes or crepitation, heart is RRR (regular rate and rhythm), no murmurs.

Differential Diagnosis

History finding(s)	Physical exam finding(s)
1. Bronchial asthma (BA)	
History of BA	
Breathing difficulties, chest wheezes	
2. Asthma exacerbation	
Breathing difficulties, chest wheezes	
Exposure to cold weather, history of common cold	
Stopped meds	

Diagnostic Studies

Chest X-ray (anteroposterior and lateral)

Pulse oximetry

Pulmonary function tests, peak flow

Role-Play 56

Doorway Information

Miss Ruth Evans, a 55-year-old female patient, came to the clinic with hearing loss.
Vital signs
- **PR:** 90/min, regular.
- **BP:** 100/60 mm Hg.
- **RR:** 16/min.
- **Temp:** 98.6°F (37°C).

Standardized Patient's Role

Throughout the encounter, act like it is difficult for you to hear the doctor. You are a 55-year-old woman, have hearing loss in both ears, and hearing people around you is difficult. This problem started gradually 5 years ago, and it has worsened over time. Nothing makes it better.

You have a problem hearing your coworkers, and hearing people over the phone.

You don't hear any buzzing sound in your ears, and have no problem with your balance while walking. You work at a grocery store that is pretty quiet.

You have high BP, which was diagnosed 15 years ago, and you take a medication named hydrochlorothiazide (HCTZ). You maintain regular checkups with your primary doctor. Your brother, who is 60 years old, has the same problem. At this time, ask your doctor:
Q1: *"Do I have the same problem that my brother has?"*

You don't smoke, do drink socially, and are not sexually active.

If the doctor examines your ear, he or she may put a tuning fork behind and in front your ears. If he or she asks in which position you hear better, answer you heard better when it was in the front of the ear.

If the doctor puts the fork on your head or on your forehead, and asks which side is better, answer that you hear the sound equally on both sides.

As your doctor finishes the encounter, ask:
Q2: *"What about hearing aid devices for me?"*

Role-Play 56 (Hearing loss) (▶Video. 11.2)

In these cases, the SP usually acts as if he or she can't hear well. Please sit down or stand close to the SP, and intentionally raise your voice and ask, *"Can you hear me better?"* For unilateral hearing loss, move close to the healthy ear (Refer to link for more details: https://www.audicus.com/causes-conductive-hearing-loss/).

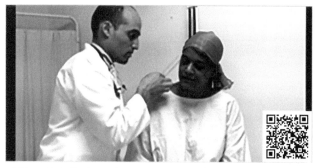

Video. 11.2 This is a real patient encounter of a 55-year-old female patient who has hearing loss. The Demo includes also patient note documentation. https://www.thieme.de/de/q.htm?p=opn/cs/20/3/11450548-345812ae

Role-Play 56: Answer Key

History

Analysis of Chief Complaint

Hearing loss:
- *When did it start? Was it sudden? Since it started, has it gotten worse?*
- *Does anything make it better?*
- *Does anything make it worse?*
- *Which ear is affected more, the right ear or the left or are they affected equally?*

Associations:
- *When it comes, do you have any ringing or buzzing sounds in your ear? Do you feel the room is spinning around you?*
- *When it comes, do you have a tendency to fall?*

More analysis:
- *Do you have a problem with hearing over the phone?*
- *Do you have to strain to hear some conversations?*
- *Do people complain when you turn up the TV volume too high?*
- *Do you have trouble with hearing when there is a noisy background?*

Analysis of DD (▶ Fig. 11.4):

- Conductive hearing loss:
  - Earwax.
  - Punctured eardrum.
  - Otitis media and fluid in the middle ear.
  - Otosclerosis.
- Sensorineural hearing loss:
  - Age-related (presbycusis).
  - Occupational-related.
  - Medication-related (HCTZ).
- Acoustic neuroma.
- Meniere's disease.

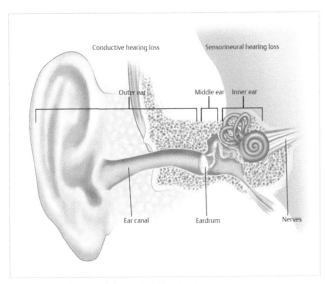

Fig. 11.4 Differential diagnosis of hearing loss.

Analysis of Differential Diagnosis

Ask the following questions:
- *Have you had any recent ear infection?*
- *Have you noticed any discharge coming from your ears?* (otitis media)
- *What do you do for work?* (occupational noise)
- *Are/were you working with a lot of noise or machines?* (Use "are" if still working and "were" if retired)
- *Has it come with new medicine use?* (ototoxicity)
- Ask about symptoms of increased intracranial pressure (ICP): headache, blurry vision, and excessive vomiting (for acoustic neuroma).

Review of the Local System

If there are symptoms suggestive of increased ICP, ask a few questions regarding the neurological system (Chapter 10, Neurology).

Review of Systems

As routine.

Past History and Others

As routine.

Physical Exam

As routine. You can do a quick LH exam in this case or it could be held till the end of the exam and done if the time permits. Stress on fundus exam, ENT (ear, nose, and throat) exam in details (▶ Fig. 11.5, ▶ Fig. 11.6, ▶ Fig. 11.7): Check for tenderness over the mastoid, at the tragus of the ear and examine the external ear with the otoscope gently. Do Rinne's and Weber's tests.

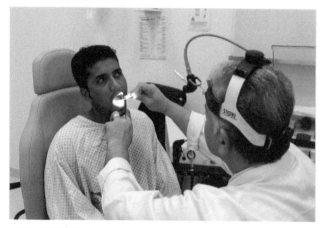

Fig. 11.5 Throat exam.

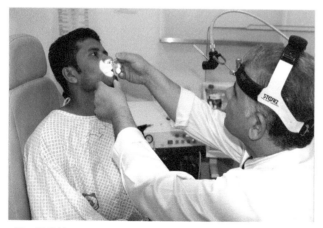

Fig. 11.6 Nose exam.

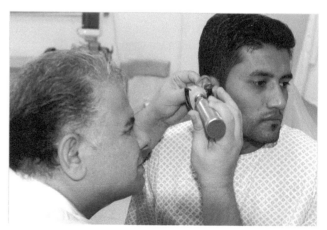

Fig. 11.7 Ear exam by otoscope.

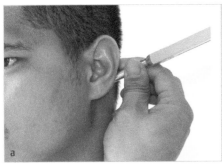
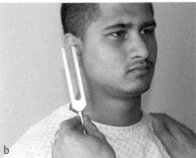

Fig. 11.8 (a,b) Rinne's test.

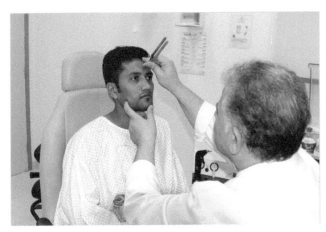

Fig. 11.9 Weber's test.

Examine the cranial nerves (CNs) and cerebellar functions quickly. Test for Romberg's sign, and finally ask the SP to walk (gait).

Rinne's test: Inform the SP that you are going to examine the ear using a tuning fork. Using a 512-Hz fork, strike it and put it first over the mastoid bone (bone conduction). While doing this, ask the SP to inform you when he or she no longer hears the sound.

Move it to the front of the ear (air conduction) and ask if he or she still hears the sound.

Normally, air conduction is better than bone conduction. Otherwise, there is conductive hearing loss. REPEAT the test again on the other side (▶ Fig. 11.8a, b).

Weber test's (▶ Fig. 11.9): Put the tuning fork in the middle of the forehead and ask the SP where the sound is coming from: the right ear, left, or both. Normally, both sides are equal; otherwise, the better one has conductive hearing loss. THE BETTER SOUND IS IN THE DISEASED EAR that has conductive hearing loss.

Communication and Interpersonal Skills Component

Suggested Closure

Standard closure.

Counseling

Advise her to keep away from noisy areas. Inform her that you are going to contact her primary doctor to discuss the possibility of stopping HCTZ, which will be replaced by another medicine for HTN.

Suggested Answers to the SP's Questions

Q1: Put your answer: As previously given.

Q2: *"It's hard to tell you for sure if you need hearing devices. We should clear up any correctable causes first, such as medication side effects. Then I'm going to recheck your hearing at your next visit."*

Patient Note

History

A 55-year-old female patient has had bilateral hearing loss for 5 years, with a gradual onset and progressive course; nothing makes it better. She has a problem hearing her coworkers over the phone. She has no history of ear infection, works at a grocery store with no noise, + family history of hearing loss, takes HCTZ for more than 10 years. She has no headache, vomiting, tingling, or any muscle weakness. She has no tinnitus, vertigo, or problems in her balance. She has normal sleep and appetite, with no urinary or bowel complaint. She is postmenopausal. **PMH:** HTN 15 years, NKDA. **FH:** Her brother, who is 60 years old, has the same problem. **SH:** denies smoking, drinks socially, and not sexually active.

Physical Exam

VS: WNL. No acute distress, alert, and oriented ×3. HEENT (head, eyes, ears, nose, and throat): AT (atraumatic), NC (normocephalic), PERRLA, intact red reflex. No tenderness over mastoid or over the ear tragus, clear TMs (tympanic membranes). Rinne's test: air conduction > bone conduction on both sides. Weber's test: no lateralization. Nose without rhinorrhea and throat without erythema. Neuro: CNs II–XII apparently normal, intact sensation on both sides, and normal gait. Romberg's test: negative. Chest: CTA/BL, normal S1 and S2.

Differential Diagnosis

History finding(s)	Physical exam finding(s)
1. Presbycusis	
Bilateral hearing loss	Clear external ear with no cerumen, TMs with light reflex bilaterally
Gradual onset over 5 y	No lateralization with Weber test
55 years with family history	
2. Medication induced	
Bilateral hearing loss	Clear external ear with no cerumen, TMs with light reflex bilaterally
Taking hydrochlorothiazide	No lateralization with Weber test

Diagnostic Studies

Audiometry

MRI brain

Role-Play 57

Mr. Peter Smith, a 40-year-old, came to the clinic because he doesn't feel well.

Vital signs:

- **PR:** 86/min, regular.
- **BP:** 120/80 mm Hg.
- **RR:** 16/min.
- **Temp:** 98.6°F (37°C).

Standardized Patient's Role

You are a 40-year-old man who came to the clinic because you don't feel well, and you can't figure out the reason. This problem started 6 months ago. It was gradual and mild, but it has grown worse with time, and affects your job performance.

You work as an accountant, and you can't concentrate for your entire work day. You feel tired and fatigued, and you lack concentration.

You were surprised when the nurse checked your weight; you have lost 6 to 8 lb over the last 3 months.

You have smoked one pack of cigarettes for 15 years, drink one to two cups of wine daily but more at parties and sometimes on the weekends. You have used marijuana since college.

You are sexually active, with both men and women, with occasional use of condoms. You've never been tested for HIV. You remember you had genital herpes 1 year ago.

As your doctor finishes the encounter, say (**Q1**): *"I heard that the treatment of HIV is expensive, and I don't have enough insurance."*

Role-Play 58

Doorway Information

Mr. Ivy Mitchell, a 50-year-old man, has fatigue.

Vital signs

- **PR:** 90/min, regular.
- **BP:** 140/100 mm Hg.
- **RR:** 16/min.
- **Temp:** 98.6°F (37°C).

Standardized Patient's Role

You are a 50-year-old male patient who came to the clinic as you have felt tired and unwell for 6 months. Your appetite has decreased, and as you eat, you feel that your stomach is full. You feel nauseous, and sometimes vomit.

You have a dull, aching abdominal pain. It's all over your abdomen, more in the upper part, sometimes traveling to the back. You would rate it as 4 out of 10. You've lost 10 lb in the last 3 months.

You don't know what is going on, since your wife died 3 months ago. You have had difficulty sleeping, feel sad, depressed, and your life isn't worth living.

You have had high BP for 20 years, and take propranolol.

Your father died from pancreatic cancer. You smoke 1 ppd/25 y, drink 2 beers/d for 30 years.

As the doctor examines you, express abdominal tenderness in the upper part. End your encounter by asking the doctor: (Q1): *"Do I have cancer, like my father had?"*

Role-Plays 57 and 58: Answer Key

Fatigue is common on the CS exam. It's a very challenging case, as it has many differential diagnoses. However, the following are the most common on the CS exam.

Common causes of fatigue on the CS exam:

- Psychiatric:
  - Posttraumatic stress disorder.
  - Depression.
- Organic:
  - Hypothyroidism.
  - Chronic diseases (anemia and DM).
  - Chronic infection (TB, HIV).
- Gastrointestinal (GI) malignancies:
  - Stomach cancer.
  - Pancreatic cancer.

History

The following are suggested questions:
- *Have you had a recent psychiatric trauma?*
- *Do you feel sad? Do you feel depressed? Do you feel like life isn't worth living?*

If yes, then go through the questions for depression (see Chapter 9, Psychiatry).

Questions for hypothyroidism: As a standard.
- *Do you drink water more than usual? Do you feel thirsty? Do you go to the bathroom more often than usual?*
- *Do you have fever or night sweating? Have you been around any sick person recently? Have you traveled outside the country recently?*
- *How is your appetite? Do you have nausea? Vomiting? Any abdominal pain?*
- *Have you noticed any dark urine? Dark stool? Any blood after brushing your teeth?*

HIV and AIDS

This case usually presents with fatigue as in the chief complaint (see fatigue cases at the end of this chapter). Rarely does it present as a case of medication refill. No matter how it appears, follow standard practice.

Ask more about the disease and its complications/medications and possible side effects.

Ask about common complications of HIV (chest infection, memory loss, peripheral neuropathy, bleeding tendencies, Kaposi's sarcoma, etc.).

The following could be asked for HIV medications side effects:
- GI symptoms, like nausea, vomiting, diarrhea and others.
- Hypersensitivity reactions, like skin rash.
- Symptoms suggestive of anemia, like fatigue and dizziness.
- Symptoms suggestive of peripheral neuropathy, like tingling and numbness.
- Upper abdominal pain and bleeding tendencies for liver toxicity.
- Vivid dreams as a side effect of efavirenz.

Please refer to your medical book for more details.

Take the social and sexual history in detail, do a quick general and local exam, ask for a genital exam, and document it in the workup. End your encounter by counseling the SP about safe sex precautions.

Suggested Counseling and Closure for HIV Cases

Provide info: *"AIDS is a sexually transmitted disease caused by HIV. The virus attacks specific cell in our immune system, named CD4, making the person much more likely to get infections.*

The workup for HIV includes a CD4 cell count and a viral load measure, which are done with special techniques. Our objective is to keep the CD4 count above a certain limit, the limit that protects you from opportunistic infections.

I have some recommendations for you; please be compliant to your meds and vaccinations (shots). I encourage you to inform your partners to take their precautions, and always use condoms as a kind of protection. The hospital has a wonderful support group. Do you have interest now to join it?"

If the SP says yes, reply: *"I'm glad to hear that."*

If the SP says no, reply: *"No problem, take your time, and when you have the interest, just give me a call. Thanks for your time. Have a good day."*

Patient Note (Role-Play 57)

History

A 40-year-old male patient complains of being tired for 6 months; onset was gradual and it's worsening with time. He suffers from lack of concentration and energy to the level that affects his job performance. He doesn't feel sad, depressed, or guilty. He denies cold intolerance, fever, night sweating, or cough; he has no polydipsia or polyuria, and there is no blood loss anywhere. **ROS:** normal sleep and normal appetite, recent loss of 6 to 8 lb in 3 months; he has no urinary or bowel issues. **PMH:** genital herpes 1 year ago, NKDA. **FH:** noncontributory. **SH:** smoker 1 ppd/15 y, drinks 1 to 2 cups of wine daily. He has been using marijuana since college. He is sexually active with multiple sexual partners, both men and women, with occasional use of condom and never tested for HIV.

Physical Exam

VS: WNL, alert, and oriented ×3, no acute distress. **Head:** normal eye, no pallor, throat without erythema. **Neck:** supple, normal thyroid, no palpable LNs (lymph nodes). **Ext:** no pallor or edema, palpable peripheral pulse. **Lung:** CTA/BL. **Heart:** normal S1 and S2. **Abdomen:** soft, Bowel sounds (BS +) no organomegaly.

Differential Diagnosis

History finding(s)	Physical exam finding(s)
1. Human immunodeficiency virus infection	
Fatigue, loss of weight	Physical exam: loss of 6–8 lb/3 mo
History of genital herpes	
Multiple sexual partners both men and women, occasional use of condom	
2. Drug abuse	
Fatigue, loss of weight	
Marijuana use since college	

Diagnostic Studies

Genital and rectal examination

Complete blood count with differential, HIV virus load, and CD4 cell count

Urine toxicology screen

Chest X-ray

A purified protein derivative (PPD) test for tuberculosis

Patient Note (Role-Play 58)

History

Please write the patient as per standard.

Physical Exam

Please write the patient as per standard.

Differential Diagnosis

History finding(s)	Physical exam finding(s)
1. Gastrointestinal malignancy	
Fatigue	Epigastric tenderness
Loss of appetite and weight	
Early satiety	
Father died from pancreatic cancer	Lost 10 lb/3 mo
2. Major depressive disorder	
Fatigue, feels sad, depressed	Blunt affect
Sense of worthlessness	Slow speech
Disturbed sleep	Normal thyroid exam
Lost his wife	

Diagnostic Studies

Rectal examination and stool analysis for occult blood

Complete blood count with differential

Thyroid-stimulating hormone and T3

CT abdomen with contrast

Upper gastrointestinal endoscopy

12 Mini Cases

Keywords: elbow pain, skin rash, tremors, vaginal discharge, penile discharge, nasal bleeding, jaundice

Case 59: Pre-employment Checkup Visit

After routine introduction, you can start your encounter with *"Mr./Mrs. ..., I so appreciate you coming in for a physical exam for your job. Do you have any complaints or health problems that you are concerned with?"*

In the cases with no complaints, go through questions for local system review (abdome n, chest, and others) and Review of Systems (ROS). Perform a quick general exam, chest and abdomen exam, and a few steps of neurological exam.

Common complaints are cough, loss of weight, symptoms that may suggest of diabetes mellitus (DM) or tuberculosis (TB). Analyze the complaint accordingly, and focus on the system affected in the history and in the physical exam.

Case 60: Hand Pain (Carpal Tunnel Syndrome)

This is a medical condition in which the median nerve is compressed as it travels through the wrist at the carpal tunnel causing pain, numbness, and tingling. It supplies the lateral 3.5 digits. In this case, do the following tests:

- Phalen's test: Ask the standardized patient (SP) to hold the dorsum on both hands together in acute flexion for 30 seconds. If there is numbness, pain, or tingling over the distribution of the medial nerve, the test is positive (▶ Fig. 12.1).
- Tinel's sign: Holding the SP's hand, press over the course of the median nerve in the carpal tunnel. The test is positive if there is numbness or tingling (▶ Fig. 12.2).

Workup: X-ray of the hand, electromyogram, and nerve conduction study.

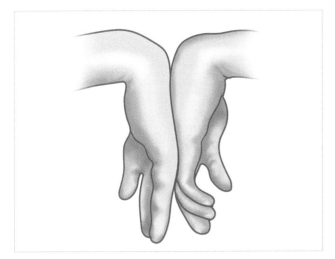

Fig. 12.1 Phalen's test.

Case 61: Elbow Pain

Lateral epicondylitis (tennis elbow): This is a condition in which the outer part of the elbow becomes sore and tender. Tennis elbow is an acute or chronic inflammation of the tendons that join the forearm muscles on the outside of the elbow (lateral epicondyle). This leads to pain and tenderness on the outside of the elbow.[1]

Do Cozen's test: While the patient is flexing the wrist with extended elbow, ask him or her to extend the wrist against gentle resistance. Pain at the lateral epicondyle area indicates a positive test (▶ Fig. 12.3).

Medial epicondylitis (golfer's elbow): This is tendinitis of the medial epicondyle of the elbow. It is in some ways similar to tennis elbow.

Workup: X-ray and MRI of the elbow.

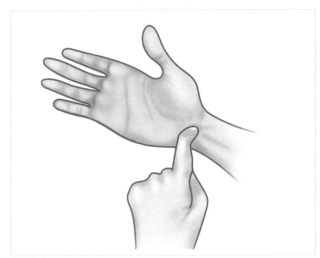

Fig. 12.2 Tinel's sign.

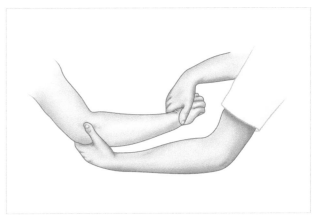

Fig. 12.3 Cozen's test.

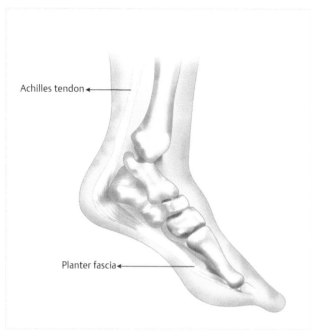

Fig. 12.4 Plantar fasciitis.

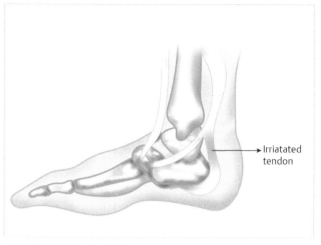

Fig. 12.5 Achilles tendinitis.

Case 62: Foot Pain

Plantar fasciitis[2-4] (▶ **Fig. 12.4**): This is a disorder that results in pain in the heel and bottom of the foot. Risk factors include overuse, such as long periods of standing, an increase in exercise, and obesity. Tenderness to palpation along the inner aspect of the heel bone on the sole of the foot may be noted during the physical examination. The foot may have limited dorsiflexion due to tightness of the calf muscles. Patients are advised to rest, change their activities, take pain medications, and stretch; if this is not sufficient, physical therapy, splinting, and steroid injections may be options. (▶ **Fig. 12.4**)[5]

Achilles tendinitis[6]: This is tendinitis of the achilles tendon, generally caused by overuse of the affected limb, and is more common among athletes training under less than ideal conditions. Symptoms are pain, burning, or swelling of the affected foot (▶ **Fig. 12.5**).

Foreign body: glass, wood, or hard objects.

Workup: X-ray and MRI ankle.

Case 63: Calf Pain[7]

The causes of calf pain vary from something as minor as muscle strain to serious problems, like deep vein thrombosis (DVT). Causes may include the following:
- **Calf injury:** It usually happens during sports, such as basketball, tennis, and running.
- **DVT:** There is usually a history of prolonged immobilization (surgery, cast, and long time of travel). A positive Homans sign (pain on dorsiflexion of the ankle) is indicative of DVT.
- **Cellulitis/myositis:** It shows all signs of inflammation.
- **Ruptured Becker's** (popliteal cyst).
- **Workup:** Doppler ultrasound (US)—lower limbs, MRI.

Case 64: Skin Rash

Questions can be divided into three groups: before the rash, character of the rash, and associations. Note that SPs can use makeup and devices to make skin rashes.

Causes of rash:
- Allergic reaction.
- Immunologic such as SLE, RA.
- Infections such as bacterial, viral, or fungal.
- Photo dermatitis, insect bite or occupational.

Before the rash:
- *Was it preceded by hiking or camping?*
- *Was it preceded by gardening? Swimming? Sun exposure?*
- *Have you been around any sick person? Any pets?*
- *Have you been exposed to any allergens? Insect bites?*
- *Has it come with any new medicine use?*

Character of the rash:
- *Where is your rash?*
- *What does the rash look like?*
- *What is the color of the rash?*
- *Have you noticed any blisters? Any crusts? Any fluid coming out?*
- *Is it itchy?/Does it itch?*

Associations:
- *What symptoms do you have besides rashes?*

Ask about symptoms that may refer to allergic or immunologic problems:
- *Have you noticed any eye redness? Sneezing? Any nasal blockage?*
- *Do you have any difficulty breathing? Any cough?*
- *Do you have any joint pain? Any fever?*

Case 65: Tremors

Tremor is rhythmic muscle contraction and relaxation of a group of muscles, commonly the hands. Types of tremor include the following:
- *Essential (benign) tremor:* Common, appears on outstretched hands, and may be familial.

- *Cerebellar tremor:* Occurs at the end of a purposeful movement (intention tremors).
  - *Parkinsonian (resting tremor):* Part of Parkinson's disease with bradykinesia and rigidity.
  - *Medication side effects:* As nicotine, theophylline, B-agonist, etc.
  - *Others:* As psychogenic and alcoholism.

Case 66: Eye/Vision Problems

Glaucoma: Headache, photophobia, and gradual loss in the peripheral visual field (▶ Fig. 12.6).

Cataract: Gradual, painless loss of vision. It is often bilateral and associated with problems with nighttime driving.

Macular degeneration: Straight lines become wavy.

Diabetic retinopathy: It is the most common cause of blindness in adults younger than 50 years. It occurs as a complication of long-standing/uncontrolled DM.

Hypertensive retinopathy: A complication of long-standing/uncontrolled hypertension (HTN).

Brain lesions: Symptoms of increased intracranial pressure (ICP; headache, blurry vision, and projectile vomiting and visual field defect).

Papilledema: Bilateral optic disc swelling due to SOL (space-occupying lesions) in the brain.

Sudden painless unilateral vision loss: It may be due to central retinal artery occlusion, central retinal vein occlusion, or retinal detachment.

Workup:
- Blood glucose, Hb A1c, 24-hour urine collection, lipid profile.

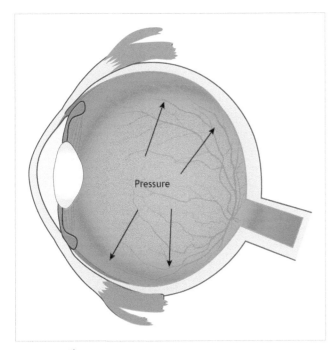

Fig. 12.6 Glaucoma.

- Slit-lamp exam for the eye.
- Tonometry (to measure intraocular pressure).
- Carotid Doppler.
- CT brain.

Case 67: Malabsorption

The hallmark of the disease is abdominal pain, bloating, and diarrhea. Among many causes, the following may encounter in the Clinical Skills exam:

Celiac disease (gluten-sensitive enteropathy): Autoimmune disease that affects and damages the small intestinal mucosa when gluten—in some grains—is eaten.

In addition to the common symptoms of malabsorption, other presentations are anemia, skin rashes, and weight loss.

Workup: Compete blood count (CBC), stool analysis, antigliadin, antitransglutaminase Ab, and small bowel biopsy.

Advise patients to avoid gluten-containing grains (wheat, rye, oats, and barley).

Lactose intolerance: Malabsorption due to deficiency of enzyme lactase with subsequent hypersensitivity to lactose sugar. Most people with lactose intolerance can manage the condition without having to give up all dairy foods.

Others are cystic fibrosis and chronic pancreatitis, rare cases, like tropical sprue and Whipple's disease.

Case 68: Dysphagia (Difficulty Swallowing)

Causes:
Achalasia of the cardia (▶ Fig. 12.7): Young age, difficult swallowing of liquid and solid (see the barium swallow study).

Esophageal cancer: Old age, difficult swallowing of solids then for semisolids, loss of weight, vomiting and regurgitation, and halitosis.

CREST syndrome (calcinosis, Raynaud's phenomenon, esophageal dysmotility, sclerodactyly, and telangiectasia).

Workup:
- Barium swallow.
- Esophageal manometry.
- Upper GI (gastrointestinal) endoscopy.

Case 69: Delayed Passage of Meconium[8]

Timely passage of the first stool is a hallmark of the well-being of the newborn infant. Failure of a full-term newborn to pass meconium in the first 24 hours may be due to the following:

Lower intestinal problems: Meconium plug syndrome can be treated with rectal stimulation and enema. Meconium ileus (cystic fibrosis) can be treated with enema with intravenous fluids, surgery.

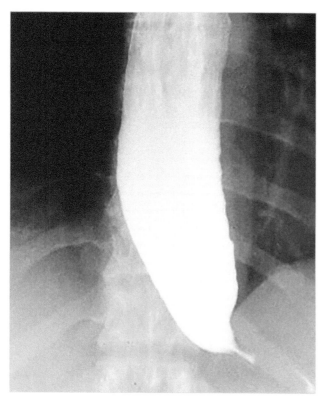

Fig. 12.7 Barium swallow showing achalasia of the cardia.

Hirschsprung's disease and imperforate anus both require surgery.

Small intestinal obstruction: Signs include refusal to eat, vomiting, and abdominal distension. Causes may include duodenal atresia, malrotation, and volvulus.

Workup: Rectal exam, X-ray abdomen.

Case 70: Epistaxis

Extra nasal (systemic): Noncontrolled hypertension and coagulation disorders.

Intranasal:
- Trauma to the nose.
- Inflammatory such as allergic rhinitis.
- Tumors such as nasopharyngeal angiofibroma.

Case 71: Sheehan's Syndrome (Panhypopituitarism)

A clinical syndrome results from ischemic necrosis to the pituitary, due to blood loss and hypovolemic shock during and after childbirth. In the CS exam, common complaints are fatigue from hypothyroidism, absence of lactation from prolactin deficiency, and cessation of menstruation (amenorrhea).

Female SPs give a positive history for significant postpartum hemorrhage.

Workup: CBC, hormonal assay (TSH [thyroid-stimulating hormone], T3, prolactin, FSH [follicle-stimulating hormone], LH [luteinizing hormone]) and MRI brain.

Case 72: Genital Discharge (▶Video. 12.1)

Analysis of the complaint (ABCD) + associations:
- *How much discharge do you have? How many pads do you use per day?*
- *Do you have to change your underwear? If yes, How many times a day?*
- *Have you noticed any blood?/What is the color of the discharge?*
- *What does the discharge smell like?/Does it have an unpleasant odor?*

Associations:
Does it burn while urinating?
Do you have any pain during sexual intercourse?

Urethral discharge in males:
- **Gonorrhea:** The discharge is profuse, yellowish, and associated with dysuria and burning.
- **Nongonococcal (chlamydial) urethritis:** Whitish, scanty with mild dysuria.

Vaginal discharge in females:
- **Candidiasis:** Cottage-cheese whitish discharge, ask about pregnancy, DM, and antibiotic use.
- **Trichomonas vaginalis:** Pale green, frothy watery discharge.
- **Gardnerella vaginalis:** Malodorous, fishy smell discharge.

Workup: Pelvic exam, high vaginal swab culture (HVS C/S), Gram stain of the smear, wet mount, KOH prep (potassium hydroxide preparation; whiff test), HIV virus load, and CD4 count.

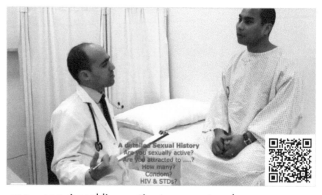

Video. 12.1 A real live patient encounter demo for a patient who has urethral discharge. https://www.thieme.de/de/q.htm?p=opn/cs/20/3/11450549-c59f24d2

Case 73: Dyspareunia[9]

It is painful sexual intercourse in female. It may be due to the following:

Entry pain: Pain during penetration may be associated with a range of factors, including the following:
- *Insufficient lubrication:* Drop in estrogen levels after menopause, certain medications as antihistamines.
- Inflammation, infection, or skin disorder.
- *Vaginismus:* It is involuntary spasms of the muscles of the vaginal wall.

Deep pain:
- **Certain illnesses and conditions:** Endometriosis, pelvic inflammatory disease, and uterine prolapse.
- Surgeries or radiotherapy.
- Emotional factors.
- **Psychological problems:** Stress, anxiety, and depression.
- History of sexual abuse.

Case 74: Jaundice

Analysis of the complaint:

Onset, course, and duration; ask for the color of skin, urine, and stool, and ask for any fever.

Analysis of the differential diagnosis:

Hematolytic jaundice:
Have you received a blood transfusion recently?
Was the yellow color preceded by any new medicine use? Any unusual food?
Do you have any chest pain? Any pain in your belly?
Do you have any blood diseases? Any blood diseases in your family?

Hepatocellular jaundice:
Have you been outside the country recently?
Have you been around anybody sick?
Have you had a fever?

Obstructive jaundice: It may be caused by gallstones or cancer head of the pancreas.
Have you been diagnosed with gallstones?

Workup: CBC, ALT, AST, bilirubin (direct and indirect), hepatitis virus serology, US—abdomen.

Case 75: Noisy/Wheezing Chest in Children

Foreign body aspiration: Sudden noisy breathing marked by gasping, like having the wind knocked out of you. In healthy kids, it may occur while the child is playing.

Noisy breathing + fever (croup): Mostly at the age 1 to 2 years, in autumn or winter. Children usually first contract upper respiratory tract (URT) infection and then develop a barking cough and stridor.

Epiglottis: Most patients are between the ages of 2 and 7 years. They appear toxic, and symptoms include high fever, drooling, and stridor.

Wheezy breathing, with past history of bronchial asthma: Bronchial asthma.

Case 76: Bronchial Asthma

Expiratory wheezing that may be triggered by RT infection. Refer to Chapter 11, Miscellaneous, Role-Play 55. Follow the same steps in case analysis after modifying to he/she questions.

Suggested Readings

1. http://orthoinfo.aaos.org/topic.cfm?topic=a00068
2. Beeson P. Plantar fasciopathy: revisiting the risk factors. Foot Ankle Surg 2014;20(3):160–165
3. Goff JD, Crawford R. Diagnosis and treatment of plantar fasciitis. Am Fam Physician 2011;84(6):676–682
4. www.galleryhip.com
5. https://en.wikipedia. org/wiki/Plantar_fasciitis - cite_note-Bee2014-1
6. http://www.md-health.com/Achilles-Tendinitis.html
7. http://www.knee-pain-explained.com/calf-muscle-pain.html
8. http://www.aafp.org/afp/1999/1101/p2043.html
9. http://www.mayoclinic.org/diseases-conditions/painful-intercourse/basics/causes/con-20033293

13 Appendix

Keywords: preventative medicine, deep tendon reflexes, muscle power grading scale, sensory levels, mnemonics, abbreviations

13.1 General Instructions to Role-Plays

13.1.1 Standardized Patient's Roles

Read your role-play for each case well; you can even keep your role-play in your hand to read it while practicing.

Try hard to act out the role-play situation, as if you are a real patient in the hospital. Act appropriately in simulating severe chest pain and shortness of breath; be anxious while informing the doctor of a family member's serious heart condition.

Simulate the clinical exam as instructed: express tenderness (over sinuses, chest, or abdomen), simulate impaired sensation or weakness on a limb, etc.

Ask the doctor the questions that are mentioned in order, while entering the room, while taking the history (Hx), while doing the exam, or at the end of the encounter. What we have mentioned are suggested ones. However, you can ask other appropriate questions according to the case.

If you are a medical student/doctor, grade the three components and the patient note (PN) as well. If you are a nonmedical professional, grade the Communication and Interpersonal Skills (CIS) and Spoken English Proficiency (SEP) checklists and leave him or her the other medical tasks.

In general, if the doctor asks you about anything other than the health matter than what is mentioned in the role-play, say that you feel fine and have had no other problems.

13.1.2 General Instructions for Medical Student's/Doctor's Roles

At the beginning of your practice and while your Standardized patient (SP) is preparing for his or her case, do a quick review of the possible differential diagnoses, history-taking questions, clinical exam steps needed, and the suggested answers for the CIS questions. Quickly read the given PN.

After you have finished, ask the SP to set up a stopwatch before showing you the doorway information, and then start your encounter.

After you finish the encounter and PN documentation, let your SP grade you, and while he or she is doing that, look again at the Suggested Answers for each case in its individual chapter. See if you asked the right history-taking questions, if you answered the SP's questions appropriately, if you did the right tests, and if you documented the case well.

13.1.3 For Telephone Encounters

Don't answer the guardian's questions until you finish taking the Hx. Remember that you can't fully answer any question because you haven't actually seen the patient yet.

Your English-language listening comprehension and speaking skills must be proficient as neither body language nor facial expressions help you communicate during encounters.

Don't be afraid to ask for clarification: ask the caller to speak up or speak slower. Also, you can ask the caller to repeat a question or paraphrase it. You can rephrase it to be sure that you have heard the question correctly.

13.2 To Avoid Redundancy in the Book

To avoid redundancy in the book, the following were suggested:

As the examinee tasks part of the "doorway information" are the same in almost all CS cases, they are only listed on the first case of each chapter.

In PN, the first row under the differential diagnosis (DD) is always for supportive info for the DD from history-taking (on the left) and the clinical exam (on the right). It was listed only on the first case of each chapter.

13.3 Preventative Medicine Notes for the Purposes of the CS Exam

Based on the gender and age of your patient, certain screening protocols may be indicated. These topics can be added to counseling SPs at the end of the encounter.

Pap smears are recommended for females at age 21, and then every 3 years thereafter. After the age of 30, Pap smears can be considered every 5 years.

Cholesterol screen should be given to males at age 35 and females at age 45, and earlier if they are at risk.

Mammograms are recommended for females at age 40, then every 2 years.

PSA (prostrate-specific antigen) screening and **colonoscopies** can be offered to males at age 50, or who are 10 years younger than the age at which the youngest first-degree relative was affected.

Note: There are some immunization protocols, but we feel they are beyond the scope of the CS exam, so they are not included here. Feel free to offer influenza vaccination to all patients in winter.

13.4 Common Medications in CS Exam Scenarios

Over-the-Counter (OTC):
- Ibuprofen.
- NSAID (Aleve).
- Acetaminophen (Tylenol).
- Antacid such as calcium carbonate (Tums).
- Antihistaminic as diphenhydramine (Benadryl) and loratadine (Claritin).

Hypertension (HTN) medications:
- Diuretics such as HCTZ (hydrochlorothiazide).
- B-blockers such as propranolol and atenolol.
- ACE (angiotensin-converting enzyme) inhibitors as lisinopril and captopril.

Medication for high cholesterol: Simvastatin (Zocor).

Diabetes mellitus (DM) medications: Insulin, metformin, sulfonylurea (glyburide, glimepiride).

Medications for depression: SSRIs (selective serotonin reuptake inhibitors) such as sertraline (Zoloft).

Medications for bronchial asthma (BA): Albuterol MDI (metered-dose inhaler).

13.5 Side Effects of Commonly Used Medicines

Aspirin: Gastritis and gastrointestinal (GI) bleeding.

B-blockers (propranolol): ↓ Bp (dizziness), chest wheezing, and sexual impairment.

Diuretic: Hypotension (syncope) and ototoxicity.

ACE inhibitors: Dry cough.

Statin drugs: Muscle ache and hepatic impairment.

Heparin (Coumadin): Bleeding as intracranial hemorrhage, and GI bleeding.

13.6 Deep Tendon Reflexes Grading Scale (▶Table 13.1)

Note: Most of the SPs will show normal deep tendon reflexes (DTR; +2). Abnormal DTRs in the CS is either (+1, hypoactive) or (+3, exaggerated).

Reflex Centers:
- Biceps (C5 and C6) and triceps (C6 and C7).
- Superficial abdominal reflexes (T8, T9, T10, T11, and T12).
- Knee (L2 and L3) and ankle (S1 and S2).

13.7 Muscle Power Grading Scale (▶Table 13.2)

Note: Most of your SPs will show normal muscle power (5/5); however, muscle weakness on the CS exam is usually expressed as 4/5.

13.8 Important Sensory Levels

Important principle dermatomes (sensory distribution) (▶Fig. 13.1) are as follows:
- Shoulder (C4).
- Outer aspect of the forearm and thumbs (C6).
- Little fingers (C8).
- Inner aspect of the forearm (T1).
- Around the umbilicus (T10).
- Front of the thighs (L2).
- Inner aspect of the leg (L4).
- Outer aspect of the leg (L5).
- Outer aspect of the foot (S1).

13.9 Mnemonics and Quick Review

HPI (history of present illness): Analysis of two (CC [chief complain], DD) and review of two (local system, review of systems [ROS]).

ROS: I SAW two (in male SPs) or three (in female SPs) systems.

Pain:
- Onset, course, and duration.
- Location and radiation.
- CSF (character, severity, and frequency) and AAA (**A**ggravating factors, **A**lleviating factors, **A**ssociations).

For any body fluids or excretions: *Onset + ABCD*.

Bleeding disorder cases: *ABCDE*.

DD for diarrhea cases: When **HIV** guy **traveled**, he got **gastroenteritis**. When he took **antibiotics**, he got **inflammatory bowel disease** and **malabsorption**.

Review of Systems (ROS):

I SAW (sleep, appetite, and weight) 2 systems (GI system and Urinary system)
In female, 3 systems (GI system, Urinary and Genital systems)

PMH (past medical history): PDS for PDA and resulted in Fast Surgery ± Scar. Past history, diseases, surgery, previous episodes, drugs, allergic history, family, social ±sexual.

General physical examination: Vital signs may change hormones (ADH + NE + LH) that are given by local shots.
Vistal signs, appearance, decubitus, head, neck, extermities, lung, heart, and local exam

Table 13.1 Deep tendon reflexes grading scale

Grade	Description
0	Absent
+1	Hypoactive (diminished)
+2	Normal
+3	Exaggerated
+4	Exaggerated with clonus

Table 13.2 Muscle power grading scale

Grade	Description
0/5	Absent muscle movement
1/5	Just flicker of movement
2/5	Movement at the joint, but not against gravity
3/5	Movement against gravity, but not against added resistance
4/5	Movement against resistance, but less than normal
5/5	Normal muscle power

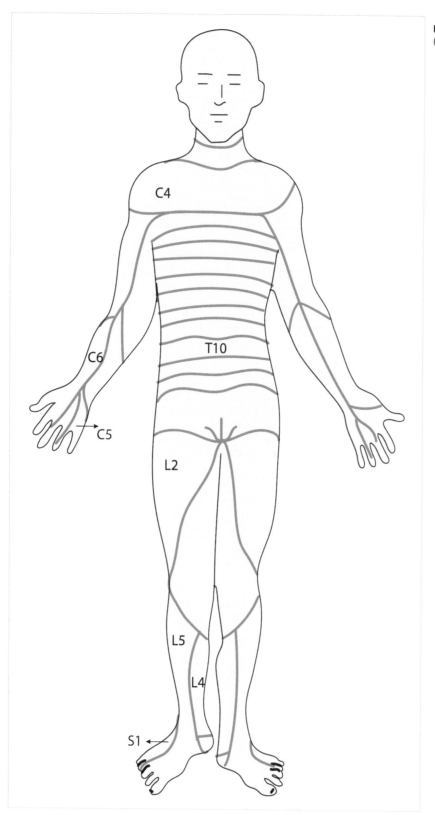

Fig. 13.1 Important principle dermatomes (sensory distribution).

Hx for *CARD*iac cases: Chest pain, Angina, Racing heart, and Dyspnea.

Hx for respiratory cases:
- **Upper:** Three in the nose (secretion out, in, and nasal allergy) and three inflammations(sinusitis, pharyngitis, and laryngitis).
- **Lower (CCD):** Chest pain, Cough, and Dyspnea.

Hx for GI cases:
- Nausea and vomiting.
- Difficulty swallowing, and heartburn.
- Abdominal pain.
- Bleeding and change in bowel habits.

For lower GI: masses and bleeding.

Gynecology and obstetrics Hx: For all CS cases other OB/Gyne cases; PPC: Period, Pap smear and Contraception.

For OB/Gyne cases:
The routine (PPC) + Bleeding (3M + C): Menarche, Menorrhagia/ Metrorrhagia/ post-Coital bleeding.

GPA (Gravida, Para, Abortion).

Pediatric Hx: *A Pregnant woman Delivered a Neonate who developed* DIC
(Pregnancy, Delivery, Neonatal Hx, Developmental Hx, Immunization and Check-up visits).

Musculoskeletal Hx: Hx of trauma, general and local complications + AND (Artery, Nerve, Disability).

Joint exam: IP AND S: Inspection, Palpation, Artery, Nerve, Disability, and Special maneuvers.

Psychiatry:
- **Major depressive disorder:** SIG E CAPS (Sleep, Interest, Guilt, Energy, Concentration, Appetite, Psychomotor agitation and Suicidal thoughts).
- **Physical/sexual abuse:** Assault happened when He hurt Her at Home.

Neurology Hx: Mini-Cranium may Sense, Move, and Walk with Special senses (Memory, Concentration, Sensory, Motor, Walking, and Special senses).

Neurological Exam: Mini Cranium may Sense, Move and Walk with Special maneuvers. (MMSE, Cranial Nerves, Sensory system, Motor system, Walking (cerebellum and gait) and Special maneuvers).

Checkup visit/medication refill cases (HTN, DM, BA, and HIV):
- Questions about the disease.
- Questions about complications of the disease.
- Questions about the medication.
- Questions about side effects of the medication.

Common abbreviations used in patient note for CS exam is given in ▶ Table 13.3.

Table 13.3 Common abbreviations used in patient note for CS exam

AIDS	Acquired immunodeficiency syndrome	JVD	Jugular venous distension
Abd	Abdomen	L	Left
Bp	Blood pressure	LMP	Last menstrual period
C	Celsius	LP	Lumbar puncture
CABG	Coronary artery bypass graft	M	Male
CBC	Complete blood count	MCA	Motor car accident
CHF	Congestive heart failure	MI	Myocardial infarction
COPD	Chronic obstructive airway disease	MRI	Magnetic resonance imaging
CT	Computed tomography	Meds	Medication
CVA	Cerebrovascular accident	Min	Minutes
CXR	Chest X-ray	NKDA	No known drug allergy
DM	Diabetes mellitus	Neg/−	Negative
DTRs	Deep tendon reflexes	Neuro	Neurology
ENT	Ear, nose, and throat	oz	Ounces
EOMI	Extraocular muscles intact	PERRA	Pupils equal, round, reactive and accommodation
ER/ED	Emergency room/department	PMH	Past medical history
EtOH	Alcohol	po	Per os/orally
Ext	Extremities	Pos/+	Positive
F	Fahrenheit	R	Right
FH	Family history	RR	Respiratory rate
GI	Gastrointestinal	SH/SHx	Social history
GU	Genitourinary	SOB	Shortness of breath
H/o	History of	SexH	Sexual history
HEENT	Head, eye, ear, nose, and throat	Temp	Temperature
HIV	Human immunodeficiency virus	UA	Urine analysis
HR	Heart rate	URT	Upper respiratory tract
HRT	Hormonal replacement therapy	UTI	Urinary tract infection
HTN	Hypertension	WBC	White blood cells
Hr	Hours	WNL	Within normal limit
Hx	History	yo	Year-old
lb	Pounds		

Checklists

Checklist for the Communication and Interpersonal Skills (CIS)			
At Entry	**Check**	**Closure**	**Check**
At the physician's entry, check if s/he:		At the physician's closure, check if s/he:	
• Knocked on the door	( )	• Provided	(/5)
• Called you by your family name	( )	A summary of history and PE	
• Greeted you	( )	Provisional diagnoses	
• Introduced her/himself to you	( )	A suggested workup	
• Asked for permission to take a medical history & perform PE	( )	• Addressed your concerns and questions	(/5)
		• Assured you that s/he will see you again	(/2)
• Smiled[1]/ shook your hand	( )	/is accessible to you at any time	
• Asked an open–ended question	( )	• Said goodbye, and smiled[1]	( )
	/7		**/13**

Throughout the Encounter			
History	**Check**	**Physical Examination (PE)**	**Check**
Determine if the physician:		During the clinical exam, check if s/he:	
• Maintained proper eye contact	(/3)	• Washed hands	( )
• Supported your emotions	(/2)	• Asked for permission to do a PE,	( )
• Was able to foster an appropriate	(/2)	• Informed you of the PE steps	( )
relationship with you	(/2)	• Warmed the stethoscope and used	( )
• Helped you make decisions		disposable tools	( )
Mark (–1) if the s/he (otherwise 1):	( )	• Did a proper draping technique	
• Interrupted you while speaking	( )	Mark (-1) if the s/he (otherwise 1):	( )
• Asked leading questions	( )	• Examined through the gown	(/2)
• Asked more than 1 question at a time	( )	• Repeated painful maneuvers	(/3)
• Gave any false assurance	( )	• Performed prohibited local exams	
• Was judgmental			
	/14		**/11**

	/5
Did the physician give proper counseling for:	
Smoking, DM, HTN, safe sex practice, medications, sleep, home situation..,..?	
Remarks	**Sum /50 = %**

[1] Smiling is not appropriate in special cases

SEP Checklist

Overall Communicating Rating

		How well did you understand the physician's speech?	How well did the physician understand you?
Completely Understood	(15)		
Mostly Understood	(10)		
Somewhat Understood	(5)		
Did not Understand	(0)		

Physician's Spoken English Proficiency

		Clarity of Speech	Necessity to Repeat Words	Word Choice
No	(15)			
Errors	(10)			
A few errors	(7)			
Some Errors	(5)			

Total Score _____ (60 possible)

ICE Checklist for Chest Cases

Name: **Age:**   **CC:**

History-taking	DD
HPI, Analysis of the CC:	
....	
....	
....	
Analysis of DD:	

History-taking	Clinical exam

General
VS

A
D
H

N
E

Local exam **(LH)**

- Lung exam
  Inspection
  Palpation + TVF
  Percussion
  Auscultation

- Heart exam
  PMI
  2 on the heart
  2 signs at the neck
  2 peripheral signs

History-taking (continued)

Analysis of DD:
....
....
....
....
....
....

Review of the affected system:
....
....

ROS (I SAW 2/3)
....

Past History

D...

S...

P...

D...

A...

F...

S...

±S...

Closure:

Counseling:

Questions:

ICE Checklist for Abdominal Cases

Name: **Age:**   **CC:**

History-taking	DD
HPI, Analysis of the CC:	

Analysis of DD:

....

....

....

....

....

....

Review of the affected system:

....

....

ROS (I SAW 2/3)

....

Past History

D...

S...

P...

D...

A...

F...

S...

±S...

Closure:

Counseling:

Questions:

DD

Clinical exam

General

VS

A

D

H

N

E

LH (Auscultation only)

Local exam (Abdomen)
Inspection
Palpation
Percussion
Auscultation

***S**pecial signs
Rebound tenderness
CVA tenderness
For appendicitis, ...
Pelvic exam (ask, then write in PN)

*Please, do the necessary steps only

ICE Checklist for OB/Gyne Cases

Name: **Age:**   **CC:**

History-taking	DD
HPI, Analysis of the CC: .... **Analysis of DD:** .... **Review of the affected system:** .... **ROS (I SAW 2/3)**	

	Clinical exam
	General **VS** **A** **D** **H** **N** **E** **LH** (Auscultation only) **L**ocal exam (Abdomen) Inspection Palpation Percussion Auscultation ***S**pecial signs Schedule pelvic and rectal exams

Past History

D..

S..

P..

D..

A..

F..

S..

±S..

Closure:

Counseling:

Questions:

ICE Checklist for Pediatrics

Name: **Age:**   **CC:**

History-taking	DD
HPI, Analysis of the CC: .... **Analysis of DD:** .... **Review of the affected system:** .... **ROS (I SAW 2/3)**	

History-taking	Clinical exam
Past History D.. S.. P.. D.. A.. F.. S.. ±S..	**None**
Closure:	
Counseling:	
Questions:	

ICE Checklist for Musculoskeletal Cases

Name: **Age:**   **CC:**

History-taking	DD
HPI, Analysis of the CC:	
....	
....	
....	
Analysis of DD:	
....	
....	**Clinical exam**
....	**General**
....	**VS**
....	**A**
....	**D**
Review of the affected system:	**H**
....	**N**
....	**E**
ROS (I SAW 2/3)	**LH** (Auscultation only)
....	Local exam **(IP AND S)**
Past History	
D..	**Joints:** Start with the healthy side, then the diseased one:
S..	**I**nspection
P..	**P**alpation
D..	**A**rtery (pulsation)
A..	**N**erve (sensation, motor, DTR)
	Disability (passive/active ROM)
F..	
S..	**S**pecial maneuver
±S..	**Spine:** The same, but **D**isabilities (leaning forwards, moving back and side to side)
Closure:	
Counseling:	
Questions:	

ICE Checklist for Neurology Cases

Name: **Age:**   **CC:**

Neurological patients with **M**ini **C**ranium may **S**ense, **M**ove and **W**alk with **S**pecial senses / maneuvers.	
Entry:	**DD**
HPI, Analysis of the CC:	
....	
....	
....	
Analysis of DD:	
....	**Clinical exam**
....	**Exam/ General**
....	**VS**
....	**A**
....	**D**
....	**H**
Review of the affected system:	**N**
....	**E**
....	
ROS (I SAW 2/3)	**L**H (Auscultation only)
....	**L**ocal exam: Neurological exam
Past History	± MMSE
D..	Cranial nerves
S..	Sensory system
	Motor system
P..	Muscle tone
D..	Muscle power
A..	DTRs
	Walk (cerebellum)
F..	
S..	**S**pecial maneuvers
± S..	
Closure:	
Counseling:	
Questions:	

303

Index

Note: Page numbers set in **bold** or *italic* indicate headings or figures, respectively.